The Short Te

Medical Microbiology
for Nurses

The Short Textbook of
Medical Microbiology
for Nurses

THIRD EDITION

Satish Gupte MD
Professor
Department of Microbiology
Kathmandu Medical College
Kathmandu, Nepal

Ex-Professor and Head
Department of Microbiology
Gian Sagar Medical College and Hospital
Patiala, Punjab, India

Ex-Professor and Head
Department of Microbiology
Adesh Institute of Medical Sciences and Research Center
Bhatinda, Punjab, India
and
Government Medical College
Jammu, Jammu and Kashmir, India

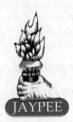

JAYPEE BROTHERS MEDICAL PUBLISHERS
The Health Sciences Publisher
New Delhi | London

Jaypee Brothers Medical Publishers (P) Ltd

Headquarters

Jaypee Brothers Medical Publishers (P) Ltd
EMCA House, 23/23-B
Ansari Road, Daryaganj
New Delhi 110 002, India
Landline: +91-11-23272143, +91-11-23272703
+91-11-23282021, +91-11-23245672
Email: jaypee@jaypeebrothers.com

Corporate Office

Jaypee Brothers Medical Publishers (P) Ltd
4838/24, Ansari Road, Daryaganj
New Delhi 110 002, India
Phone: +91-11-43574357
Fax: +91-11-43574314
Email: jaypee@jaypeebrothers.com

Overseas Office

J.P. Medical Ltd
83 Victoria Street, London
SW1H 0HW (UK)
Phone: +44 20 3170 8910
Fax: +44 (0)20 3008 6180
Email: info@jpmedpub.com

Website: www.jaypeebrothers.com
Website: www.jaypeedigital.com

© 2021, Managing Editor: Mrs Jyotsna Gupte and Jaypee Brothers Medical Publishers

Inquiries for bulk sales may be solicited at: jaypee@jaypeebrothers.com

The Short Textbook of Medical Microbiology for Nurses

First Edition: 2011

Second Edition: **2018**

Third Edition: **2021**

ISBN: 978-93-90595-23-5

Printed at: Sterling Graphics Pvt. Ltd.

Preface to the Third Edition

Essentially nurses now are expected to have sufficient knowledge and proper training in medical microbiology. This shall enable today's nurses to become qualified to perform many roles within clinical nursing practice, such as administering antibiotics, collection and transportation of specimen to clinical laboratories, education of patients and families, proper communication of results to healthcare team, etc. Most attention inviting topics for nurses are infection control, hospital-acquired infections, infectious diseases transmission, collection, handling plus transportation of patient specimens and sterilization, etc.

Overwhelming response to second edition to *The Short Textbook of Medical Microbiology for Nurses* and revision of syllabus has prompted us to bring out third edition absolutely revised strictly according to new syllabus prescribed. Description of text is simple, lucid, easy to understand. Hand-drawn illustrations, multicolored photographs, flowcharts and tables are placed appropriately in between text.

The text has nine sections namely General Microbiology, Bacterial Genetics, Immunology, Systemic Bacteriology, Virology, Mycology, Parasitology and Medical Entomology, Clinical Microbiology, and Practical Microbiology. Special attention is provided in discussing collection and transportation of clinical specimens to clinical laboratory. Also discussed hospital/laboratory waste, control of infection, hand hygiene and practical suggestions in dealing with day-to-day hospital infection problems. A new chapter on Infectious Diseases and their Prevention is added. Highlights of COVID-19 is also incorporated.

We are grateful to Dr EM Warke of HiMedia Laboratory, Mumbai, Maharashtra, India, for kind permission to use some photographs. I am immensely grateful to all my family members including my wife Mrs Jyotsna Gupte and dear son Anubhav Gupte, for their great contribution in compiling the manuscript. Many many thanks to Faculty of Microbiology, Kathmandu Medical College, Kathmandu, Nepal, for their cooperation and well wishes. It is my pleasure to acknowledge with thanks, the help rendered by my dear postgraduates Dr Anjita and Dr Sita in typing and searching material required in the preparation of this volume.

I take opportunity to thank Shri Jitendar P Vij (Group Chairman), Mr Ankit Vij (Managing Director), Mr MS Mani (Group President) and his great studious team of M/s Jaypee Brothers Medical Publishers (P) Ltd, New Delhi, India, for their joint efforts for bringing out this book in so impressive form. Suggestions and healthy criticism is invited from students, teachers, readers towards improvement and additions in future editions.

Satish Gupte

Preface to the First Edition

Noble profession of nursing is attracting students of high ranks in the qualifying examination. To be successful, nurses must have good grasp of specialty of medical microbiology. Nursing students are expected to acquire basic knowledge to the best of their ability especially of sterilization, aseptic invasive procedures, control and spread of infection, etc. As a matter of fact, a student entering nursing profession is in a dilemma that how much information is needed to remember to practice microbiology in day-to-day work in the hospital.

There are a number of books available on microbiology addressed to nursing students. *The Short Textbook of Medical Microbiology for Nurses* is an attempt to fulfill the actual needs and requirement of nursing students. Material is presented in simple, hand-drawn illustrations and clear meaningful photographs adjusted appropriately between text.

The volume is divided into General Microbiology, Bacterial Genetics, Immunology, Systemic Bacteriology, Virology, Mycology, Parasitology and Clinical Microbiology. More emphasis is given to collection and transportation of clinical specimen to laboratory, laboratory diagnosis of important infectious diseases, hospital infection, disposal of laboratory and hospital wastes, prevention and control of infection, hand hygiene plus nurses and microbiology.

Professor AS Sekhon, Principal and Dean, Gian Sagar Medical College and Hospital, Ram Nagar, Banur, Patiala, Punjab, is kind enough to shower his blessings and write foreword of this book.

I am grateful to Dr GM Warke of HiMedia Laboratory, Mumbai, India, for kind permission to use some photographs and Dr Suruchi Bhagra of Indira Gandhi Medical College, Shimla, India, for her contribution of photographs on dermatophytes.

I am immensely thankful to all family members including my wife Mrs Jyotsna Gupte (Managing Editor) and son Anubhav Gupte for their help and support.

Many many thanks to Shri Jitendar P Vij (Chairman and Managing Director), of M/s Jaypee Brothers Medical Publishers (P) Ltd and his team for their cooperation in bringing out this volume speedily and in impressive form.

I am grateful to Mr Gurpreet Singh and Ms Kavita Malik for performing the secretarial work diligently and intelligently.

I look forward to our esteemed readers to communicate their critical comments, suggestions and shortcomings towards improvement of subsequent editions of this volume.

Satish Gupte

Contents

Section 9   Practical Microbiology

Syllabus

Placement: First Year   **Time:** 60 Hours (Theory 45 hours + Lab 15 hours)

Course Description: This course is designed to enable students to acquire understanding of fundamentals of microbiology and identification of various microorganisms. It also provides opportunities for practicing infection control measures in hospital and community settings.

Unit	Time (Hours) Theory	Time (Hours) Practical	Learning objectives	Content	Teaching learning activities	Assessment methods
I	5		• Explain concepts and principles of microbiology and their importance in nursing	**Introduction:** • Importance and relevance to nursing • Historical perspective • Concepts and terminology • Principles of microbiology	• Lecture discussion	• Short answers • Objective type
II	10	5	• Describe structure, classification morphology and growth of bacteria • Identify micro-organisms	**General characteristics of microbes:** • Structure and classification of microbes • Morphological types • Size and form of bacteria • Mortility • Colonization • Growth and nutrition of microbes – Temperature – Moisture – Blood and body fluids • Laboratory methods for identification of microorganisms • Staining techniques, Gram staining, acid fast staining, hanging drop preparation • Culture; various medias	• Lecture discussion • Demonstration	• Short answers • Objective type

Unit	Time (Hours)		Learning objectives	Content	Teaching learning activities	Assessment methods
	Theory	Practical				
III	10	2	• Describe the methods of infection control • Identify the role of nurse in hospital infection control program	**Infection control:** • Infection: Sources, portals of entry and exit, transmission • Asepsis • Disinfection; Types and methods • Sterilization; Types and methods • Chemotherapy and antibiotics • Standard safety measures • Biomedical waste management • Role of nurse • Hospital acquired infection • Hospital infection control program – Protocols, collection of samples, preparation of report and status of rate of infection in the unit/hospital, nurse's accountability, continuing education, etc.	• Lecture discussion • Demonstration • Visits to CSSD • Clinical practice	• Short answers • Objective type

IV	12	4	Describe the different disease producing organisms	**Pathogenic organism:**
				• Microorganisms
				  – Cocci—Gram positive and Gram negative
				  – Bacilli—Gram positive and Gram negative
				  – Spirochaete
				  – Mycoplasma
				  – Rickettsiae
				  – Chlamydiae
				• Viruses
				• Fungi—superficial and deep mycoses
				• Parasites
					• Lecture discussion
					• Demonstration
					• Clinical practice
						• Short answers
						• Objective type

Unit	Time (Hours) Theory	Practical	Learning objectives	Content	Teaching learning activities	Assessment methods
				• Rodents and vectors, characteristics, source, portal of entry, transmission of infection, identification of disease producing microorganisms, collection, handling and transportation of various specimens		

V	8	4	Explain the concept of immunity, hyper-sensitivity and immunization	**Immunity:**
				• Immunity—types, classification
				• Antigen and antibody reaction
				• Hypersensitivity—skin test
				• Serological tests
				• Immunoprophylaxis
				  – Vaccines and sera—types and classification, storage and handling, cold chain
				  – Immunization for various diseases
				  – Immunization schedule
					• Lecture discussion
					• Demonstration
					• Clinical practice
						• Short answers
						• Objective type

General Microbiology

SECTION OUTLINE

- ❖ Microbiology and Nurses
- ❖ History and Scope
- ❖ Morphology of Bacteria
- ❖ Nutritional Requirements of Bacteria
- ❖ Media for Bacterial Growth
- ❖ Classification and Identification of Bacteria
- ❖ Sterilization and Disinfection
- ❖ Infection
- ❖ Chemotherapeutic Agents

SECTION 1

Microbiology and Nurses

In fact medical microbiology discipline forms the foundation for nurses capability to the followings:

1. Development of infection control program.
2. Participation in the appropriate application of techniques to reduce or prevent the incidence of hospital infection.
3. Reduce the opportunity for the development of antibiotic resistance.

The daily problems faced in patient health-care and clinical decision made by nurses are quite difficult and require broadest foundation of knowledge possible. In this regard medical microbiology remains a vital part of foundation. Moreover, it is compulsory that nurses have a working knowledge of principles of epidemiology, surveillance and outbreak management of infections to provide ongoing quality care in special situations.

It is important to understand main elements of medical microbiology. The way they can affect the health of a person, the family and community, is vital requisite in blocking the transmission of diseases.

INFECTION CONTROL TEAM

The team consists of:

1. Physician (Infection Control Officer)
2. Nurse (Infection Control Nurse)
3. Medical Microbiologist

Infection Control Nurse

She supervises the infection control program and provides intermediate care facilities, etc.

ROLE OF NURSES IN PREVENTION OF HOSPITAL ACQUIRED INFECTION

Nurses play an important role to prevent hospital acquired infection. In this regard their responsibilities include:

1. By explaining the importance of hand-washing to patients and all those who come in contact with patients. It really reduces the load of bacteria and thus reducing the chances of transfer of infection from one patient to others.
2. Isolation of infected patients in private room, e.g., chickenpox, measles, typhoid fever, meningitis, etc.
3. Considering all blood and body fluids samples as infectious and thus handle them with utmost care.
4. Handling of blood, fluids, secretions, excretions, etc., using sterilized gloves.
5. Wearing of mask, gown, eye protecter during any procedure likely to cause splash of body fluids, secretions, etc.
6. Ensure the single use items proper disposal.
7. Proper sterilization of reusable items.
8. Practical knowledge and its application regarding disposal of biomedical wastes infections.
9. Practically following the policies of Infection Control Committee (ICC) of the hospital regarding use of disinfectants and hygiene practices.
10. Carefully handling of soiled linen and body fluids. This is done to avoid transmission of microorganisms to other patients and environment.

11. Must arrange placing of cards on the doors of the patients, mentioning the type of isolation and instructions for visitors and nursing staff.

12. Making the patients to understand to avoid the over use of antibiotics. This is possible by explaining to them about infection, differences between viruses and disease causing organisms, bad effects of antibiotic over use and body immunity.

13. Restricting the entry of number of attendants of patient.

14. Teaching of infection control isolation, etc., to employees at all levels.

15. Identification of areas of hospital showing infection risk and act to remove hazards of infections.

16. Assist in identifying carriers, tracing source of infection and preventing transmission of disease.

17. Review of microbiological data and note the significant findings.

18. Maintaining records of all environmental culturing and surveillance.

History and Scope

INTRODUCTION

The first simple forms of life appeared on earth more than three billion years ago. Their descendants have changed and developed into the several million types of animals, plants and microorganisms recognized today. Of course, thousands more remain to be discovered and officially described.

Microscopic forms of life are present in vast numbers in nearly every environment known, i.e., soil, water, food and air. Since, the conditions that favor the survival and growth of many are the same as those under which people normally live. It is not unusual to find out these microscopic forms on the surface of our bodies and in mouth, nose, portions of the digestion tract and other body regions. Fortunately, the majority of these microorganisms are not harmful to humans.

Many microscopic microorganisms or microbes occur as single cell, others are multicellular, and still others such as viruses, do not have a true cellular appearance. Some organisms called anaerobes are capable of carrying out their vital functions in the absence of free oxygen; whereas other organisms can manufacture the essential compounds for their physiological needs from atmospheric sources of nitrogen and carbon dioxide. Other microorganisms, such as viruses and certain bacteria are totally dependent for their existence on the cells of higher forms of life. The branch of science known as microbiology embraces all of these properties of microorganisms and many more.

As we progressed towards conquering over many infectious diseases like smallpox, anthrax, plague, etc., and campaign is in progress with varied vaccines and other efforts on war footing hopes we dashed to the ground with reemergence of diseases like malaria, influenza, tuberculosis, plague, dengue and many more. Not only this, but we were further discouraged with the appearance of new microbes causing disastrous diseases like AIDS (1981), Lyme's disease, Ebola fever, Marburg disease, Hepatitis C, Hepatitis E, Hepatitis F, Hepatitis G, SARS bird flu, swine flu, etc.

On the positive side microbiology has its share in contributing as a model in studies of genetics, molecular biology in addition to suggesting diagnostic methods, prevention and control of various diseases of microbes origin. Genetic engineering is another magnificient gift of microbes with other technique of genetic manipulations.

Historical Events

Long before the discovery of microorganisms certain processes caused by their life activities, such as fermentation of wine juice, milk, yeast, etc., were known to mankind. In ancient times at the beginning of civilization, man by using these processes learned to prepare koumurs, sour milk and other products.

In the works of Hippocrates (460–377 BC), Verona (2nd century BC), Lucretins (95–55 BC), Pliny (23–79 AD), Galen (131–211 AD) and other scientists of that time, the hypotheses of living nature (contagium vivum) of contagious diseases was described.

Varo and Columella (first century BC) suggested that diseases were caused by invisible organisms (animalia minuta) inhaled or ingested.

Fracastorius of Verona (1546) felt that contagium vivum may be the cause of infectious disease.

Kircher (1659) could find minute worms in the blood of a plague patient. It is more likely that he observed perhaps only blood cells with the apparatus which he had at his disposal at that time.

Antoni van Leeuwenhoek (1683) could give description of various types of bacteria. He also invented the simple microscope.

As microbes are not visible to the unaided eye, the observation had to wait till microscopes were developed. Jensen (1590) happened to be the first fortunate person who successfully magnified object using hand lens. The credit for observation and description of bacteria is attached to Antoni van Leeuwenhoek of Holland (1683). An amateur lens grinder and was first person to make glass lenses powerful enough for observation and description of bacteria. He suggested that population of increase of animalcules were progeny of few parenteral organisms and described many different living and parasitic protozoa, filamentous fungi and globular bodies (yeast cells) from human and animal stools. He introduced meat and vegetable infusions in culture medium and 250 single lensed microscopes. Robert Hook, a contemporary of Leeuwenhoek developed compound microscope in 1678 and confirmed Leeuwenhoek's observation.

Von Plenciz (1762) proposed that each disease was caused by a separate agent.

Augustino Bassi (1835) proposed that muscardine disease of silk worm was caused by fungus.

Oliver Wendell Holmes (1843) and Ignaz Semmelweis in Vienna (1846) independently put forward the view that puerperal sepsis was transmitted by the contaminated hands of obstetricians and medical students. Washing of hands in antiseptic solution was suggested for its prevention.

Pasteur (1857) established that fermentation was the result of microbial activity. Different types of fermentation were associated with different kinds of microorganisms. He introduced techniques of sterilization and developed steam sterilizer, hot air oven and autoclave. He started his work on pebrine, anthrax, chickenpox, cholera and hydrophobia. He attenuated culture of anthrax bacilli by incubation at high temperature (42°C to 43°C) and proved that inocculation of such culture in animal induced specific protection against anthrax. Pasteur's development of vaccine for hydrophobia was the greatest breakthrough in medicine. He is remembered as a man who laid the foundation of microbiology. He is also known as father of microbiology.

Robert Koch (father of bacteriology) perfected bacteriological techniques during his studies on the culture of anthrax bacillus (1876). He introduced staining techniques and also methods of obtaining bacteria in pure culture using solid media. He discovered bacillus tuberculosis (1882), *Vibrio cholerae* (1883) and also demonstrated Koch's phenomena which is the expression of hypersensitivity phenomena of *Mycobacterium tuberculosis.*

He also suggested criteria before blaming the organism responsible for disease. It goes by the name of Koch's postulate, according to which:

1. Organism should be present in the pathological lesion and its demonstration from this lesion.
2. We must be able to culture the organism from the lesion.
3. These cultured organisms must be able to produce same lesion when injected into animals.
4. Again these organisms should be cultured from animal lesion.
5. Antibodies against these organism should be demonstrable (added subsequently).

Lord Lister (1854) used carbolic acid spray on wound during operation. He is also called father of antiseptic surgery.

Hansen (1874) described leprosy bacillus.

Neisser (1879) described *Gonococcus*.

Ogston (1881) discovered *Staphylococcus*.

Loeffler (1884) isolated diphtheria bacillus.

Nicolaier (1884) observed tetanus bacilli in soil.

Fraenkel (1886) described *Pneumococcus*.

Schaudin and Hoffman discovered the spirochaete of syphilis.

Roux and Yersin (1888) described mechanism of pathogenesis when they discovered diphtheria toxin.

Loeffler and Frosch (1898) observed that foot and mouth disease of cattle was caused by a microbe, i.e., filter passing virus.

Walter Reed (1902) observed that yellow fever was caused by filterable virus and that it was transmitted through the bite of mosquitoes.

Landsteiner and Popper (1909) showed poliomyelitis was caused by filterable virus.

Towert (1951) and Herelle (1917) discovered lytic phenomenon in bacterial culture. The agent responsible was termed as bacteriophage (viruses that attack bacteria).

Fleming (1925) made the accidental discovery that the fungus penicillium produces a substance which destroys staphylococci.

Ruska (1934) introduced electron microscope and hence detailed study of morphology of virus was possible.

Jerne (1955) proposed natural selection theory of antibody synthesis.

Burnet (1957) put forward clonal selection theory.

Burnet (1967) introduced concept of immunological surveillance.

New agent of infectious diseases continue to emerge, e.g., HIV (identified in 1980). The outbreaks of plague in 1994, cholera in 1995, and dengue hemorrhage fever in 1996.

As such many workers in medicine have been awarded Nobel Prizes for their outstanding contributions in microbiology **(Table 2.1)**.

The methods of many infectious diseases and vaccine production have been revolutionized, e.g., recombine DNA technology, PCR, nuclear anaprobes, radioimmunoassay, ELISA, etc.

MICROBIOLOGY

In short this is the science dealing with the study of microorganisms.

Branches of Microbiology

1. Medical microbiology
2. Industrial microbiology
3. Food microbiology
4. Soil microbiology
5. Plant microbiology

Here we are concerned with medical microbiology. It is studied under following headings:

a. Parasitology deals with the study of parasites causing diseases in human being.

b. Mycology deals with the study of fungi causing diseases in human beings.

c. Immunology is concerned with mechanism involved in the development of resistance by body to infectious diseases.

d. Bacteriology deals with the study of bacteria.

e. Genetics is the study of heredity and variations.

f. Virology is the study of viruses.

Scope of Microbiology

1. Diagnostic, e.g., isolation and identification of causative organism from the pathological lesions. We can also diagnose typhoid fever by doing Widal's test.

2. Prognosis of disease, e.g., in Widal's test rising titer signifies active disease and ineffective treatment. Falling titer means effective treatment and curing of disease.

Table 2.1: Nobel prize winners in microbiology.

1901	Behring	Antitoxins
1902	Ross	Malaria
1905	Koch	Bacteriology
1907	Laveran	Malaria
1908	Ehrlich and Metchnikoff	Theories of immunology
1913	Richet	Anaphylaxis
1919	Bordet	Immunology
1928	Nicolle	Typhus fever
1930	Landsteiner	Blood groups
1939	Domagk	Sulfonamide
1945	Fleming, Florey and Chain	Penicillin
1951	Theiler	Yellow fever vaccine
1952	Waksman	Streptomycin
1954	Ender	Cellular culture of polio virus
1958	Lederberg, Tatum and Beadle	Genetics
1959	Ochoa, Kornberg	Genetics RNA
1960	Burnet and Medawar	Theories of immunity
1962	Watson and Crick	Genetic code, structure of DNA
1965	Jacob, Monod and Lwoff	Genetic episome and prephage
1966	Rous	Viral etiology of cancer
1968	Nirenberg, Holley and Khurana	Synthesis of DNA
1969	Hershey, Luria and Delbruck	Genetics, mutations
1972	Porter and Edelman	Structure of immunoglobulin
1974	Christian	Lysosomes
1975	Dulbeco, Baltimore and Temin	Genetics and mutations
1976	Gajdusek and Blumberg	Slow virus and Australia antigen
1977	Rosalyn Yalow	Radioimmunoassay
1978	Arber, Nathans and Smith	Restriction enzyme
1980	Snell, Dausse and Benacerraf	Major histocompatibility complex (MHC) and genetic control of immune response
1983	Barbara McClintock	Mobile genetic element
1984	Georges Koehler and Danish Niels Jerne	Monoclonal antibodies
1987	Tonegawa Susumu	Generation of immunoglobulin diversity
1988	Gertrude Elion, George Hitchings and James Black	Discoveries of important principles that have resulted in the development of a series of new drugs including Acyclovir for herpes and AZT for treating AIDS
1989	Michael Bishop and Harold Varmus	Discovery of cellular origin of viral oncogenes
1993	Richard J Robert	Split genes
1997	Stanley B Prusiner	Prion
2005	Barry J Marshal and Robin Warren	*Helicobacter pylori* as causative agent of gastritis and peptic ulcer
2006	Andrew Fire and Craig Mello	RNA interference—gene silencing by DS RNA

3. Guidance in treatment, e.g., by culturing the organism in pure form and then performing drug sensitivity test we can suggest the effective drug for the treatment of that particular infection.
4. Source of infection, e.g., in sudden outbreak of infectious disease we can find out the source of infection.
5. Detection of new pathogens and then development of vaccines.

BIOLOGICAL WEAPONS

Now it is quite clear and understandable that biological warfare is not new at all. Biological warfare was resorted by early Romans who polluted water sources of their enemies by dumping animal carcasses. Then British distributed blankets to Indians in 1763. These blankets had been used by smallpox patients. Hence, Indian users contracted smallpox. British had detonated an experimental anthrax bomb in Gruinard Island in second world war. In 1984, 750 people fell ill to food poisoning in Oregaon because of spread of *Salmonella* that had been cultured in the laboratory.

Biological warfare may be defined as intentional use of doses to harm or kill an adversary military forces, population, food or livestock and includes any living, or nonliving organisms or its bioactive substance (toxin). Hence, germ warfare can be spearheaded by bacteria, viruses, fungi, toxins, etc.

Some of the characteristics of biological warfare agents include low infective dose, high virulence, short incubation period, little immunity in target population, ease of production, ease of delivery, rebustness, stability and availability with aggressor, etc.

Organisms which can be used for biological war are *Bacillus anthracis* (causing pneumonia with a mortality rate 95%, if untreated), smallpox (contagious with high mortality rate), *Yersinia pestis* (plague causing bacteria), *Francisella tularensis* (tularemia), Ebola and Marburg viruses (hemorrhage fever), *Clostridium botulinum* (botulinism), etc.

Since organisms are capable of infecting widespread illness together with their low cost, their use as biological war weapons seems to be next possibility. The organisms likely to be used for this purpose may be rendered resistant to antibiotic agents, or even to vaccine by genetic means, etc.

Morphology of Bacteria

▆ INTRODUCTION

Bacteria are unicellular free living organisms without chlorophyll having both DNA and RNA. They are capable of performing all essential processes of life, e.g., growth, metabolism and reproduction. They have rigid cell wall containing muramic acid. They were originally classified under plant and animal kingdoms. This being unsatisfactory a third kingdom Protista was proposed by Hackel in 1866 for them. Protista is again divided into two groups: (a) Prokaryotes, and (b) Eukaryotes. Bacteria and green algae (photosynthetic and possess chlorophyll which can exhibit gliding movement like photosynthetic bacteria) are prokaryotes while fungi, algae, slime molds and protozoa are eukaryotes. It is worth mentioning to enumerate the differences between prokaryotic and eukaryotic cells **(Table 3.1)**.

Size of bacteria: Most of bacteria are so small that their size is measured in terms of micron.
1 micron (μ) or micrometer (μm) =
    One-thousandth of millimeter.
1 millimicron (mμ) or nanometer (nm) =
    One-thousandth of micron.
1 Angstrom units (Å) =
    One-tenth of nanometer.
    Generally, cocci are about 1 μ in diameter and bacilli are 2 to 10 μ in length and 0.2 to 0.5 μ in width. The limit of resolution with unaided eye is about 200 μ. Obviously bacteria can be visualized only under magnification.

Shape of bacteria: On the basis of shape, bacteria are classified as under:

Table 3.1: Differences between prokaryotic cell and eukaryotic cell.

Character	Prokaryotic cell	Eukaryotic cell
I. Nucleus		
Nuclear membrane	Absent	Present
Nucleolus	Absent	Present
Histones	Absent	Absent
Chromosome	One	More
Mitotic division	Absent	Present
DNA	Circular	Linear
II. Cytoplasm		
Cytoplasmic streaming	Absent	Present
Cytoplasmic ribosome	70s	80s
Pinocytosis	Absent	Present
Mitochondria	Absent	Present
Lysosomes	Absent	Present
Golgi apparatus	Absent	Present
Endoplasmic reticulum	Absent	Present
III. Chemical composition		
Sterol	Absent	Present
Muramic acid	Present	Absent
Diaminopimelic acid	May be present	Absent
IV. Miscellaneous		
Diameter	1 µm	10 µm
Oxidative phos-phorylation site	Cell membrane	Chloro-plast
Cilia	Absent	Present
Pili	Present	Absent

A. Cocci (from kakkos, meaning berry): They are spherical. On the basis of arrangement of individual organisms, they are described as staphylococci (clusters like bunches of grapes), streptococci (arranged in chains), diplococci (forming pairs), tetrads and sarcina are cocci arranged in groups of four and cubical packet of eight cell respectively (**Figs. 3.1A to E**).

B. The cylindrical or rod shaped organisms are called *bacilli* (from baculus, meaning rods). They are of following types (**Figs. 3.2A to F**):

1. In some of the organisms length may approximate the width of the organisms. These are called coccobacilli, e.g., brucella.
2. Chinese letter arrangement is seen in corynebacteria.
3. Vibrio: These are comma shaped, curved rods and derive the name from their characteristic vibratory motility.
4. Spirochaetes (from speria meaning coil, chaete meaning hair). They are relatively longer, thin, flexible organisms having several coils.
5. Actinomycetes (actis meaning ray, mykes, meaning fungus) are branching filamentous bacteria, so called because of resemblance to radiating sunrays.
6. Mycoplasma are organisms which lack cell wall and so do not possess a stable morphology. They are round or oval bodies with interlacing filaments.

Many a time cell wall synthesis becomes defective either spontaneously or as a result of drug, e.g., in presence of penicillin bacteria lose their distinctive shape. Such organisms are called protoplast spheroplast or L forms.

Bacterial Anatomy

The outermost layer consists of two components—(a) a rigid cell wall, and (b) cytoplasmic membrane or plasma membrane. Inside this there is protoplasm comprising of the cytoplasm, cytoplasmic inclusions, such as ribosomes, mesosomes, granules, vacuoles and nuclear body. The cell may be enclosed in a viscid layer which may be loose slime layer or organized as a capsule. Nowadays all substances containing polysaccharides lying external to cell wall (both slime layer and capsule) are called glycocalyx. Apart from this some bacteria carry filamentous appendages protruding from cell surface; the flagella, organ of locomotion and the fimbriae which seem to be organ of adhesion.

The important structural features of bacterial cell as found under electron microscope are described below (**Figs. 3.3 and 3.4**).

■ SLIME LAYER

Some bacteria secrete viscid substance which may diffuse out into surrounding media or remain outside cell wall. This viscid

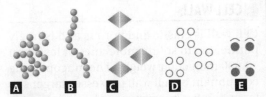

Figs. 3.1A to E: Arrangement of bacilli (A) Cocci in cluster—staphylococci; (B) Cocci in chain—streptococci; (C) Cocci in pair—diplococci; (D) Cocci in groups of four—tetrad; (E) Cocci in group of eight—sarcina.

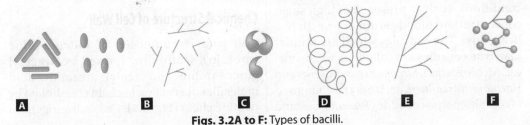

Figs. 3.2A to F: Types of bacilli.

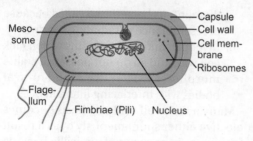

Fig. 3.3: Structure of bacterium.

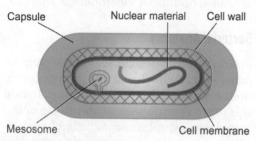

Fig. 3.4: Capsulated bacterium showing nuclear material, a mesosome and relation of cytoplasmic membrane to cell wall.

carbohydrate material is called slime layer. Its presence can be shown only on immunological ground. Bacteria secreting large amount of slime produce mucoid growth on agar with stringy consistency when touched with loop, e.g., *Klebsiella*. Slime has little affinity for basic dye and so not visible in Gram stained smear.

▌CAPSULE (FIG. 3.4)

It is the gelatinous secretion of bacteria which gets organized as a thick coat around cell wall and is known as capsule. Capsulated bacteria are usually nonmotile as flagella remains unfunctional in the presence of capsule. Development of capsule is dependent on the existence of favorable environmental conditions, such as presence of high sugar concentration, blood serum or growth in a living host. The capsules which are thinner than true capsules are called microcapsule, e.g., Meningococci, *Streptococcus pyogenes* and *Haemophilus influenzae*. It may be composed of complex polysaccharide (*Pneumococci* and

Klebsiella) or polypeptide (*Bacillus anthracis*) or hyaluronic acid (*Streptococcus pyogenes*). Capsules have no affinity for dyes and so they are not seen in stained preparations.

Demonstration of Capsule

a. Negative staining with India ink: In this procedure, bacterial bodies and spaces in between are filled with India ink and capsule is seen as halo around cell.
b. Special capsule staining technique using copper salt as moderant.
c. Serological methods: If suspension of capsulated bacterium is mixed with its specific serum and examine under microscope, capsule becomes prominent and appears swollen due to increase in refractivity (Quellung reaction).

Functions

1. Protection against deleterious agents, e.g., lytic enzymes.
2. Contribute to the virulence of pathogenic bacteria by inhibiting phagocytosis.
3. Capsular antigen is hapten in nature and specific for bacteria.

▌CELL WALL

Cell wall is elastic and porous and is freely permeable to solute molecules of less than 10,000 molecular weight. The mucopeptide component of cell wall possesses target site for antibiotics lysozymes and bacteriophages. The cell wall is the outermost supporting layer which protects the internal structure. It is about 10 to 25 nm in thickness and shares 20 to 30% of dry weight of the cells.

Chemical Structure of Cell Wall

Cell wall is composed of mucopeptide (muerin), scaffolding formed by N-acetyl glucosamine and acetyl muramic acid molecules alternating in chain crosslinked by peptide chain (**Fig. 3.5**). Cell wall antigens of

Gram-negative organisms act as endotoxin. A comparison of cell walls of Gram-positive and Gram-negative bacteria is enumerated in **Figure 3.7** and **Table 3.2**.

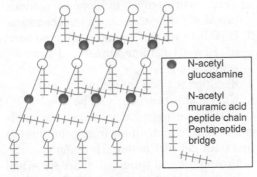

Fig. 3.5: Chemical structure of bacterial cell wall.

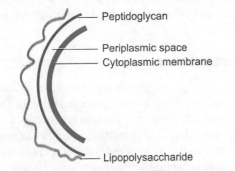

Fig. 3.6: Cell wall (Gram-negative bacteria).

Gram-negative Cell Wall

It is a complex structure **(Fig. 3.6)** comprising of:

  i. Lipoprotein layer which connects outer membrane to peptidoglycan.
 ii. Outer membrane is a phospholipid bilayer containing specific proteins. These specific proteins form porins and hydrophilic molecules are transported through these porins. Other proteins are target sites for phages, antibiotics and bacteriocins.
iii. Lipopolysaccharide consists of a complex lipid, called lipid A, to which is attached a polysaccharide. Lipopolysaccharide is the endotoxin of Gram-negative bacteria—the toxicity is associated with lipid portion (lipid A) and the polysaccharide represents a major surface antigen, the O antigen. The polysaccharide consists of a core and a terminal series of repeat units. These terminal repeat units confer antigenic specificity to the bacterium.
 iv. The periplasmic space is the space in between the inner and outer membranes and contain a number of important proteins (such as enzymes and binding proteins for specific substrates) and

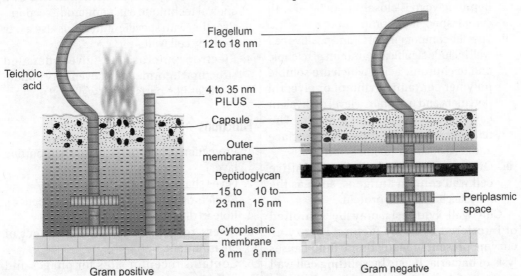

Fig. 3.7: Difference between Gram-positive and Gram-negative organisms.

Table 3.2: Comparison of cell walls of gram-positive and gram-negative bacteria.

	Gram-positive	Gram-negative
• Thickness	15 to 25 nm	10 to 15 nm
• Variety of amino acid	Few	Several
• Aromatic and sulfur containing amino acids	Absent	Present
• Lipids	Low 2 to 4%	High 15 to 20%
• Teichoic acids	Present	Absent
• Periplasmic space	Absent	Present
• Result of enzyme digestion	Protoplast	Spheroplast

oligosaccharides (which play an important role in osmoregulation of the cells).

Gram-positive Cell Wall

i. The peptidoglycan layer of Gram-positive bacteria is much thicker (15 to 25 nm) than that in Gram-negative (10 to 15 nm). The periplasmic space is absent and the peptidoglycan is closely associated with cytoplasmic membrane.

ii. Specific components of Gram-positive cell wall include significant amount of teichoic and teichuronic acids which are soluble polymer containing ribotol or glycerol polymers and maintain a level of divalent cations outside cell membrane. The teichoic acids constitute major surface antigens of Gram-positive bacteria.

iii. Other components of Gram-positive cell wall contain antigens, such as the polysaccharide and protein.

Cell wall synthesis may be inhibited or interfered by many factors. Lysozyme enzyme present in many tissue fluid causes lysis of bacteria. It acts by splitting cell wall mucopeptide linkages. When lysozyme acts on Gram-positive organism in hypertonic

solution, a protoplast is formed consisting of cytoplasmic membrane and contents. Characteristic features of protoplast are:

1. Unstable structures.
2. Very sensitive to the influence of osmotic pressure, mechanical action and aberration.
3. Unable to synthesize the component parts of cell wall (diaminopimelic and muramic acids).
4. Resistant to phage infection.
5. Not capable of active motility.

With Gram-negative bacteria the result is spheroplast which differs from protoplast in that some cell wall material is retained.

Protoplast and spheroplast are spherical regardless of original shape of the bacterium. Such organisms might have a role in certain persistent chronic infections, such as pyelonephritis.

Demonstration

1. When intact bacteria are placed in a solution of very high solute concentrations and osmotic pressure, protoplast shrinks thus retracting the cytoplasmic membrane from cell wall. The process is called plasmolysis and is useful in demonstrating cell wall.
2. Cell wall may also be demonstrated by a special technique called microdissection.
3. Reaction with specific antibody is also a way to study cell wall.
4. Electron microscope gives detailed structural information of even very minute particles like parts of cell wall.

Functions

1. Protection of internal structure (supporting layer).
2. Gives shape to the cell.
3. Confers rigidity and ductility (mucopeptide).
4. Role in division of bacteria.
5. Offers resistance to harmful effect of environment.
6. Contains receptor sites for phages and colicin.
7. Provides attachment to complement.

CYTOPLASMIC MEMBRANE

It is thin semipermeable membrane which lies just beneath the cell wall. The whole bacterial cytoplasm is bound peripherally by a very thin, elastic and semipermeable cytoplasmic membrane also known as cell membrane. It is 5 to 10 nm in width. Electron microscope shows the presence of three layers constituting a unit membrane structure. Chemically, the membrane consists of phospholipid with small amount of protein. Sterol is absent except in mycoplasma (**Figs. 3.8 and 3.9**).

Demonstration

1. The separation of membrane from the cell wall is achieved readily in Gram-negative bacteria when they are suspended in medium of high osmotic tension. Such a phenomenon is called plasmolysis.
2. Electron microscope.

Functions

1. It controls inflow and outflow of metabolites to and from protoplast.

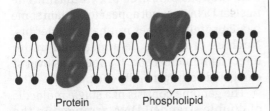

Protein   Phospholipid

Fig. 3.8: Chemical structure of cytoplasmic membrane.

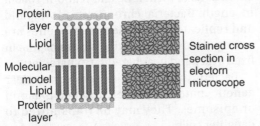

Protein layer

Lipid

Molecular model

Lipid

Protein layer

Stained cross-section in electorn microscope

Fig. 3.9: A unit cell membrane with a lipid bilayer with hydrophilic regions towards a protein layer at each surface with characteristic appearance of stained cross-section in electron microscope.

2. Presence in the membrane of specific enzyme (permease) which plays important role in passage through membrane of selective nutrients.
3. The cytoplasmic membrane contains some other enzymes, e.g., respiratory enzymes and pigments (cytochrome system), certain enzymes of tricarboxylic acid cycle and perhaps, polymerizing enzymes that manufacture the substance of cell wall and extracellular structure.
4. It provides little mechanical strength to bacterial cell.
5. It helps DNA replication.
6. It concentrates sugar, amino acids and phosphatase creating 300 to 400 fold gradient across osmotic barrier.

CYTOPLASM

The bacterial cytoplasm is suspension of organic and inorganic solutes in viscous watery solution.

It does not exhibit protoplasmic streaming (internal mobility) and it lacks endoplasmic reticulum or mitochondria. It contains ribosomes, mesosomes, inclusions and vacuoles.

Ribosomes: Ribosomes appear as small granules and pack the whole cytoplasm. These are strung together on strands of mRNA to form polymers. The code of mRNA is translated into peptide sequence at this place. The ribosomal particles become linked up and travel along the mRNA strand. It determines the sequence of amino acids brought to the site on tRNA molecule and build up the polypeptide.

Ribonucleoprotein granules measure 10 to 20 nm units in diameter and their sedimentation coefficient is 70 svedberg units. The 70s ribosome is composed of two smaller units of 50s and 30s.

Functions: They are the sites of protein synthesis.

Polysomes: They are groups of ribosomes linked together like beads of chain by messenger RNA.

Mesosomes: They are vesicular, convoluted or multilaminated structures formed as invaginations of plasma membrane in the cytoplasm. They are prominent in Gram-positive bacteria. There are two types of mesosomes, i.e., septal mesosome and lateral mesosome. The septal mesosome is attached to bacterial chromosome and is involved in DNA segregation and in the formation of cross walls during cell division. They are also called chondroids and are visualized only under electron microscope. They are more prominent in some Gram-positive bacteria.

Functions

1. They are the sites of respiratory enzymes in bacteria.
2. Coordinate nuclear and cytoplasmic division during binary fission.
3. Responsible for compartmenting DNA at sporulation.

Intracytoplasmic Inclusions

Three types of cytoplasmic granules are encountered, i.e., glycogen (enteric bacteria), Poly-beta-hydroxybutyrate (Bacillus and *Pseudomonas*) and Babes-Ernst (*Coryne-bacterium, Yersinia pestis*).

a. **Volutin granules** (Metachromatic or Babes-Ernst granules) are highly refractive, basophilic bodies consisting of polymetaphosphate.
   Demonstration: Special staining techniques, such as Albert, or Neisser, demonstrate the granules more clearly. They are characteristically present in diphtheria bacilli and *Yersinia pestis*.
   Function: They are considered to represent a reserve of energy and phosphate for cell metabolism.
b. **Polysaccharide granules** may be demonstrated by staining with iodine. They appear to be storage products. These granules are used as carbon sources when protein and nucleic acid synthesis is resumed.

Table 3.3: Cytoplasmic granules in bacteria.

Granules	Bacteria
• Glycogen	• Enteric bacteria
• Poly-beta-hydroxylbutyrate	• Bacillus and *Pseudomonas*
• Babes-Ernst	• *Corynebacterium, Yersinia pestis*

c. **Certain sulfur oxidizing bacteria** convert excess H_2S from environment into intracellular granules of element sulfur.
d. **Lipid inclusion** are storage product and demonstrated with fat soluble dyes, such as sudan black.
e. **Vacuoles** are fluid containing cavities separated from cytoplasm by a membrane. Their function and significance is uncertain **(Table 3.3)**.

NUCLEUS

It is a long filament of DNA tightly coiled inside the cytoplasm. The bacterial nucleus is not surrounded by nuclear membrane and is Feulgen positive. It is an ill-defined homogenous pale area of cytoplasm. The nuclear DNA does not appear to contain some basic protein. It does not have nucleolus. Nucleus cannot be demonstrated under direct light microscope. It appears as oval or elongated body, generally one per cell.

The genome consists of a single molecule of double stranded DNA arranged in the form of circle. It may open under certain conditions to form long chain about 1000 µ in length. Bacterial chromosome is haploid and replicates by simple fission. Genes are arranged along the length of chromosome in fixed order and bear hereditary characters.

Bacteria may sometimes have extranuclear genetic material. These are called plasmid or episomes. They may be transmitted to daughter cells:

a. During binary fission
b. By conjugation or
c. Through agency of bacterial phages.

Plasmids are not essential for the life of cell. They may confer certain properties like toxigenicity virulence and drug resistance.

FLAGELLA

These are long, sinnous contractile filamentous appendages known as flagella. These are organs of locomotion, e.g., *Escherichia coli, Salmonella, Vibrio, Pseudomonas*, etc. The number of flagella varies up to 10 to 20 per cells according to species of bacteria. *Escherichia coli* has a motility of about 30 μ and that of *Vibrio cholerae* about 60 μ per second. These are extremely thin 12 to 30 nm, helical shaped structure of uniform diameter throughout their length. These are 3 to 20 μ long. Each flagellum **(Fig. 3.10)** consists of hook and basal body. It originates in a spherical body (basal granule) located just inside cell wall. These are antigenic and are composed of protein called flagellin which has properties of fibrous protein, keratin and myosin. Around 40 gene products are involved in its assembly and function.

The number and arrangement of flagella are characteristic of each bacteria. Flagella may be arranged on bacterial body in following manner **(Fig. 3.11)**.

Monotrichate: One flagellum at one end of the organism, e.g., *Vibrio, Pseudomonas, Spirillum*, etc.

Amphitrichate: One flagellum at both poles, e.g., *Alcaligenes fecales*.

Lophotrichate: A tuft of flagella at the end, e.g., *Pseudomonas*.

Peritrichate: Several flagella present all over the surface of bacteria, e.g., *Escherichia coli, Salmonella*.

Function: It is responsible for bacterial motility. Motility may be observed microscopically (hanging drop preparation) or by detecting the spreading growth in semi-solid agar medium. It has been suggested that heat formed as a result of metabolism is given off

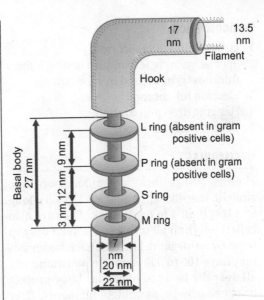

Fig. 3.10: Basal structure of bacterial flagella.

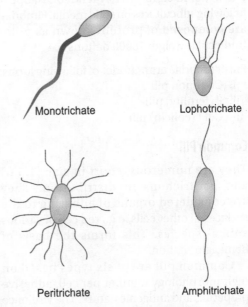

Fig. 3.11: Arrangement of flagella in bacteria.

to the environment through the flagella, while ATP serves as an energy source. The created difference in temperature causes a stream of water along the flagella, and the bacterium moves in an opposite direction.

Demonstration

1. Dark ground microscopy
2. Special staining techniques in which their thickness is increased by mordanting
3. Electron microscope
4. Hanging drop preparation
5. Craigie's tube method.

FIMBRIAE

Fimbriae (fringes) are filamentous, short, thin, straight, hair-like appendage 0.1 to 1.5 µ long and less than 4 to 8 nm thick. They are also called pili (hair). Fimbriae are seen only in some Gram-negative bacteria. Each bacterium may have 100 to 500 fimbriae peritrichously all over the body of bacteria. They project from cell surface, as straight filaments. They are best developed in freshly isolated strains and in liquid culture. They tend to disappear following subcultures on solid media. Fimbriae are composed of protein known as pillin (molecular weight 18000 daltons).

Pili or fimbriae are as under of following forms:
  i. Common pili
 ii. F (fertility) pili
iii. Col I (colicin) pili

Common Pili

They are numerous, short in size (1.5 µ) and peritrichous in distribution. They are considered organs of adhering to the surfaces of other cells, e.g., red cell of various animal species. This forms the basis of hemagglutination.

Common pili are of six types based on their morphology number per cell, adhesive properties and antigenic nature. The virulence of certain pathogenic bacteria depends both on toxins as well as "colonization antigens (pili)" which provide adhesive properties.

F Pili

They are associated with fertility (F+) and help in bacterial conjugation processes. They are longer (20 µ length) than common and Col I pili.

Col I Pili

They are about 2 µ in length and associated with colicin factor I.

Demonstration

1. Electron microscope
2. Hemagglutination
3. Fimbriated bacteria form pellicle in liquid media.

Functions

1. Organ of adhesion
2. Hemagglutination
3. Conjugation tube through which genetic material is transferred from the donor to recipient cell
4. They are antigenic
5. Agglutination and pellicle formation.

Table 3.4 lists the differences between flagella and fimbriae.

Table 3.4: Differences between flagella and fimbriae.

Flagella	Fimbriae
Size larger and thicker	Smaller and thinner
Arise from the cytoplasm or cytoplasmic membrane but not attached to the cell wall	Attached to the cell wall
Organ of movement	Organ of adhesion and conjugation
They are never straight	They are always straight
Not required for conjugation	Required for conjugation

SPORES (FIG. 3.12)

They are highly resistant dormant state of bacteria found in certain genera, e.g., *Bacillus, Clostridium, Sporosarcina* (Gram-positive coccus) and *Coxiella burnetii*. They are not destroyed by ordinary methods of boiling for several hours. They are killed when autoclaved at 15 lb pressure per square inch at 121°C for 20 minutes. The spores are characterized by the presence of 5 to 20% dipicolinic acid which is not found in vegetative cell and by

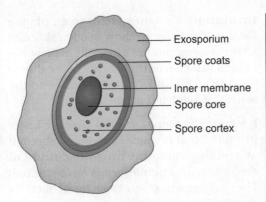

- Exosporium
- Spore coats
- Inner membrane
- Spore core
- Spore cortex

Fig. 3.12: Structure of bacterial spore.

their high calcium content. The resistance to destruction by physical or chemical method is ascribed to factors like impermeability of spores, cortex and coat, low contents of water, low metabolic activity, low enzymatic activity and high contents of calcium and dipicolinic acid. Spores of different species of bacteria are antigenically distinguishable. Spores are highly refractile and require special staining for demonstration, e.g., (1) Modified Ziehl–Neelsen method, (2) Gram stain, (3) Moller stain.

Function: They make survival of certain organisms possible under unfavorable condition like dry state. Spores are resistant to heat, drying, freezing and toxic chemicals.

Laboratory application: Can be used as sterilization control.

i. *Bacillus stearothermophilus* is killed at 121°C in 15 to 30 minutes.
ii. *Bacillus subtilis* may be destroyed at 105°C in 5 minutes.

Formation of Spores (Fig. 3.13)

Exact stimulus for sporulation is not known. Perhaps it is related to depletions of exogenous nutrient. Sporulation involves the production of many new structures, enzymes and metabolites along with the disappearance of many vegetative cell components. Sporulation can be induced by depleting PO_4, S, C, N and Fe from culture medium. A series of genes whose products determine the formation and final composition of spore are activated. Another series of genes involved in vegetative function are inactivated. These changes involve alterations in the transcriptional specificity of RNA polymerase, determined by the support of the polymerase core protein with promoter specific protein called sigma factor. Different sigma factors are produced during vegetative growth and sporulation. During the process of sporulation, some bacteria may release peptide antibiotics which may play a role in regulating sporogenesis.

Sporulation is initiated by appearance of clear area near one end of cell which gradually becomes more opaque to form forespore. The fully developed spore **(Fig. 3.12)** has its core nuclear body surrounded by spore wall, a delicate membrane (future cell wall). Outside this is spore cortex which in turn is enclosed by multilayered spore coat. Spore cortex contains an unusual type of peptidoglycon sensitive to lysozyme. The spore coat is formed by keratin like protein which is imprevious to antibacterial chemical agents. Exosporium is a lipoprotein membrane with some carbohydrate residue. Young spores remain attached to parent cell. Some spores have an additional outer covering called exosporium having ridges and grooves. Spores may be **(Fig. 3.14)**:

1. Spherical central
2. Oval central
3. Oval subterminal not bulging
4. Oval subterminal bulging
5. Oval terminal bulging
6. Terminal spherical bulging

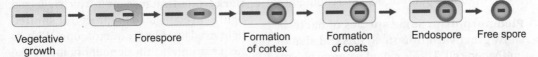

Vegetative growth   Forespore   Formation of cortex   Formation of coats   Endospore   Free spore

Fig. 3.13: Formation of spore.

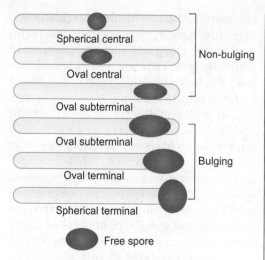

Fig. 3.14: Types of bacterial spores.

Spore Forming Bacteria

a. Gram-positive bacilli
1. Obligatory aerobic
   - *Bacillus anthracis*
   - *Bacillus subtilis*
2. Obligatory anaerobic
   - *Clostridium tetani*
   - *Clostridium perfringens*
   - *Clostridium botulinum*
3. Other bacteria
   - Gram-positive coccus—spore sarcina
   - Gram-negative Bacillus—*Coxiella burnetii*

When transferred to favorable conditions of growth, spores germinate. The spore loses its refractility and swells. The spore wall is shed and germ cell appears by rupturing the spore coat. The germ cell elongates to form vegetative bacterium.

Germination of Spore

It is the process of conversion of spore into a vegetative cell under suitable condition. It occurs in about 2 hours under ideal conditions.

Pleomorphism: Some species of bacteria show great variation in shape and size of undivided cell. This is called pleomorphism. It may be due to defective cell wall synthesis.

Involution: Certain species (e.g., plague *Bacillus*, *Gonococcus*) show swollen aberrant forms in aging cultures especially in presence of high salt concentration. It may be due to defective cell wall synthesis or due to the activity of autolytic enzymes.

L forms: The name L form is after the Lister Institute, London where swollen and aberrant morphological forms from the culture of *Streptobacillus moniliformis* were studied. They are seen in several species of bacteria developing either spontaneously or in the presence of penicillin or other agents that interfere with cell wall synthesis.

L form resembles *Mycoplasma* in several ways including morphology, type of growth on agar and filterability. Possibly *Mycoplasma* represent stable L forms of as yet unidentified parent bacteria. L form of bacteria have been isolated from patients of chronic urinary and suppurative infections. Yet their role is not clarified.

Study of Morphology of Bacteria

It is of considerable importance that identification of bacteria be made. For this purpose following methods are employed:

Optical Methods

a. **Light microscopy** is useful for the motility, size, shape and arrangement of bacteria. Due to lack of contrast, details cannot be appreciated.
b. **Phase contrast microscopy** makes evident structure within cells that differs in thickness and refractive index. In the phase contrast microscope "phase" differences are converted into differences in intensity of light producing light and dark contrast in the image.
c. **Dark ground microscopy** in which reflected light is used instead of direct transmitted light used in ordinary microscope. With its help extremely thin slender organism like spirochaetes can clearly be seen.

Table 3.5: Morphological properties of bacteria as seen in light and electron microscope.

Properties	Light microscope	Electron microscope
• Image formation	Visible light	Electron
• Medium through which radiation travels	Air	Vacuum
• Specimen mounting	Glass slides	Thin film of collodion
• Nature of lenses	Glass	Electrostatic lenses or magnetic fields
• Focussing	Mechanical	Electrical
• Magnification	Changing of objectives	Changing the current of the projector lens cool
• Mean of providing specimen contrast	Light absorption	Electron scattering

d. **Oil immersion microscopy** in which magnification produced by oil immersion objective of light microscope makes visible majority of bacteria.

e. **Fluorescence microscope** in which bacteria are stained with auramine dye or rhodamine dye. Dye changes the wavelength of bacteria stained with above dye and become visible as shining objects against a dark background. Here ultraviolet light is used as a source of light.

f. **Electron microscope** where beams of electron is used instead of beams of light used in optical microscope. The electron beam is focussed by circular electromagnets, analogous to the lenses in light microscope. The object which is kept on path of beam scatters the electrons and produces an image which is focussed on fluorescent viewing screen. **Table 3.5** depicts some points of difference between light microscope and electron microscope. Resolving power of electron microscope is 0.1 nm. Scanning electron microscope is a recent development and provides a three-dimensional image of the surface of the object.

g. **Interference microscope** can reveal cell organelles and also enable quantitative measurement of chemical constituents of cell, e.g., lipids, protein, nucleic acid, etc.

h. **Polarization microscope** enables the study of intracellular structure using differences in birefringence.

i. **Autoradiography** where cells that have incorporated radioactive atoms are fixed on a slide, covered with photographic emulsion, and stored in the dark for a suitable period of time, and then tracks appear in the developed film emanating from the sites of radioactive disintegration. If the cells are labelled with a weak emitter, such as tritium, the tracks are sufficiently labelled. This procedure, called autoradiography, has been particularly useful in following replication of DNA, using tritium labelled thymidine as a specific tracer.

Other types of microscope available are scanning electron microscope, X-ray, dissecting microscope, laser microscope (vaporize minute part of tissue in vivo or in vitro or biopsy specimen which is then subjected to emission spectrography) and operation microscope for conducting delicate surgical operations.

UNSTAINED PREPARATIONS

The wet preparations of bacterial suspensions are mainly used for (a) bacterial motility, and (b) for demonstration of spirochaetes.

Four to eight hours growth in fluid media is examined in hanging drop preparation or cover slip preparation. For the study of spirochaete, e.g., *Treponema pallidum*, dark ground microscopic examination is done.

STAINING OF BACTERIA

The bacterial nucleic acid contains negatively charged phosphate group which combines with positively charged basic dye. Acidic dye does not stain bacterial cells and are used to stain background material. Most commonly used stains to study bacterial morphology are as below:

Gram's Stain

First described by Gram in 1884. It is used to study morphologic appearance of bacteria. Gram's stain differentiates all bacteria into two distinct groups:

1. Gram-positive organisms.
2. Gram-negative organisms.

Principle: Some organisms are not decolorized and retain color of basic stain, e.g., gentian violet (Gram-positive organisms) while the others lose all gentian violet when treated with decolorizing agent and take up the counterstain, e.g., dilute carbol fuchsin or safranin (Gram-negative organisms).

Procedure: Bacterial suspension is spread in the form of thin films on the surface of clean glass slide and allowed to dry in air. It is called smear. Smear is fixed by passing the slide over the flame two or three times. Now proceed as follows:

1. Cover the slide with gentian violet for 1 to 2 minutes.
2. Wash the smear with Gram's iodine and keep Gram's iodine on the slide for 1 to 2 minutes.
3. Decolorize the slide with acetone or alcohol carefully and immediately wash the smear with water.
4. Counter stain with 0.5 percent aqueous safranin solution or dilute carbol fuchsin (1:20) for 1 to 2 minutes.
5. Finally wash the smear, allow it to dry in air and put a drop of oil and see under oil immersion lens.

Mechanism of Gram Staining: Different theories are put forward regarding mechanism of Gram reaction as exact mechanism is not known. They are:

1. **Acidic protoplasm theory:** As per this theory, Gram-positive bacteria have more acidic protoplasm as compared to Gram-negative bacteria. So, Gram-positive bacteria tend to retain the primary stain (basic in nature) more than Gram-negative bacteria. Additionally because of iodine, the cytoplasm becomes more acidic and acts as mordant. Hence, it enhances the attraction of the primary stain to the cell cytoplasm. As a result it helps to fix the stain in bacterial cell.

2. **Cell wall permeability:** Gram-positive bacterial cell wall contains more mucopeptide. It makes the cell wall thicker and stronger. As a result due to iodine complex cannot come out of Gram-positive cell wall. On the contrary, Gram-negative cell wall contains less mucopeptide and so its cell wall is thin and less strong. It is the reason that dye iodine complex diffuses out of cell and color of the counterstain is taken up.

3. **Magnesium ribonucleate theory:** As per the theory, magnesium ribonucleate is present in Gram-positive bacteria. Hence, there is formation of magnesium ribonucleate dye iodine complex which is isoluble in alcohol. In Gram-negative bacteria, magnesium ribonucleate is absent. And so only dye iodine complex is formed which is soluble in alcohol.

Acidic Acridine Orange Stain

Routine Gram stains require at least 10^5 bacilli/mL (almost close to the limit of visible turbidity in liquid media) to make its detection microscopically possible. Acidic acridine orange stain may detect bacteria much earlier with bacilli count much less. Bacteria fluoresce under ultraviolet light as red orange forms against greenish leukocytes and unstained erythrocytes. In short, this stain may be substituted for early detection of bacilli.

Albert Stain

Some bacteria may have metachromatic black granules, e.g., *Corynebacterium diphtheriae* which stain dark bluish or black with methylene blue or a mixture of taludine blue and malachite green.

Procedure: Heat fixed smear is covered with Albert stain I. After 5 to 7 minutes it is replaced by iodine solution (Albert stain II) and is kept there for 5 minutes. Smear is washed with water and studied under oil immersion lens. The body of bacilli look green while granules take bluish-black color.

Ziehl–Neelsen Stain

This is also called acid-fast stain.

Principle: Some organisms retain carbol fuchsin even when decolorized with acid. Such organisms are called acid-fast organism. However, mycolic acid is thought to be responsible for acid fastness.

Procedure: Take heat fixed smear and add concentrated carbol fuchsin. Now gently heat it till steam comes out. Do not allow the stain to boil or dry. Keep it up for 8 to 10 minutes. Now decolorize the smear with 3% solution of hydrochloric acid in 95% ethyl alcohol or 20% aqueous sulfuric acid. Now wash the slide with water and counterstain it with methylene blue or melachite green. Acid fast organisms take red stain. Acid-fast organisms are:

1. Mycobacteria (*tubercle bacilli, leprabacilli*)
2. Bacterial spores
3. Nocardia
4. Ascospore of certain yeast

5. Actinomyces club
6. Inclusions in lungs from cases of lipid pneumonia
7. Ceroids in liver of rat
8. Exoskeleton of insects **(Table 3.6)**.

Spore Stain

Spores are resistant to ordinary method of staining. In Gram stain spores appear as clear areas in deeply stained body of bacilli. Methods of spore staining are:

1. **Modified acid-fast stains:** Treat the heat fixed smear with steaming carbol fuchsin for 3 to 6 minutes. Decolorize with 0.5 percent sulfuric acid or 2% nitric acid in absolute alcohol. Wash and counter stain with 1% aqueous methylene blue. Wash with water and study it under oil immersion lens. Spores are stained bright red and vegetative part of bacilli blue.

2. **Moller methods:** Here heat fixed smear is kept over beaker with boiling water. As soon as steam starts condensing over under surface of slide, add malachite green. Keep it up for 1 to 2 minutes. Wash it and counterstain it with dilute carbol fuchsin.

Capsular Stain

They are not stained with ordinary aniline dyes. In Gram stain they are shown as area of halo around bacterium. Methods of capsule staining are:

1. **India ink method:** Emulsify small amount of culture in a loopful of India ink on a slide

Table 3.6: Examination of exoskeleton of insects.

Examination	Result	Grading	No. of fields to be examined
• More than 10 AFB per oil immersion field	Positive	3+	20
• 1–10 AFB per oil immersion field	Positive	2+	50
• 10–99 AFB per 100 oil immersion fields	Positive	1+	100
• 1–9 AFB per 100 oil immersion fields	Positive	Scanty 1–9 (Record exact number seen)	100
• No AFB per 100 oil immersion fields	Negative	–	100

and cover it with coverslip. Capsule is seen as clear halo between refractile outline of cell wall and greyish background of India ink. It is the best and rapid method of capsule demonstration.

2. **Hiss's method:** Treat thin freshly prepared smear with hot crystal violet for one minute. Now wash with 20% solution of copper sulfate and blot.

The capsule is stained blue and the body of the bacteria stains deep purple.

BIOFILM

Definition: Biofilm is obiquitous and medically important complex structure consisting of microbial associated cells embedded in self-produced extracellular matrix of hydrated extra polymeric substances which are irreversibly attached to biological or nonbiological surface. Microbes that reside as biofilms are resistant to traditional antibiotics.

Formation of biofilms: Basically biofilms formation comprises of:
a. Initial attachment of microbes and microcolony formation.
b. Maturation of attached microbes into differentiated biofilm.
c. Detachment and dispersal of planktonic cells, from biofilm.

Clinical importance of biofilm:
1. Biofilm persisters are well protected from host defense because of exopolysaccharide matrix.
2. Biofilm is relevant because the mode of growth is associated with chronicity and persistence of diseases.
3. Biofilm associated diseases are periodontitis, bacterial keratitis, chronic lung infections in cystic fibrosis.
4. Nosocomial infections connected with use of central venous catheters, urinary catheters, prosthetic heart valves, intraocular lenses and orthopedic devices are in fact closely associated with biofilms that adhere to biometrical surfaces.
5. Microbes in biofilm evade host defenses and withstand antimicrobial agents.
6. Important microorganisms capable of forming biofilms are: *Staphylococcus epidermidis; Staphylococcus aureus, Pseudomonas aeruginosa, Vibrio cholerae, Bacillus subtilis* etc.
7. Biofilm can easily be, studied in a better way using atomic force microscope. Thus, application of new microscopic and molecular techniques has revolutionized our understanding of biofilm structure, composition, organization and activities resulting in significant advances in prevention and treatment of biofilm related diseases.

Nutritional Requirements of Bacteria

Bacteria may require adequate nutrition, optimum pH, temperature and oxygen for multiplication and growth. Bacteria can be classified into following types on the basis of nutritional requirement:

1. On the basis of energy sources:
   a. *Phototrophics* which get energy from photochemical reaction.
   b. *Chemotrophics* which get energy from chemical reaction.
2. On the basis of their ability to synthesize essential metabolites.
   a. *Autotrophic:* These are the organisms in which all essential metabolites are synthesized from inorganic sources. They use carbon dioxide as the main source of carbon and simple inorganic salts, e.g., nitrates, nitrites, ammonium sulfate, phosphates, etc., to form new protoplasm of the cell.
   b. *Heterotrophic:* Here some of the essential metabolites are not synthesized. Organic compounds, e.g., protein, peptones, amino acids, vitamins and growth factors are supplied from outside. Most of the bacteria producing disease in man are heterotrophic.

GROWTH REQUIREMENTS

Nutritional Requirements

1. **Essential elements**: The essential elements required for synthesis of bacterial structural components (carbohydrate, lipid, protein nucleic acid) are hydrogen, carbon and nitrogen. Of course, phosphorous and sulfur are also required for bacterial growth.

   Hydrogen and oxygen are made available from water added to culture medium. Heterotrophic bacteria require organic carbon for growth in a suitable form and can be assimilated by the bacteria. Carbohydrate is principal source of carbon which is degraded by the bacteria either by oxidation or by fermentation. Thus providing energy in the form of adenosine triphosphate.

   Nitrogen is a major component of protein and nucleic acids and its main source is ammonia usually in the form of ammonium salt. The ammonium salt is made available either from environment or it may be produced by deamination of amino acids by bacteria.

   Sulfur forms part of the structure of several coenzymes cysteinyl and methionyl side chains of proteins. Most bacteria use sulfate (SO_4) as a sulfur source and reduce it to hydrogen sulfide.

   Phosphorus is required as a component of nucleic acid ATP coenzyme NAD, and flavins. It is always assimilated as free inorganic phosphate.

2. **Mineral salts**: They are potassium, calcium, magnesium, iron, copper, manganese, molybdenum and zinc required in traces for enzyme function and can be provided in tap water or as contaminant of other medium ingredients.

3. **Growth factor**: These may be essential for some who do not grow in their absence. Following a gene mutation of bacterium, there results in failure of one of the enzymes to synthesize amino acids or purines or pyrimidines from simpler compounds. In such case exogenous supply of relevant factor is required called accessory growth factors.

The other nutritional requirements are as follows:

Gas Requirements

a. **Oxygen:** The capacity of bacteria to grow in the presence of oxygen and to utilize it depends on possession of a cytochrome oxidase system.

Aerobes: The aerobe organisms grow only in the presence of oxygen, e.g., pseudomonadaceae, *Bacillus, Nitrobacter, Sarcina,* etc. They require oxygen as hydrogen acceptor.

Facultative anaerobes: They are the organisms that can live with or without oxygen, e.g., *Vibrio, Escherichia coli, Salmonella, Shigella* and *Staphylococcus.* The microaerophilic organisms grow well with relatively small quantities of oxygen, e.g., *Hemophilus.*

Obligate anaerobes: The strict anaerobes multiply only in the absence of oxygen, e.g., *Bacteroides, Clostridium.* They require a substance other than oxygen as hydrogen acceptor.

The toxicity of oxygen results from its reduction by enzymes in the cell (e.g., flavoprotein) to hydrogen peroxide and even more toxic free radical superoxide. Aerobes and aerotolerant anaerobes are protected from these products by the presence of superoxide dismutase, an enzyme and the presence of catalase. There is one exception to this rule, i.e., lactic acid bacteria; aerotolerant anaerobes that do not contain catalase. This group, however, relies instead on peroxidases. All strict anaerobes lack superoxide dismutase, catalase and peroxidase. Superoxide dismutase is indispensable for survival in presence of oxygen.

Hydrogen peroxide owes much of its toxicity to the damage it causes to DNA. DNA repair deficient mutants are exceptionally sensitive to hydrogen peroxide. The rec A gene product has the function of both genetic recombination and repair. It is said to be more important than either catalase or superoxide dismutase in protecting *Escherichia coli* against hydrogen peroxide toxicity.

b. **Carbon dioxide:** The metabolic activities of some organisms like *Neisseria gonorrhoeae, Brucella abortus* are greatly enhanced by the presence of extra amount of carbon dioxide (capnophilic bacteria) in atmospheric air.

Moisture

Bacteria require water for their growth. Desiccation may kill most of bacteria.

Accessory Nutritional Requirements

Most often the accessory growth factors are vitamins. The requirement of growth factors differ widely in various bacteria, e.g.

Organisms	Growth factors
Neisseria gonorrhoeae	Glutathione
Corynebacterium diphtheriae	B-alanine
Staphylococcus aureus	Nicotinic acid, thiamine
Haemophilus influenzae	Hematin (Coenzyme I)

They are not synthesized by bacteria and so supplied in media.

Bacterial growth *in vivo* depends upon:
- ❖ Availability of nutrition with human body
- ❖ Generation time of bacteria
- ❖ Cellular and humoral defence of host, i.e., human body
- ❖ Redox potential
- ❖ pH.

GROWTH CURVE

When organisms are cultured in appropriate fluid media, there would be increase in the size of bacteria without any multiplication for some time (lag phase). This is followed by multiplication and increase in number of bacteria to the extent that media look turbid to the naked eye (log phase). After some time growth rate becomes stationary and later on declines **(Table 4.1)**. Counting of bacteria at different periods after inoculation and then events of sequences are represented on a graph which is called growth curve **(Fig. 4.1)**.

Lag Phase

It has short duration (1 to 40 hours) and during this phase there occurs:

1. Increase in size of cell.
2. Increase in metabolic rate.
3. Adaptation to new environment and necessary enzymes plus intermediate

Table 4.1: Bacterial changes during growth curve.

Bacterial changes	Phase of growth curve
• Maximum size	• End of lag phase
• Uniform staining and bacteria are more sensitive to antibiotics	• Log phase
• Irregular staining, variable Gram reaction, exotoxin production and sporulation	• Stationary phase
• Involution form	• Phase of decline

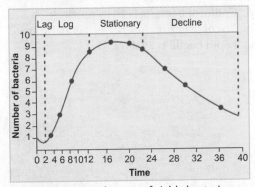

Fig. 4.1: Growth curve of viable bacteria.

metabolites are built up for multiplication to proceed.

The length of lag phase depends upon:
a. Type of bacteria
b. Better the medium, shorter the lag phase
c. The phase of culture from which inoculation is taken
d. Size of inoculum
e. Environmental factors like temperature.

Log Phase

Following lag phase (8 hours duration) the cells start dividing and their number increase by geometric progression with time. Logarithms of viable count plotting time gives straight line. During this period:

1. Bacteria have high rate of metabolism.
2. Bacteria develop best morphologically with typical biochemical reactions.
3. Bacteria are more sensitive to antibiotics. Control of log phase is brought about by:
   a. Nature of bacteria
   b. Temperature
   c. Rate of penetration of the medium depends on the concentration of material in the medium.

Stationary Phase

After some time (few hours to few days) a stage comes when rate of multiplication and death becomes almost equal. It may be due to:
a. Depletion of nutrient
b. Accumulation of toxic products. Sporulation may occur during this stage.

Decline Phase

During this phase (few hours to few days) population decreases due to death of cells. Factors responsible for this phase are:
  i. Nutritional exhaustion
 ii. Toxic accumulation
iii. Autolytic enzymes. Involution is common in phase of decline.

Survival Phase

When most organisms have died, a few survive for several months or years.

Factors Influencing Growth

1. **Temperature:** The temperature range at which an organism grows best is called optimum temperature. In human parasitic organisms, optimum temperature ranges between 30° and 37°C.

   There are three groups of bacteria related to regards the temperature of growth.

   a. *Psychrophilic:* These are the organisms growing between 0 and 25°C. They are mostly soil and water bacteria.

   b. *Mesophilic:* They grow between 20 and 44°C. This group includes bacteria producing disease.

   c. *Thermophilic:* Some organisms grow between 50 and 60°C, e.g., bacillus and algae. The upper range of temperature tolerated by them correlates well with the thermal stability of the species protein as measured in cell extract.

2. **Hydrogen ion concentration:** Most of pathogenic bacteria grow best at pH 7.2 to 7.6. However, *Lactobacillus* and *Thiobacillus thiooxidans* grow at acidic pH while *Vibrio cholerae, Alcaligenes fecalis* grow at alkaline pH.

3. **Moisture:** Water is quite essential for the growth of bacteria. Organism like *Neisseria gonorrhoeae* and *Treponema pallidum* die almost at once on drying. However, *Mycobacterium tuberculosis* and *Staphylococcus aureus* survive for quite a long time even on drying.

4. **Osmotic pressure:** Bacteria are usually resistant to changes of osmotic pressure. However, 0.5% sodium chloride is added to almost all culture media to make environment isotonic.

5. **Light:** Darkness is usually favorable for the growth and viability of all the organisms. Direct light exposure shortens the survival of bacteria. Photochromogenic mycobacteria form pigment on exposure to light. Organisms are sensitive to ultraviolet and other radiations.

6. **Mechanical and sonic stress:** Bacteria have tough cell walls. Vigorous shaking with glass beads, grinding and exposure to ultrasonic vibration may cause rupture or disintegration of cell wall.

▌BACTERIAL REPRODUCTION

The bacteria reproduce by a sexual binary fission. The DNA is a double helix with complementary nucleotide sequences in the two strands. At replication the strands separate and new complementary strands are formed on each of the originals so that two identical double helices are produced. Each of them has the same nucleotide sequence and so the same genetic information as the original one. The sequence of cell division includes:

a. Formation of initiator of chromosome replicator.

b. Chromosome duplication.

c. Separation of chromosomes.

d. Formation of septa and cell division.

▌GENERATION TIME

Time required for bacterium, to give rise to two daughter cells under optimum condition is called generation time or generation gap. Generation time of:

a. Coliform bacteria is 20 minutes

b. *Mycobacterium tuberculosis* is 20 hours

c. Lepra bacilli is 20 days.

Media for Bacterial Growth

Culture media gives artificial environment simulating natural conditions necessary for growth of bacteria. The basic requirement of culture media are:

1. Energy source.
2. Carbon source.
3. Nitrogen source.
4. Salts like sulphates, phosphates, chlorides and carbonates of sodium, potassium, magnesium, ferric, calcium and trace elements like copper, etc.
5. Satisfactory pH 7.2 to 7.6.
6. Adequate oxidation-reduction potential.
7. Growth factor like tryptophan for *Salmonella typhi*, glutathione for gonococci, X and V factors for *hemophilus*.

The characteristics of an ideal culture medium are:

1. Must give a satisfactory growth from single inoculum.
2. Should give rapid growth.
3. Should be easy to grow.
4. Should be reasonably cheap.
5. Should be easily reproducible.
6. Should enable to demonstrate all characteristics in which we are interested.

Media used for obtaining the growth of bacteria are:

▌FLUID MEDIA

Bacteria grow very well in fluid media in 3 to 4 hours. Hence, they are used as enriched media before plating on solid media. They are not suitable for the isolation of organism in pure culture. We cannot study colony characters as well. Examples of fluid media are nutrient broth, peptone water, etc.

Types of Fluid Media (Table 5.1)

Broth

It is a clear transparent straw colored fluid prepared from meat extract or peptone. Following types of broth are in common use:

a. **Infusion broth:** Fat free minced beef meat is added to water and kept in refrigerator overnight. Fluid obtained after removal of meat is boiled for 18 minutes. To it peptone and 0.5% sodium chloride is added.

b. **Meat extract broth:** This is commercially available as Lab Lemco.

c. **Digest broth:** It is prepared from meat by enzymatic action. Nutritionally, it is more rich than infusion and extract broth. Addition of peptone is not required in digest broth. Hence, it is more economical. Enzymes used are trypsin, pepsin, etc.

Peptone

It is a protein partially digested with hydrolytic enzymes like pepsin, trypsin, papain, etc. Peptones supply nitrogenous material and also act as a buffer. Several bacteria can grow in 1% peptone water. Constituents of peptone are proteoses, polypeptides and amino acids.

Yeast extract: It is prepared by extracting autolyzed yeast with water. It has high contents of vitamin B.

The other examples of fluid media are sugar media (1% sugar in peptone water), glucose

Table 5.1: Fluid media.

Medium	Uses
• Peptone water	Routine culture
	Demonstration of motility
	Sugar fermentation
	Indole test
• Nutrient broth	Routine culture
	Methyl red test
	Voges Pauskaur test
• Glucose broth	Blood culture
	Culture of bacteria like streptococci, etc.
• Enrichment media	
– Glycerole alkaline peptone water	Transport media for stool samples
– Selenite F broth	Culture of stool for *Salmonella* and *Shigella*
– Tetrathionate broth	Culture of stool for *Salmonella*
– Robertson cooked meat broth	Culture of anaerobic bacteria

Table 5.2: Solid media.

Medium	Uses
• Nutrient agar	• Routine culture
	• Antibiotic sensitivity test
• Blood agar	• Routine culture
• Chocolate agar	• Culture of fastidious bacteria like *Neisseria*, *H. influenzae*, etc.
• Loeffler serum slope	• Culture of *C. diphtheriae*
• Deoxycholate citrate agar	• Culture of *Salmonella* and *Shigella*
• MacConkey's medium	• Culture of intestinal bacteria
• Bile salt agar	• Culture of *Vibrio cholerae*
• TCBS	• Culture of *Vibrio cholerae*
• Lowenstein-Jensen medium	• Culture of *Mycobacterium tuberculosis* and atypical *Mycobacterium*

broth (1% glucose in nutrient broth), bile broth (0.5% bile salts in nutrient broth), Hiss serum (1 part serum and 3 parts glucose broth), liquid MacConkey, glycerol saline and enrichment media (tetrathionate and selenite).

SOLID MEDIA (TABLE 5.2)

They are used to study colonies of individual bacteria. They are essential for isolation of organism in pure form.

a. **Agar:** It is important constituent of solid media. It is complex polysaccharide obtained from seaweeds (Algae geledium species). It melts at 80 to 100°C and solidifies at 35 to 42°C. It does not provide any nutrition to the bacteria. It acts only as solidifying agent. It is not metabolized by any pathogenic bacteria.

b. **Gelatin:** It is protein prepared by hydrolysis of collagen with boiling water. It is in liquid

form at 37°C. It forms transparent gel below 25°C. The main use of gelatin is to test the ability of bacteria to liquefy it. This feature is important in the identification and classifications of bacteria. Blackening of media indicates hydrogen sulfide production.

Classification of Media

Media have been classified in many ways:
A. i. Solid media
   ii. Liquid media
   iii. Semisolid media.
B. i. Simple media
   ii. Synthetic media or defined media
   iii. Complex media
   iv. Semidefined media
   v. Special media.

Special medias are further divided as under:
   i. Enriched media
   ii. Enrichment media
   iii. Selective media
   iv. Indicator and differential media
   v. Sugar media
   vi. Transport media.
C. Aerobic media and anaerobic media.

1. **Simple media:** It is also called basal media. It consists of meat extract, peptone, sodium chloride and water.
   a. *Peptone water:* It is prepared by adding 1 Gram peptone, 0.5 Gram sodium chloride to 100 mL of distilled water.
   b. *Nutrient agar:* Addition of 2% agar in nutrient broth constitute nutrient agar.
2. **Complex media:** These are ingredients for special purposes or for bringing out certain characteristics or providing special nutrient required for the growth of certain organisms.
3. **Synthetic or defined media:** These media are prepared solely from pure chemical substances and the exact composition of medium is known. They are used for research purposes.
4. **Special media**
   a. *Enriched media:* In these media substance like blood, serum or egg is added to basal medium, e.g., blood agar, chocolate agar, egg media and Loeffler serum slope.
   b. *Enrichment media:* Some substances are added to liquid media with the result that wanted organism grow more in number than unwanted organism. Such media are called, enrichment media, e.g., selenite F broth, tetrathionate broth.
   c. *Selective media:* This is like enrichment media with the difference that inhibiting substance is added to solid medium, e.g., deoxycholate citrate medium which contains nutrient agar, sodium deoxycholate, sodium citrates lactose and neutral red.
   d. *Indicator media:* The media contain an indicator which changes color when bacterium grow in them, e.g., *Salmonella typhi* reduces sulphite to sulphide in Wilson and Blair medium (colonies of *Salmonella typhi* have black and metallic sheen).
   e. *Differential media:* A medium which has substance enabling it to bring out differing characteristic of bacteria thus helping to distinguish between them, e.g., MacConkey's medium (peptone, lactose, agar, neutral red and taurocholate). It shows lactose fermenter as red colonies while nonlactose fermenter as pale colonies **(Figs. 5.1A and B).**

Blood agar is an enriched medium but also differentiates between hemolytic organisms and nonhemolytic organisms. So it also acts as a differential medium.
   f. *Sugar media:* The usual sugar media consist of 1% sugar concerned, in peptone water along with appropriate indicator. A small tube (Durham's tube) is kept inverted in sugar tube to detect gas production **(Fig. 5.2).**
   g. *Hiss's serum* (25% serum) is used for organisms which are exacting in their growth requirement, e.g., pneumococci.
   h. *Transport media:* Delicate organisms like gonococci which may not survive the time taken for transporting the specimen to the laboratory or may be overgrown by nonpathogen (dysentery or cholera organism) special medium is required called transport medium, e.g., Stuart medium for gonococci and glycerol saline for stool.

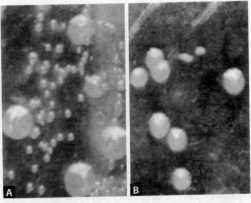

Figs. 5.1A and B: (A) Lactose fermenter colonies on MacConkey media; (B) Nonlactose fermenter colonies on MacConkey media.

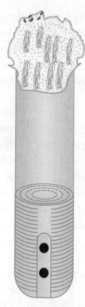

Fig. 5.2: Sugar media with inverted Durham's tube.

Anaerobic media: These media are used to grow anaerobic organisms, e.g., Robertson's cooked meat medium.

Anaerobic indicators used is reduced methylene blue and it contains NaOH, methylenes blue, glucose.

Storage media: Lyophilization (freeze drying in vacuum) is the best method of preservation and storage of bacteria Dorset egg and semisolid agar may be used to preserve and store bacteria for a few months. For this loop charged with bacteria is inoculated on these media. After giving adequate incubation bacterial growth appears on the media which can be stored in the refrigerator. Robertson cooked meat media can also be used for preservation.

Culture Techniques

In clinical laboratory indications for culture are:

a. Isolation of bacteria in pure culture.
b. To demonstrate their properties.
c. To obtain sufficient pure growth for preparation of antigen and for other tests.

d. For typing of bacterial isolate by method like bacteriophage and bacteriocin susceptibility.
e. To determine sensitivity to antibiotics.
f. To estimate viable count.
g. To maintain stock culture.

METHODS OF ISOLATING PURE CULTURE

1. Surface plating.
2. Use of enriched and selective media.
3. Pretreatment of specimens with appropriate bacteriocidal agents.
4. By heating liquid medium.

Methods of Culture

1. **Streak culture** (surface plating) is the method routinely employed for the isolation of bacteria in pure culture. A platinum loop with 2½" long wire and loop with diameter 2 mm **(Fig. 5.3)** is charged with specimen to be cultured and is placed on the surface of dried plate of solid media towards peripheral area **(Fig. 5.4)**. The inoculum is spreaded thinly over the plate in series of parallel lines in different segment of the plate. On incubation we may find confluent growth at the site of primary inoculum. Well-separated colonies are obtained over the final series of streaks.

2. **Lawn or carpet culture:** Lawn cultures are prepared by flooding the surface or plate with suspension of bacteria. It provides uniform surface growth of bacteria. It is useful for bacteriophage typing and antibiotic sensitivity test.

3. **Stroke culture:** It is made in tubes containing agar slopes. It is used for providing a pure growth of bacterium for slide agglutination.

4. **Stab culture:** It is prepared by puncturing with charged long, straight wire (4" long). Stab culture are employed mainly for demonstration of gelatin liquefactions and for maintaining stock culture.

5. **Pure plate culture:** 15 mL of agar medium is melted and left to cool in water bath at 45

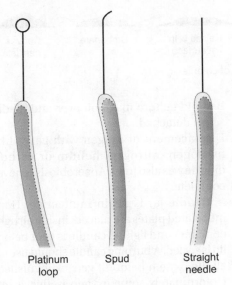

Platinum   Spud   Straight
loop   needle

Fig. 5.3: Types of inoculation loops.

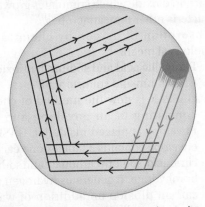

Fig. 5.4: Method of streaking culture plate.

to 50°C. Appropriate dilution of inoculum is added in 1 mL volume to molten agar and mixed well. Content of tube is poured in Petri dish. It is allowed to set and after incubation colonies will be seen distributed throughout the depth of medium. This method gives viable bacterial count in a suspension. It is the recommended method for quantitative urine culture.

6. **Liquid culture** in a tube, bottle or flask may be inoculated by touching with a charged loop. Liquid cultures are preferred when large and quick yield is required. The major

disadvantage of liquid culture is that it does not provide pure culture from mixed inocula.

Description of colonies of bacteria: Colonies of bacteria are described as follows:

Shape: Circular, irregular, radiate or rhizoid.

Surface: Smooth, rough, fine or coarsely granular, papillate, glistening, etc.

Size: Surface of colony is measured in millimeter. It measures 2 to 3 mm and if very small then 0.5 to 1 mm.

Elevation: Raised, low convex dome, umbilicate **(Fig. 5.5)**.

Some bacteria produce spreading growth, e.g., proteus, clostridia, etc.

Edges: Mostly edges are entire, e.g., *Klebsiella, Escherichia coli, Staphylococcus.* Sometimes edges may be crenated, fimbriated (*B. subtilis*) or effuse **(Fig. 5.6)**.

Color: Some organisms may produce pigmented colonies, e.g., staphylococci, *Pseudomonas aeruginosa.*

Opacity: Colonies on nutrient agar may be transparent, translucent or opaque.

Consistency: Colonies may be hard or firm, e.g., *Mycobacterium tuberculosis,* friable and membranous, e.g., *B. subtilis.* Mostly they are soft and butyrous, e.g., *Escherichia coli.*

Changes in the medium: Some organisms produce beta type of hemolysis around the colony, e.g., *Staphylococcus aureus* and *Streptococcus pyogenes.* Few bacteria produce soluble pigment that diffuses into the medium, e.g., *Pseudomonas aeruginosa.*

Emulsifiability: Growth of bacteria like *Escherichia coli, Salmonella* is easily emulsifiable whereas growth of *Neisseria catarrhalis* is not emulsifiable.

Growth in liquid media is described as:
1. *Turbid*
2. *Deposit:* Growth of *Streptococcus pyogenes* is characterized by deposits at the bottom of tube.

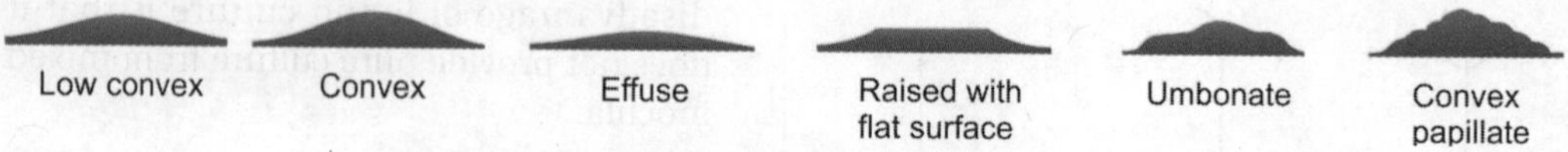

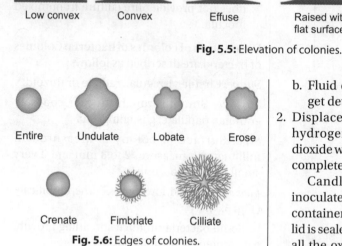

Fig. 5.5: Elevation of colonies.

Fig. 5.6: Edges of colonies.

3. *Surface growth:* Surface growth is related to aerobic, nature of organism.
4. *Color changes:* Some organisms produce water soluble pigment which after diffusion change the color of medium, e.g., *Pseudomonas aeruginosa.*

METHODS OF ANAEROBIC CULTURE

Obligate anaerobes grow only in absence of free oxygen. These bacteria lack mechanism of oxidation through respiratory enzymes like cytochrome oxidase, catalase and peroxidase resulting in H_2O_2 accumulation. This H_2O_2 is toxic for the growth of anaerobic bacteria.

Clostridium tetani are strictly anaerobic. A number of methods are described for achieving anaerobiosis on the basis of following principles:
a. Exclusion of oxygen.
b. Production of vacuum.
c. Displacement of oxygen with other gases.
d. Absorption of oxygen by chemical or biological means.
e. Reduction of oxygen.

1. Cultivation in vacuum was tried by incubating culture in vacuum desiccator. It has disadvantages:
   a. Some oxygen is always left behind.
   b. Fluid culture may boil over and media get detached.
2. Displacement of oxygen with gases like hydrogen, nitrogen, helium or carbon dioxide was also tried. Anaerobiosis is never complete.

   Candle jar is again ineffective. Here inoculated plates are placed, inside airtight container and lighted candle is kept before lid is sealed. A burning candle should use up all the oxygen before it gets extinguished. Unfortunately some oxygen is always left behind. It also provides concentration of carbon dioxide which stimulates growth of bacteria other than anaerobes.
3. Absorption of oxygen by chemical or biological mean:
   a. Pyrogallic acid and sodium hydroxide.
   b. Chromium and sulfuric acid.
   c. GASPAK is now the method of choice consisting of an envelope and jar. Envelope is placed inside jar. GASPAK envelope contains 3 tablets, one each of citric acid, sodium carbonate and sodium borohydrate. It generates hydrogen and carbon dioxide on addition of water. Hydrogen combines with oxygen to produce water, and thus creation of anaerobiosis.
   d. McIntosh and Fildes anaerobic jar (**Fig. 5.7**): It consists of glass or metal jar with metal lid which can be clamped airtight with screw. The lid has two tubes, one acts as a gas inlet and the other one as outlet. Additionally lid has two terminals which can be connected to electrical supply.

      Inoculated culture plates are placed inside jar. Outlet tube is connected to vacuum pump and air inside is evacuated. The outlet tap is closed and inlet tube is connected with hydrogen gas

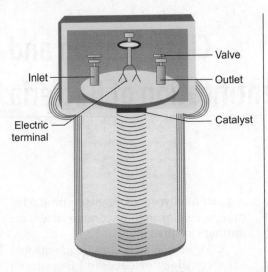

Fig. 5.7: McIntosh and Fildes jar.

cylinder. After filling of jar with hydrogen, electric terminals are connected so that palladinised asbestos is heated. This acts as catalyst for combination of hydrogen and residual oxygen. It ensures complete anaerobiosis. At the same time, it also carries risk of explosion.

An indicator should also be kept for verifying anaerobic condition in jar. Reduced methylene blue is used for this purpose. It is colorless anaerobically and regains blue color on exposure to oxygen.

4. *Anaerobic glove box:* This is a self-contained anaerobic system with provisions of circulation of hydrogen, nitrogen and carbon dioxide within it and catalytic conversion of residual oxygen to water. It is expensive. It is recommended for total anaerobic gut flora studies.

5. *Reduction of oxygen* in medium is achieved by using various reducing agents:
   a. 1% glucose.
   b. 0.1% thioglycolate.
   c. 0.1% ascorbic acid.
   d. 0.05% cystine.
   e. Broth containing iron pieces flamed red hot.
   f. Broth containing fresh animal tissue, e.g., rabbit kidney, spleen, etc.
   g. Robertson cooked meat medium produces anaerobiosis as under:
      i. Unsaturated fatty acids present in meat utilize oxygen for autoxidation.
      ii. Glutathione and cystein are reducing agents of meat and use oxygen.
      iii. Sulfahydryl compounds of cystein also precipitate for reduced oxidation reduction.

It consists of fat free minced meat in broth. It permits growth of even strict anaerobes. The meat itself contains reducing substances, particularly glutathione, which helps in the growth of anaerobes. Further fresh entry of oxygen into the medium is prevented by layering the top with sterile liquid paraffin. It indicates sacchrolytic (meat being red) and proteolytic (meat being black) activities.

Chapter 6

Classification and Identification of Bacteria

Bacterial classification presents special problem. A number of criteria have been employed to group them, e.g.

a. *Energy source:* Phototrophic, chemotrophic, autotrophic and heterotrophic.
b. *Nutrient requirement:* Simple or complex.
c. *Ability to grow* in living tissue—saprophytes and parasites.
d. *Temperature of growth:* Psychrophilic, mesophilic and thermophilic.
e. *Oxygen requirement:* Aerobic and anaerobic.

None of these seem satisfactory. Following systems are used to classify bacteria:

BIOLOGICAL CLASSIFICATION

It is based on observable characters like physiological, immunological and ecological.

Division Protophyta

Class: Schizomycetes.
Orders:
1. Pseudomonadales.
2. Eubacteriales.
3. Actinomycetales.
4. Spirochaetales.
5. Mycoplasmatales.

On the basis of main characters of each order, further families and genera are classified.

MORPHOLOGICAL CLASSIFICATION

All the organisms are classified into two groups:

A. Higher bacteria: They are filamentous and grow by branching to form mycelium, e.g., antinomycetes. Organisms producing true mycelium among actinomycetales are further classified into:

a. Vegetative mycelium fragments into bacillary or coccoid element. Of course they are Gram-positive. They may be of following types:
   i. Anaerobic, acid fast, e.g., nocardia.
   ii. Anaerobic non-acid fast, e.g., *Actinomyces israelii, Actinomyces bovis.*
b. Vegetative mycelium does not fragment into bacillary or coccoid form. Conida are formed in chain from aerial hyphae, e.g., streptomyces.

B. Lower or true bacteria: They are unicellular and never form mycelium. They are grouped on the basis of their shape.
a. Cocci—spherical
b. Bacilli—rod shaped
c. Vibrio—comma shaped
d. Spirilla—spiral twisted non-flexous rods
e. Spirochaetes—thin spirally twisted, flexous rods

Cocci: Following types of arrangement is seen:

❖ **Diplococcus:** Binary fission occurs in one plane, e.g., pneumococci.
❖ **Streptococcus:** Cocci are arranged in chain, e.g., *Streptococcus pyogenes, Streptococcus viridans.*
❖ **Staphylococcus:** Cocci are arranged in cluster, e.g., *Staphylococcus aureus, Staphylococcus albus.*
❖ **Tetracoccus:** Arrangement of cocci in group of four, e.g., *Micrococcus tetragena.*

Flowchart 6.1: Classification of cocci.

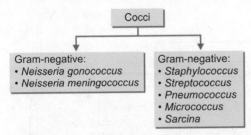

The cocci are further classified into Gram-positive and Gram-negative **(Flowchart 6.1)**. Gram positive are again divided on the basis of arrangement of cells.

Vibrio: They are curved, non-flexible, Gram-negative, highly motile, e.g., *Vibrio cholerae.*

Spirilla: Consists of coiled, non-flexous motile cells, e.g., *Spirilum minus.*

Bacilli: They may be Gram-positive or Gram-negative **(Flowchart 6.2)**. Gram-positive may be acid fast on the basis of staining reaction to Ziehl-Neelsen stain. Gram-negative organism are further identified on the basis of biochemical reaction and antigenic analysis.

Spirochaetes: They are slender, refractile and spiral filaments. The pathological species are classified into 3 genera.
a. Treponema, e.g., *Treponema pallidum.*
b. Leptospira, e.g., *L. icterohemorrhagica.*
c. Borrelia, e.g., *Borrelia recurrentis.*

IDENTIFICATION OF BACTERIA

For the identification of organism we proceed as under:

1. *Microscopic examination:* It helps to find out whether the bacteria is cocci, bacilli, vibrio, spirillum or spirochaete. On Gram staining we can have two groups of organism: Gram-positive and Gram-negative organisms.
2. *Motility* **(Flowchart 6.3):** Pathogenic cocci are nonmotile. Among Gram-negative bacilli, *Salmonella, Escherichia coli, Proteus, Pseudomonas, Alcaligens fecalis, Vibrio cholerae* are motile. Among Gram-positive bacilli clostridia and bacillus are motile. Hanging drop preparation, dark ground microscopy, phase contrast, electron microscope help in their study.

Common Staining Techniques

1. Simple stains where watery solution of single basic dye such as, methylene blue or basic fuchsin are used as simple stain.
2. Negative staining bacteria are mixed with dyes (India ink nigrosin). The background gets stained leaving the bacteria contrastingly colorless. The technique is useful in demonstration of bacterial capsule.
3. Impregnation methods where bacterial cells and appendages that are too thin and

Flowchart 6.2: Classification of bacteria.

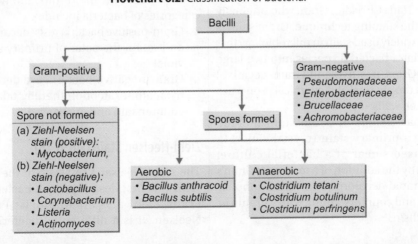

Flowchart 6.3: Identification of bacteria based on motility.

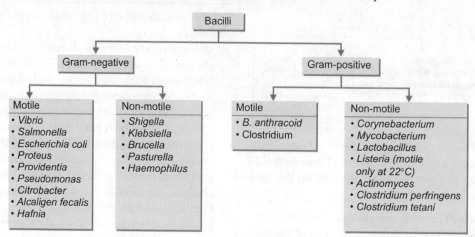

Bacilli

Gram-negative

Gram-positive

Motile	Non-motile
• Vibrio	• Shigella
• Salmonella	• Klebsiella
• Escherichia coli	• Brucella
• Proteus	• Pasturella
• Providentia	• Haemophilus
• Pseudomonas	
• Citrobacter	
• Alcaligen fecalis	
• Hafnia	

Motile	Non-motile
• B. anthracoid	• Corynebacterium
• Clostridium	• Mycobacterium
	• Lactobacillus
	• Listeria (motile only at 22°C)
	• Actinomyces
	• Clostridium perfringens
	• Clostridium tetani

delicate cannot be seen under ordinary microscope. These delicate structures are thickened by impregnation of silver on the surface to make them visible under light microscope, e.g., demonstration of spirochaetes and bacterial flagella.

4. Differential stains impart different colors to different bacteria or their structures. In a stained film, bacterial shape, arrangement and presence of other cells (pus cells) are noted. The two commonly used differential stains are Gram's stain and acid fast stain (**Figs. 6.1A and B**).

Gram Stain (Fig. 6.1A)

The Gram stain is named after the Danish scientist, Hans Christian Gram who originally devised the staining technique. Gram stain is the most widely used stain in microbiology that differentiates bacterial species into two large groups (Gram-positive and Gram-negative) based on the physical and chemical properties of their cell walls.

The basic steps of Gram stain include applying a primary stain (crystal violet) to a heat-fixed smear of a bacterial culture, followed by the addition of a mordant (Gram's iodine), rapid decolorization with alcohol or acetone, and counterstaining with safranin or basic fuchsin.

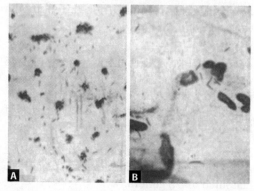

Figs. 6.1A and B: (A) Gram-stained smear showing Gram-positive cocci (cluster) and Gram-negative bacilli; (B) Ziehl-Neelsen stained smear showing acid-fast bacilli.

Depending on the results, the two broad categories of bacteria include:
❖ Gram-positive bacteria resist decolorization and retain the color of primary stain, i.e. violet
❖ Gram-negative bacteria are decolorized by acetone/alcohol, thereby take up the counterstain and appear red.

Ziehl-Neelsen Stain (Fig. 6.1B)

The Ziehl-Neelsen (ZN) stain or the acid fast stain was first described by a bacteriologist, Franz Ziehl and a pathologist Friedrich Neelsen. It is a differential bacteriological stain used to identify acid fast bacteria, especially *Mycobacterium*. The reagents used are Ziehl-Neelsen carbol fuchsin (primary stain), acid alcohol and methylene blue (counterstain). 5% sulphuric acid is used for staining *Mycobacterium leprae* and 20% for *Mycobacterium tuberculosis*.

A positive smear typically contain pink colored, rod shaped bacteria that are slightly curved, sometimes branching, sometimes beaded in appearance, present singly or in small clumps against a blue background of other cells. Acid fastness of a bacterium is attributed to the high content of lipids, fatty acids and higher alcohols found in the cell wall. Mycolic acid, acid fast, waxy material is present in all acid fast bacteria. Apart from lipids, integrity of the cell wall also contributes to the acid fastness of a bacterium.

Staining Reaction

Ziehl-Neelsen stain into acid fast and non-acid fast bacilli, Albert stain for the demonstration of metachromatic and fluorescent dye to bring out special character.

Study of morphology and staining characteristics helps in preliminary identification.

Culture character: Growth requirement and colonial characteristics in culture are useful for the identification of organism, e.g., *Staphylococcus aureus* shows beta type hemolysis with pinhead colonies whereas *Staphylococcus albus* is without any hemolysis. *Streptococcus pyogenes* are pinpoint colonies with b hemolysis whereas *Streptococcus viridans* show a type hemolysis.

Resistance: Resistance to heat, concentration of disinfectant, antibiotic, chemotherapeutic agent and bacitracin help in differentiating and identification, e.g., resistance of *Streptococcus fecalis* to heat at 60°C for 30 minutes and clostridial spores to boiling for various period.

Metabolism: Requirements of oxygen, need of carbon dioxide, capacity to form pigment and power of hemolysis is helpful for classification of bacteria and to differentiate species.

Biochemical Reactions

The more important and widely used tests are as under:

1. **Sugar fermentation:** This is tested in sugar media having Andrade's indicator. Acid production changes the color of medium into pink. Gas produced collects in Durham's tube.

2. **Indole production:** This test demonstrates production of indole from tryptophane. This tryptophane is present in peptone water. In 48 hours peptone water culture 0.5 ml Kovac reagent is added. Red colored ring indicates positive test.

3. **Methyl red test:** It is to detect the production of acid during fermentation of glucose and maintenance of pH below 4.5. Glucose phosphate culture is taken and few drops of 0.04% methyl red are added. Red color is positive while yellow color means negative test.

4. **Voges-Proskauer test:** It depends on production of acetyl methyl carbinol from pyruvic acid. 48 hours growth of glucose phosphate culture is taken. To it we add 40% KOH (1 vol.) and 3 volumes of a naphthal. Deep pink color in 2.5 minutes which deepens into magenta or crimson color means positive tests.

5. **Citrate utilization:** Some organisms use carbon as sole source of energy. Koser citrate medium (liquid) is taken for this test. Turbidity in this medium means citrate has been used up. In Simmon's medium (solid) after overnight incubation color of medium changes from green to blue if citrate is used up by the organism.

6. **Nitrate reduction:** Organism is grown in broth containing 1% KNO_3 for 5 days. To it is added 1 to 2 drops of mixture of sulfanilic acid and naphthalamine (mixed in equal proportion). Red color appears within few minutes if test is positive.

7. **Urease test:** It is done in Christensen's urease medium. Inoculate heavily the slope and incubate at 37°C. Urease producing organism produce pink color.

Urease producing bacteria reduce urea to ammonia and hence pink color.

8. **Hydrogen sulfide production:** Some of the organisms decompose sulphur containing amino acid producing H_2S among the products. It turns lead acetate paper strip into black. Instead of lead acetate we may use ferrous acetate or ferric ammonium citrate.

9. **Catalase production:** Pour a drop of 10 vol H_2O_2 on glass slide. Now touch straight wire charged with bacterial colony. In positive reaction gas bubbles are produced.

10. **Oxidase reactions:** The reaction is due to cytochrome oxidase. One percent solution of tetra methyl-p-phenylene diamine hydro-chloride is made. The colony to be tested is smeared (5 mm line) overpaper soaked in above-mentioned solution. Smeared area turns dark purple in 5 to 10 seconds in positive cases.

Bacteriophage typing: Viruses that parasitize bacteria are called bacteriophage or phage. Phage brings about lysis of susceptible bacterial cells. Phage typing is useful in distinguishing strain among *Salmonella* and *Staphylococcus*. There is correlation between bacteriophage type and epidemic source.

Pathogenicity: For pathogenicity test commonly used laboratory animal models are guinea pig, rabbit, rat and mouse. The route used may be subcutaneous, intramuscular, intraperitoneal, intracerebral, intravenous, oral or nasal spray.

Resistance to antibiotic and other agents: Information about sensitivity pattern of strain is useful for selecting choice of drug. This may be useful as an epidemiological marker in tracing hospital infection, e.g., *Staphylococcus aureus* sensitivity to mercury salt.

In other cases sensitivity of bacteria to agents help in identification of organism, e.g., *Streptococcus pyogenes* are sensitive to bacitracin and *Pneumococcus* to optochin.

Plasmid profile and bacitracin typing also further help in identification of bacteria.

Sterilization and Disinfection

The process of sterilization finds application in microbiology for prevention of contamination by extraneous organisms, in surgery for maintenance of asepsis, in food and drug manufacture for ensuring safety from contaminating organism and many other situations.

Sterilization: It is a process by which articles are freed of all microorganisms both in vegetative as well spore state.

Disinfection: It is a process of destruction of pathogenic organisms capable of giving rise to infection.

APPLICATION OF DISINFECTANTS

In Bacteriology

❖ For disposal of culture (3% Lysol)
❖ For preservation of sera, agar or phenol agar, vaccine, etc.

In Surgical Procedures

❖ Washing the hand
❖ To prepare and clean the area of operation
❖ To collect the blood under aseptic precautions
❖ For safe disposable of excreta and surgical dressing
❖ Cleaning of infected wounds
❖ For disinfection of used instrument.

In Hospitals

❖ To disinfect the operation theaters

❖ To disinfect costly equipments like endo-scopes and cystoscopes etc.
❖ To control the spread of cross infection
❖ To disinfect linen and surgical dressing.

In Public Health Services

❖ For providing safe drinking water (e.g. chlorinated water)
❖ For disinfection of sewage before its disposal into the fields.

Antiseptic: It means prevention of infection by inhibiting growth of bacteria.

Bactericidal agents: These are those which are able to kill bacteria.

Bacteriostatic agents: Only prevent multi-plication of bacteria and they may remain alive.

Mainly there are two methods of sterilization.

Physical

1. Sunlight
2. Drying
3. Dry heat
4. Moist heat
5. Filtration
6. Radiation
7. Ultrasonic vibrations.

Chemicals

1. Acids
2. Alkalies

3. Salts
4. Halogens
5. Oxidizing agents
6. Reducing agents
7. Formaldehyde
8. Phenol
9. Soap
10. Dyes
11. Aerosol, etc.

Physical Methods

1. **Sunlight:** It possesses appreciable bacterio-cidal activity. The action is due to ultraviolet rays. This is one of the natural methods of sterilization in case of water in tanks, river and lakes.
2. **Drying:** Drying in air has deleterious effect on many bacteria. Spores are unaffected by drying. Hence, it is a very unreliable method.
3. **Heat:** The factors influencing sterilization by heat are:
   i. Nature of heat:
      (a) Dry
      (b) Moist
   ii. Temperature and time.
   iii. Number of organisms present.
   iv. Whether organism has sporing capacity.
   v. Type of material from which organism is to be eradicated.

Dry Heat

Killing by dry heat is due to:
1. Protein denaturation.
2. Oxidative damage.
3. Toxic effect of elevated levels of electrolytes.
   a. *Red heat:* It is used to sterilize metallic objects by holding them in flame till they are red hot, e.g., inoculating wires, needles, forceps, etc.
   b. *Flaming:* The article is passed over flame without allowing it to become red hot, e.g., mouth of culture tubes, cottonwool plugs and glass slides.
   c. *Incineration:* This is an excellent method for rapidly destroying material, e.g., soiled dressing, animals carcasses, bedding and pathological material, etc.

On the negative side incinerators send toxic material like dioxin and mercurial products into the environment and cause pollution. Dioxin is released from half burnt chlorin based plastics, e.g., PVC. The source of mercury and its products may be broken thermometers, blood pressure apparatus and other diagnostic products. Mercury is known to cause irreversible poisoning. Dioxin may cause cancer and hormone mimicking, i.e. it replaces the natural hormones and can cause serious disturbances in reproductive process.

   d. *Hot air oven* (**Fig. 7.1**)*: Sterilization by hot air oven requires temperature of 160°C for one hour. We can sterilize all glass syringes, petridishes, test tubes, flask, pipettes, cotton swabs, scalpel, scissors, liquid paraffin, dusting powder, etc.

Precautions in Use of Hot Air Oven

1. It must be fitted with fans to ensure distribution of hot air.
2. It should not be overloaded.
3. Oven must be allowed to cool for about 2 hours before opening the doors otherwise glasswares are likely to get cracked.

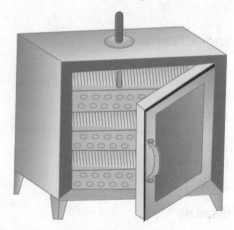

Fig. 7.1: Hot air oven.

Sterilization Control of Hot Air Oven

1. The spores of non-toxigenous strain of *Clostridium tetani* are used to test dry heat efficiency.
2. Browne's tube (green spot) is available for sterilization by dry heat. A green color is produced after 60 minutes at 160°C.
3. Thermocouples may be used.

Moist Heat

The lethal effect of moist heat is by denaturation and coagulation of protein.

Temperature below 100°C

i. *Pasteurization of milk:* Temperature employed is either 63°C for 30 minutes (holder method) or 72°C for 15 to 20 seconds (flash method). Heating is always followed by sudden and instant cooling of milk. Organisms like *Mycobacterium, Salmonellae* and *Brucellae* are killed. *Coxiella burnetii* is relatively heat resistant and hence, may survive the holder method.
ii. *Vaccine bath* (**Fig. 7.2**)*:* It is used for killing non-sporing bacteria which may be present in vaccine. In vaccine bath the

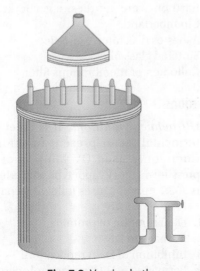

Fig. 7.2: Vaccine bath.

vaccine is treated with moist heat for one hour at 60°C.

iii. *Inspissation:* The slow solidification of serum or egg is carried out at 80°C in an inspissator, e.g., serum slopes, Lowenstein-Jensen's medium, etc.

Temperature at 100°C

i. *Tyndallization:* This is the process by which medium is placed at 100°C in flowing steam for 30 minutes each on 3 successive days. The mechanism underlying this method is that vegetative cells get destroyed at 100°C and remaining spore which germinate during storage interval are killed on subsequent heating. This method may be used for sterilization of egg or serum containing media.
ii. *Boiling:* Most of vegetative form of bacteria, fungi and viruses are killed at 50 to 70°C in short time. For needles and instruments boiling in water for 10 to 30 minutes is sufficient to sterilize them. Addition of little acid, alkali, or washing soda, markedly increases the sterilizing power of boiling water. Spores and hepatitis viruses are not readily destroyed by such procedure.
iii. *Steam at atmospheric pressure* (100°C): Here free steam is used to sterilize culture media which may decompose if subjected to higher temperature. A Koch or Arnold steamer (**Fig. 7.3**) is used. This is a cheap method of sterilization.

Temperature above 100°C

Steam under pressure: For bacteriological and surgical work boiling is not sufficient because spores survive boiling. Hence high pressure sterilizer or autoclave is used.

AUTOCLAVE (FIG. 7.3)

In this apparatus, material for sterilization is exposed to 121°C for 15 to 20 minutes at 15 lb pressure per square inch. Saturated

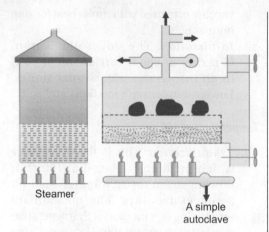

Steamer

A simple
autoclave

Fig. 7.3: Steamer and autoclave.

steam heats the article to be sterilized rapidly by release of latent heat. On condensation 1600 mL of steam at 100°C and at atmospheric pressure condenses into 1 mL of water and liberates 518 calories of heat. The condensed water ensures moist conditions for killing bacteria.

Air is poor conductor of heat and must be removed from chamber. The contents must be so packed that free circulation of steam occurs.

Autoclave is used for culture media, rubber goods, syringes, gowns and dressing, etc.

Sterilization Control

1. Bacillus stearothermophilus
2. Browne's tube
3. Autoclave tapes
4. Thermocouples.

Types of Autoclave

1. Simple iron jacketed.
2. Low pressure/low temperature.
3. High pressure high vacuum type having facility to expel 98% of air rapidly by an electric pump and hence sterilization is done quickly.

Sterilization by Filtration

This is a method of sterilization useful for antibiotic solutions, sera, carbohydrate solution, etc. We may also get bacteria free filtrates of toxin and bacteriophages. It is also useful when we want to separate microorganisms which are scanty in fluid.

Other Uses of Filter

❖ Separation of soluble products of bacterial growth, e.g., toxins.
❖ Sterilization of hydatid fluid
❖ Sterilization of serum
❖ Sterilization of antibiotic solution
❖ Sterilization of blood products
❖ Purification of water.

Membrane filter: They may be comprised of cellulose esters. They can be used as under:
1. Water analysis
2. Sterility testing of solution
3. Preparation of parenteral solution.

Nitrocellulose membrane filter is commonly used. It is also called multipore. Membrane filters are available in pore sizes of 0.015 um, 0.12 um and 0.22 um.

Drawback of filtration: Viruses and mycoplasma may pass through filter. Hence in filtered serum is not safe for clinical use as it may be containing viruses or mycoplasma.

Various types of filters are:
   i. Earthen-ware candles, e.g., Berkefeld, Chamberland.
  ii. Asbestos disk filter, e.g., Seitz.
 iii. Sintered glass filters.
  iv. Collodion or membranous filter.

Radiations

   i. *Ultraviolet radiations:* It is chief bacteriocidal factor present in sunlight. Commonly used UV lamp is of low pressure mercury vapor type whose length is 253.7 mm. It causes following changes in cell:
   1. Denaturation of protein.
   2. Damage to DNA.
   3. Inhibition of DNA replication.
   4. Formation of H_2O_2 and organic peroxide in culture media.

5. Induction of colicin production in colicinogenic bacteria by destruction of cytoplasmic repressor.

Ultraviolet lamps are used in:

a. Killing of organisms
b. Making bacterial and viral vaccines
c. Prevention of airborne infection in operation theater, public places and bacteriological laboratories.

   Gram-positive bacteria show a little more resistance than Gram-negative bacteria to ultraviolet radiations. Spores are highly resistant to UV radiations.

ii. *X-rays and other ionizing radiations:* Ionizing radiations have greater capacity to induce lethal changes in DNA of cell. They are useful for the sterilization of disposable material like catgut, disposable syringes, adhesive dressing, etc.

iii. Gamma radiations: X-ray are utilized using two types of mechanics.

   i. Linear accelerator for X-ray
   ii. Cobalt-60 for gamma rays.

A dose of 2.5 M rad is sufficient to kill both vegetative and spore form of bacteria. They are used to sterilize rubber or plastic syringes, surgical catgut, bone tissue graft, adhesive dressings, etc.

Ultrasonic and Sonic Vibrations

They are bactericidal causing mechanical agitation and rupture of bacteria.

Chemical Methods

The chemical substances act as bacteriocidal agent as under:

a. Coagulation of bacterial protoplasm, e.g., heavy metals.
b. Disruption of cell membrane by chemical substances. They may alter physical and chemical property of cell membrane thus results in killing or inhibiting the bacterial cell growth.
c. Oxidation or burning out the bacterial proto-plasm, e.g., halogens.

d. By affecting bacterial enzymes or coenzyme system thus causing interference of bacterial metabolism.

Following chemicals are of common use:

1. *Acids and alkalies:* They are inhibitory to the growth of bacteria. Mycobacteria are more resistant to acid than alkalies. Boric acid is weak antiseptic.
2. *Distilled water:* It causes loss of viability. This action may be due to traces of metal in distilled water.
3. *Metallic ions:* $HgCl_2$ and $AgNO_3$ prevent the growth of many bacteria in concentration less than 1 part per million. This action is due to affinity of certain protein for metallic ions.
4. *Inorganic anion:* They are much less toxic to bacteria. Potassium tellurite is inhibitory to gram-negative bacteria. Fluoride inhibits many enzymes of bacteria.
5. *Halogens:* Halogen derive their name from Greek word "halos" meaning salt. Hence, halogen means salt former. Three of the halogens, i.e. chlorine, iodine and bromine are among the best bactericidal agents. They act mainly by forming protein halogen (salt like) compounds in living cells and they get killed quickly. Because of both toxicity and high cost bromine is not used. Halogens kill vegetative bacteria, fungi, viruses but not tubercle bacillus or bacterial spores. Iodine is used chiefly for skin. Chlorine combines with water to form hydrochloric acid which is bactericidal.
6. *Oxidizing agents:* They are weak antiseptic, e.g., H_2O_2, potassium permanganate.
7. *Formaldehyde:* It is useful in sterilizing bacterial vaccine and in inactivating bacterial toxin without affecting their antigenicity. 5 to 10% solution in water kills many bacteria. It is bactericidal, sporicidal and lethal to viruses also.
   Uses:
   i. Disinfection of woolen blankets, wool hides to destroy bacterial spores.

ii. Footwear of person with fungal infection (atheletic foot).
iii. Wards and operation theater.
Fumigation: For sterilization of 100 cubic feet of air space in a room, 50 ml of 40% formalin is required. This gives vapor of 2 mg gas per liter of air. Formalin with sufficient water is heated in the room with its windows and doors closed and sealed. Articles and rooms are exposed to fumes for 4 hours. Alternatively, diluted formalin (50%) can be sprayed which also liberates formaldehyde gas. Ideally, humidity of air of room should be attained up to 60% to increase the sterilization power.

8. *Phenol:* It is used for sterilizing surgical instruments, and for killing culture accidentally split over in the laboratory. It is generally used in 3% solution.

Table 7.1: Sterilization methods and their applications.

Article	Methods of sterilization
Disposable syringes	• Gamma radiations • Ethylene oxide
Nondisposable syringes	• Autoclavation • Hot air oven • Infra-red radiation • Boiling at 100°C
Glasswares	• Autoclavation • Hot air oven
Metal instruments	• Autoclavation • Hot air oven • Infrared radiation
Cystoscope, endoscope and other anesthetic equipment	• Ethylene oxide • Glutaraldehyde
Heart lung machine	• Ethylene oxide
Disposable instrument	• Gamma rays • Ethylene oxide
Thermometer	• Glutaraldehyde
Disposable catheter, gloves and transfusion sets	• Gamma rays • Ethylene oxide
Nondisposable catheter, gloves and transfusion sets	• Autoclavation
Powder, fat and oil	• Hot air oven
Surgical dressing, bowl and linen	• Autoclavation
Antibiotic solutions and toxins	• Filtration
Sealed bottles, ampoules of aqueous solutions	• Autoclavation
Culture media containing sugars, gelatin, etc	• Tyndallization • Autoclavation at low pressure
Other culture media without sugar or gelatin	• Autoclavation • Steam at 100°C, for 90 minutes
Serum	• Filtration
Operation theater, inoculation hood and cubical entrance	• Ultraviolet radiation
Hospital blankets, etc.	• Exposure to formalin followed by autoclavation.

9. *Soap and detergents:* They are bacteriocidal and bacteriostatic for Gram-positive and some acid fast organisms. Detergent acts by concentrating at cell membrane and thus disrupting its normal function or it may denaturate protein and enzyme.

10. *Alcohol:* Ethyl alcohol is most effective in 70% solution than 100% alcohol. It is so because 70% alcohol has better penetration power than 100% alcohol. It does not kill spores.

11. *Dyes:* Gentian violet and malachite green, etc. are active against Gram-positive bacteria. They have poor penetration and hence action is bacteriostatic. Acriflavin is bacteriostatic for *Staphylococcus* in 1:3000,000 concentration.

12. *Aerosols and gaseous disinfectant:* SO_2, chlorine and formalin vapors have been used as gaseous disinfectant. Propylene glycol is powerful disinfectant.

13. *Vapor phase disinfectants:* Examples of vapor phase disinfectant are ethylene oxide and formaldehyde. Ethylene oxide can kill all kinds of microbes (Spores and tubercle bacilli). It is useful to sterilize material likely to be damaged by heat, e.g., plastics and rubber items, drugs powder, heart lung machine, etc.

Hydrogen peroxide vapors: These vapors are oxidizing by nature and so they are effective sterilants. They may be used to sterilize instruments. Hydrogen peroxide is vaporized producing reactive free radicals either with microwave frequency or radiofrequency energy. There are many variations of hydrogen peroxide vapor or gas sterilization available, e.g., plasma gas sterilization, 100s sterilizer, etc. It is felt that in near future ethylene oxide may be replaced by above mentioned methods.

Other sterilant gases are chlorine dioxide, peracetic acid, glutaraldehyde, etc.

Sterilization and their appropriate uses are shown in **Table 7.1**.

Table 7.2: Spaulding classification of items/equipment.

Sl. No.	Items/equipment	Definition	Examples	Disinfection/sterilization
1.	Critical devices	Entry to normal site	• Surgical instruments • Cardiac instruments • Urinary catheter • Implants • Eye instrument, etc.	• Heat sterilization • Chemical sterilant • High level disinfectant (glutaraldehyde)
2.	Semi-critical devices	Contact with mucous membrane or skin	• Respiratory treating equipment • Anesthesis equipment • Endoscope • Larynogoscope	High level disinfectant (glutaraldehyde or formalin)
3.	Noncritical devices	In contact with normal skin	• Blood pressure cuff • ECG electrodes • Bedpans • Crutches • Stethoscope • Thermometer	• Intermediate or low level disinfectant (isopropyl alcohol or phenol)
4.	Noncritical environmental surfaces	Not frequently coming in contact with patient	• Examination table • Computer	Low level disinfectant (quaternary ammonium compounds)

Uses of Disinfectant

In practice disinfectant is useful and necessary for:

1. Contaminated disposable material before incineration.
2. Surfaces like table and trolley top.
3. Cleaning material when contaminated material has been split.
4. Disinfection of instruments, not amenable to heat.
5. Disinfection of skin.

▌SPAULDING PRINCIPLES OF DISINFECTION

They are used by infection control workers for disinfection of sterilization of items requirement used in the care of carious categories of patients. It also depends on degree of risk for infection involved in the used items or equipments (**Table 7.2**).

Infection: The lodgement and multiplication of organism in the tissue of host constitutes infection.

■ CLASSIFICATION OF INFECTION

1. *Primary infection:* Initial infection with organism in host constitutes primary infection.
2. *Reinfection:* Subsequent infection by same organism in a host is called reinfection.
3. *Secondary infection:* When in a host whose resistance is lowered by pre-existing infectious disease, a new organism may set-up an infection.
4. *Focal infection:* It is a condition where due to infection at localized sites like appendix and tonsil, general effects are produced.
5. *Cross infection:* When a patient suffering from a disease and new infection is set-up from another host or external source.
6. *Nosocomial infection:* Cross infection occurring in hospital is called nosocomial infection.
7. *Subclinical infection:* It is one where clinical affects are not apparent.

Saprophytes: They are free living organisms which live on decaying organic matter. They fail to multiply on living tissue and so are not important in infectious disease.

Parasites: They are organisms that can establish themselves and multiply in hosts. They may be pathogens or commensal. Pathogens are those which are capable of producing disease in a host. On the contrary, commensal microbes can live in a host without causing any disease.

Sources of Infection in Man

1. *Man:* Man is himself a common source of infection from a patient or carrier. Healthy carrier is a person harboring pathogenic organism without causing any disease to him. A convalescent carrier is one who has recovered from disease but continues to harbor the pathogen in his body.
2. *Animals:* Infectious diseases transmitted from animals to man are called zoonosis. Zoonosis may be bacterial (e.g., plague from rat), rickettsial (e.g., murine typhus from rodent), viral (e.g., rabies from dog), protozoal (e.g., leishmaniasis from dogs), helminthic (e.g., hydatid cyst from dogs) and fungal (zoophilic dermatophytes from cats and dogs).
3. *Insects:* The disease caused by insects are called arthropod borne disease. Insects like mosquitoes, fleas, lice that transmit infection are called vector. Transmission may be mechanical (transmission of dysentery or typhoid bacilli by housefly) and these are called mechanical vector. They are called biological vector if pathogen multiplies in the body of vector, e.g., anopheles mosquito in malaria.
4. Some vectors may act as reservoir host (e.g., ticks in relapsing fever and spotted fever).
5. *Soil:* Soil may serve as source of parasiting infection like roundworm and hookworm. Spores of tetanus bacilli remain viable in soil for a long time, fungi like *Histoplasma*

capsulatum and higher bacteria like *Nocardia asteroides* also survive in soil and cause human infection.

6. *Water: Vibrio cholerae*, infective hepatitis virus (Hepatitis-A), guinea worm may be found in water.
7. *Food:* Contaminated food may be source of infection. Presence of pathogens in food may be due to external contamination (e.g., food poisoning by *Staphylococcus*).

Methods of Transmission of Infection

1. *Contact:* Syphilis, gonorrhea, trachoma.
2. *Inhalation:* Influenza, tuberculosis, smallpox, measles, mumps, etc.
3. *Infection:* Cholera (water), food poisoning (food) and dysentery (hand borne).
4. *Inoculation:* Tetanus (infection), rabies (dog), arbovirus (insect) and serum hepatitis, i.e. Hepatitis-B (infection).
5. *Insects:* They act as mechanical vector (dysentery and typhoid by housefly) or biological vector (malaria) of infectious disease.
6. *Congenital:* Congenital syphilis, rubella, *Listeria monocytogenes,* toxoplasma and cytomegalic inclusion disease.
7. *Laboratory infection:* Infection may be transmitted during procedures like, injection, lumbar puncture, catheterization, etc. if proper care is not taken.

Characters of Pathogens

1. Bacteria should be able to enter the body.
2. Organism should be able to multiply in the tissue.
3. They should be able to damage the tissue.
4. They must be capable to resist the host defence.

Factors Predisposing to Microbial Pathogenicity

Before discussing factor it is worthwhile to make fine distinction between the terms pathogenicity and virulence.

Pathogenicity: It is referred to the ability of microbial species to produce disease.

Virulence: It is referred to the ability of microbial strains to produce disease, e.g., polio virus contains strain of varying degree of virulence.

Virulence is the sum of the following factors:

A. **Invasiveness:** It is the ability of organism to spread in a host tissue after establishing infection. Less invasive organisms cause localized lesion, e.g., staphylococcal abscess. Highly invasive organisms cause generalized infection, e.g., streptococcal septicemia.

B. **Toxigenicity:** Bacteria produce two types of toxins—

  a. *Exotoxin:* It has following characters.
    1. Heat labile proteins.
    2. Diffuse readily into the surrounding medium.
    3. Highly potent, e.g., 3 kg botulinum can kill all the inhabitants of world whereas 1 mg of tetanus toxin is sufficient to kill one million guinea pigs.
    4. They are generally formed by Gram-positive organism and also by Gram-negative organisms like *Shigella, Vibrio cholerae* and *Escherichia coli.*
    5. Exotoxin are specifically neutralized by antitoxin.
    6. Can be separated from culture by filtration.
    7. Action is enzymatic.
    8. It has specific tissue affinity.
    9. It is highly antigenic.
    10. Specific pharmacological effects for each exotoxin.
    11. Can be toxoided.
    12. Cannot cause pyrexia in a host.

  b. *Endotoxin:* Endotoxin (Lipid a portion of lipopolysaccharide) has biological activities causing fever, muscle proteolysis, uncontrolled intravascular coagulation and shock. These may be mediated by production from mononuclear cells of IL-I, TNFX α 2 probably IL-6. It has following characters.

1. Proteins polysaccharide lipid complex heat stable.
2. Forms part of cell wall and will not diffuse into the medium.
3. Obtained only by cell lysis.
4. They have no enzymatic action.
5. Effect is nonspecific action.
6. No specific tissue affinity.
7. Active only in large doses 5 to 25 mg.
8. Weakly antigenic.
9. Neutralization by antibody ineffective.
10. Cannot be toxoided.
11. Produce in Gram-negative bacteria.
12. Can cause pyrexia in a host.

C. **Communicability:** This is ability of parasite to spread from one host to another. It determines the survival and distribution of organism in a community. Highly virulent organism may not exhibit a high degree of communicability due to rapid lethal effect on hosts. Infections in which pathogen is shed in secretions as in respiratory and intestinal diseases are highly communicable.

D. **Other bacterial products**

1. Coagulase *(Staphylococcus aureus)* which prevents phagocytosis by forming fibrin barrier around bacteria.
2. Fibrinolysin promotes the spread of infection by breaking down the fibrin barrier in tissues.
3. Hyaluronidase split hyaluronic acid (component of connective tissue) thus facilitating spread of infection along tissue spaces.

4. Leukocidins damage polymorphonuclear leukocytes.
5. Hemolysin is produced by some organisms capable of destroying erythrocytes.
6. Ig A1 proteases: Gonococci, meningococci, *Hemophilus influenzae* pneumococci, may produce IgA1 protease which splits IgA and inactivates its antibody activity.

E. **Bacterial appendages:** Capsulated bacteria like pneumococcus, *Klebsiella pneumoniae* and *Hemophilus influenzae* will stand phagocytosis. Surface antigen, e.g., Vi antigen of *Salmonella typhi* and K antigen of *Escherichia coli* resist phagocytosis and lytic activity of complement.

F. **Infecting dose:** The minimum infection dose (MID) or minimum lethal dose (MLD) is the minimum number of organisms required to produce clinical evidence of infection or death of susceptible animal.

G. **Route of infection:** *Vibrio cholerae* is effective orally. No effect when it is introduced subcutaneously. Streptococci can initiate infection whatever be the mode of entry. They also differ in ability to produce damage to different organs in different species, e.g., tubercle bacilli injected into rabbit cause lesion mainly in kidney and infrequently in liver and spleen. In guinea pig, main lesion is in liver and spleen whereas kidney is spared.

Chemotherapeutic Agents

These are the agents which have lethal or inhibitory effect on the microbes responsible, but in therapeutic concentration have little or no toxic action on the tissues.

However, these agents used in chemotherapy are of very diverse chemical structure. They can be divided into two categories:

a. Relatively simple compounds obtained by laboratory synthesis, e.g., sulfonamides, isoniazid, PAS, trimethoprim, etc.

b. Antibiotics are the substances produced by living organisms and which are active against other living organisms. Most of them are produced by soil actinomycetes.

Antibacterial agents are divided into two classes on the basis of type of action they exhibit against bacteria:

1. Bacteriostatic drugs are drugs which, in the concentration attainable in the body, only inhibit bacterial growth, e.g., chloramphenicol, sulfonamides, tetracyclines, etc.

2. Bactericidal drugs are the drugs which kill the bacteria by virtue of their rapid lethal action, e.g., penicillins, cephalosporins, aminoglycosides, fucidin, nalidixic acid, etc. Bactericidal drugs are more effective therapeutic agents than bacteriostatic drugs.

Mode of Action

The problem can be considered from two aspects:

1. Identification of site of action of drug.
2. Its precise mechanism of action.

Site of Action

There are four major loci of action.

1. Inhibition of synthesis of cell wall peptido-glycon, e.g., penicillins, cephalosporin, cyclo-serine, vancomycin, ristocetin and bacitracin.

2. Damage to the permeability of the cytoplasmic membrane, e.g., tryocidin, gramicidin, polymyxin and antifungal polyene antibiotics.

3. Inhibition of protein synthesis, e.g., amino-glycosides (amikacin, netilmicin, tobra-mycin, gentamicin, kanamycin, neomycin, streptomycin, etc.), tetracyclines, chlor-amphenicol. They bind to and inhibit the function of 30 S.

4. Inhibition of nucleic acid synthesis, e.g., rifampicin inhibits the synthesis of messenger RNA by its action on the RNA polymerase whereas nalidixic acid inhibits DNA replication. Other examples, are novobiocin, pyrimethamine, sulfonamide, etc.

Mechanism of Action

There are three general mechanisms of action.

1. Competition with a natural substrate for the active site of enzyme, e.g.,
   a. Action of sulfonamides to interfere competitively with the utilization of para-amino benzoic acid (PABA).
   b. Action of para-amino benzoic acid with para-amino salicylic acid (PAS).

2. Combination with an enzyme at a site sufficiently close to the active site as to

interfere with its enzymatic function, e.g., vancomycin, ristocetin and bacitracin.

3. Combination with nonenzymatic structural components, e.g., drugs which inhibits protein synthesis and drugs which act by damaging cytoplasmic membrane.

Laboratory Uses of Antibiotics

1. They may be incorporated as selective agents in culture media, e.g., penicillin may be used for isolation of *Hemophilus influenzae* from material taken from upper respiratory tract (penicillin inhibits the growth of Gram-positive bacteria and Neisseriae). Neomycin is used in Willis and Hobb's medium for the isolation of clostridia.

2. They are used for the control of bacterial contamination in tissue cultures used for virus isolation, e.g., penicillin, streptomycin, nystatin, etc.

3. The pattern of sensitivity of an organism to a battery of antibiotics constitute a simple method of typing which is of considerable epidemiological value.

Antibiotic Sensitivity Tests

Drug sensitivity tests are also important in studies of the epidemiology of resistance and in studies of new antimicrobial agents. Mueller-Hinton agar media (4 mm thickness plate) is considered best because:

   i. Acceptable batch to batch reproducibility for susceptibility testing
  ii. It is low in sulfonamide, trimethoprim and tetracycline inhibitors
 iii. It gives satisfactory growth of most non-fastidious pathogens
  iv. A large body of data and experience has been collected concerning susceptibility tests performed with the medium.

This medium should contain as low as possible thymidine or thymine (reverse the inhibitory effect of sulfonamide and trimethoprim) **(Fig. 9.1)**.

Zones of inhibition are measured to the nearest whole millimeter using sliding calipers,

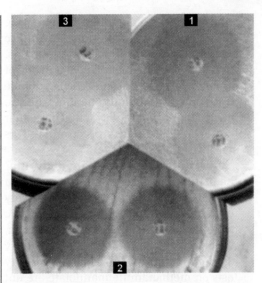

Fig. 9.1: Mueller Hinton agar. Clear zones of inhibition for combination of Trimethoprim and sulpha. *(1) Escherichia coli; (2) Staphylococcus aureus; (3) Streptococcus faecalis*

ruler or template prepared for this purpose which is held on the back of inverted petri plate.

These are applied to determine the susceptibility of pathogenic bacteria to antibiotics to be used in treatment. Antibiotic sensitivity tests are very useful for clinician and hence constitute important routine procedure in diagnostic bacteriology.

Mainly sensitivity test are of three types:

1. *Diffusion tests:* The principle of it is to allow the drug to diffuse through a solid medium, concentration of drug being highest near the site of application of drug and decreasing with distance.

There are many methods for implementation of this diffusion test. The most common, simple and easy method is to use filter paper disks impregnated with antibiotics (disk diffusion method). Here filter paper disks 6 mm in diameter are charged with required concentration of drugs and are stored dry in the cold. Inoculation of pure bacterial growth in liquid medium, may be done by spreading with swabs on solid medium. After drying the plate at 37°C for ½ hour antibiotic discs are applied with sterilized forceps. After overnight incubation at 37°C, zone of inhibition of growth around each antibiotic disc is noted. Inhibition zone shows degree of sensitivity of antibiotic for that particular bacteria. The results are reported as sensitive or resistant.

Disk diffusion test is done only after the pathogenic bacteria are isolated from clinical specimen in pure form. Sensitivity tests should be done only with pathogenic bacteria and not with commensals. Further, nitrofurantoin need to be tested only against urinary pathogens. Sensitivity tests on methanamine mandelate are not relevant as the drug is active only *in vivo*.

In case we require the drug sensitivity test sooner, clinical material is directly inoculated uniformly on the surface of solid media plate and disks are applied. This is done only in emergency and results are subsequently verified by testing the pure isolates.

2. *Dilution tests:* These are quite laborious for routine use. However, these are useful where therapeutic dose is to be regulated accurately, e.g., in treatment of bacterial endocarditis and to find out small degree of resistance in slow growing bacteria like tubercle bacilli. In dilution test, serial dilutions of drug are prepared and are inoculated with test bacterium. It may be done by tube dilution or agar dilution methods.

3. *E. test:* It is known as epsilometer test. Here antibiotic with known gradient of concentration in length on absorbent strip may be used. Now above mentioned strip is kept on the petridish containing nutrient agar seeded with test micro-organism. The antibiotic diffuses into nutrient agar medium. The minimum inhibitory concentration (MIC) is noted by recording the lowest concentration of the gradient which, in fact, inhibits growth of microorganisms.

ANTIBIOTIC STEWARDSHIP

It is a program that promotes the use of antibiotics

It improves patients outcome, reduces antibiotic resistance and decreases the spread of infections caused by multidrug resistance microbes.

This improves further:
1. Safety of patient
2. Ensure the continuous efficacy of antibiotic.

Bacterial Genetics

SECTION OUTLINE

❖ **Bacterial Genetics**

Bacterial Genetics

STRUCTURE OF DNA

Essential material of heredity is DNA which is the storehouse of all information for protein synthesis except some viruses where genetic material is RNA instead of DNA. Unit of code consists of sequences of three bases, i.e. code in triplet. Each codon specifies for single amino acid. More than one codon may exist for same amino acid. Thus, triplet AGA codes for arginine whereas AGG, CGU, CGC, CGA and CGG also code for same amino acid. Three codons (UAA, UAG, UGA) do not code for any amino acid and are called nonsense codons. They act as a mark, terminating the message for the synthesis of polypeptides. The transfer of genetic information from DNA to RNA is called transcription and from RNA to DNA (Protein synthesis) is called translation.

The genes are made of DNA. The structural components of a DNA molecule **(Fig. 10.1)** are arranged in two chains of nucleotides spiralled round a common axis. The chains are interconnected with pairs of bases at regular interval like the crossbars of a ladder. The sequence of their bases in DNA constitutes the genetic code. DNA molecules are chains of nucleotide. The four nucleotides present in DNA contain nitrogenous bases, purines (adenine, guanine) and pyrimidine (cytosine, thymine). There is a backbone of alternating deoxyribose and phosphate while purine and pyrimidine are attached to sugar. Two DNA strands are bound together to form double helix **(Fig. 10.2)**.

Double stranded nature of the molecule is stabilized by hydrogen bonding between the

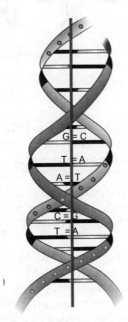

Fig. 10.1: DNA double helix.

bases on the opposite strands. They are held in such a manner that adenine is always linked to thymine forming a complementary base pair as do guanine and cytosine. There is equal amount of adenine and thymine in DNA and so also of guanine and cytosine. Ratio of each pair A+T/G+C varies widely from one bacterial species to another. However, this ratio is fixed for any given species. The DNA molecule replicates by first unwinding at one end to form a fork. Each strand of the fork acts as template for the synthesis of complementary strand with which it forms double helix.

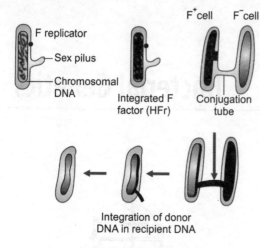

Fig. 10.2: Conjugation.

RNA is structurally similar to DNA except for two major differences:
1. It contains the sugar ribose (deoxyribose in DNA).
2. One of pyrimidine base is uracil instead of thymine in DNA. There are 3 distinct types of RNA on the basis of structure and function.
   i. Messenger RNA (mRNA).
   ii. Ribosomal RNA (rRNA).
   iii. Transfer RNA (tRNA).

DNA acts as the template for the synthesis of mRNA. Adenine, guanine, cytosine and uracil in RNA will be respectively complementary to thymine, cytosine, guanine and adenine in the DNA.

PLASMID

It consists of DNA situated in the cytoplasm in the free state and reproducing independently. Plasmids may be conjugative (e.g., R, F or bacteriocinogen plasmids) and nonconjugative (determinants).

Features of Bacterial Plasmids

❖ They are double stranded, circular DNA exist autonomously within a cell.

❖ Contain genes for self-replication.
❖ Plasmids are lost spontaneously or by curing agents.
❖ Two members of same group of plasmids cannot coexist in the same cells.
❖ Some plasmids are self transferable.
❖ Some plasmids can integrate with host chromosome (episome).
❖ Self-transferable plasmid can mobilize chromosomal gene or other plasmid by integration.
❖ They are not essential for cell survival.

TRANSMISSION OF GENETIC MATERIAL

Genetic material transmission occurs by the following ways:

Transformation

It is the transfer of genetic information through the agency of free DNA. This process, originally discovered in *Pneumococcus* has now been also observed in *Hemophilus, Neisseria* and *Bacillus*. Pieces of DNA involved in transformation may carry 10 to 50 genes. The frequency and significance of transformation in bacteria is not known.

Pneumococci are capsulated bacteria and can be divided into large number of types according to the chemical composition of their capsule. Descendents of type 1 *Pneumococcus* would always have type 1 capsule unless they lose ability to form capsule at all. The possibility of type transformation was demonstrated by Griffith in 1928 and its mechanism elucidated by Avery, McLeod and McCarty in 1944 that transforming principle was actually DNA. Griffith injected living type II (R) bacteria mixed with large number of killed type III (S) into mice. Many of the mice died and from heart blood he obtained pure live type III (S) bacteria. Something must have passed from dead type III bacteria and change type II (R) strain into virulent type III (S) which killed mice. This process is called transformation.

There are three mechanisms of transformation:

i. In Gram-positive bacteria like pneumococci the invading DNA fragment is cut to 7 to 10 kb by endonuclease of membrane and only one strand enters the cell.

ii. In Gram-negative bacteria like *Haemophilus*, a membrane protein binds a sequence of about 10 nucleotides and DNA enters as double strand inside the cell.

iii. In case of enteric group of bacteria, transformation takes place after modification of cell envelope by conversion to spheroplasts or otherwise. The modified cell surface permits taking up double stranded DNA fragments.

Transduction

It is the transfer of a portion of DNA from one bacterium to other by bacteriophages (viruses that parasitize in bacteria). Transduction is not confined to transfer of chromosomal DNA. Episomes and plasmids may also be transduced. The plasmid determining penicillin resistance in *Staphylococcus* is transferred from cell-to-cell by transduction.

Transduction may be generalized when it involves any segment of donor DNA. It may be restricted when specific bacteriophage transduces only a particular segment of DNA.

Several properties may be transduced.

a. Antigenic.
b. Nutritional requirements, drug resistances between *Salmonella, Shigella, Escherichia coli* and *Staphylococcus aureus.*

Lysogenic Conversion

Some strain may get infected with temperate bacteriophage. This phage confers new properties to bacterial host. These properties are retained so long as the bacteria remain infected with phages, e.g., nonvirulent strain of *C. diphtheriae* may acquire toxigenicity (capacity to produce exotoxin responsible for virulence) by infection and lysogenization with phage derived from virulent strain. This process by which prophage DNA confers genetic information to bacterium is called lysogenic conversion.

Conjugation (Fig. 10.2)

It is the process by which a male or donor bacterium makes contacts with female or recipient bacterium and transfers genetic elements into it. The capacity of a strain to act as a donor is determined by sex or fertility factor F in the cytoplasm. Such cells are called (F+) or male. The strain lacking this factor acts as recipient and this is known as female.

Before conjugation F factor migrates from cytoplasm to chromosome and becomes integrated with it. Such male cells are called (HFr). When in contact with F+ cell genetic material passes to F- cell through conjugate tube and F- is converted to F+ due to transfer of F+ factor. This phenomena is seen in *Escherichia coli, Shigella, Salmonella, Pseudomonas* and *Vibrio cholerae.* F factor however confers certain properties such as:

1. Cell produces a specific surface antigen. Such cells tend to adhere to F- cells.
2. It controls production of sex pilus.
3. It mobilizes F+ chromosomes for transfer.

Protoplast Fusion

Survival of protoplast may occur in osmotically buffered environment. This facilitates protoplast fusion by uniting together cell membrane and generation of cytoplasmic bridges through which genetic material is exchanged. Fusion may occur amongst members of various kingdoms as well as unrelated cells. The gene transfer by this method is also named as genetic transfusion.

Drug Resistance

During treatment with drugs, bacteria may acquire resistance to them. Following are the various mechanisms of drugs resistance:

1. *Mutation:* All bacteria contain drug resistant mutants arising spontaneously

once in 107 to 1010 cell divisions. It is again of two types.

a. Stepwise mutation in which series of small step mutations result in high levels of resistance, e.g., penicillin, chloramphenicol, tetracycline, sulfonamides, etc. However, this type of resistance can be prevented by using adequate dosage of drugs.

b. One step mutation in which case resistance develops suddenly even with first exposure of drug. This type of resistance is seen in tubercle bacilli developing resistance to streptomycin and isoniazid.

2. Resistance transfer by transformation may be demonstrated experimentally but its role in nature is not known.

3. Drug resistance by transduction is very commonly found in staphylococci. Penicillinase plasmid carrying determinant for resistance to mercuric chloride and erythromycin may be transmitted by transduction.

4. Drug resistance may be mediated by R factor. This is a very important mode of transferable drug resistance. There is evidence that many time R factor may lead to enhanced virulence. By this way there is simultaneous transfer of resistance to number of drugs, e.g., multiple resistance to chloramphenicol, streptomycin, tetracycline and sulfonamides, etc. Multiple drug resistance was initially seen in bacteria causing diarrhea, typhoid, urinary tract infection and so on.

5. Biochemical methods of drug resistance are:

a. Increased destruction of the drug by bacterial products, e.g., penicillinase produced by penicillin resistance bacteria.

b. Decreased permeability of bacterial cell to the drug.

c. Increased formation of metabolites with which drug competes for an enzyme, e.g., increased PABA synthesis by sulfonamide resistance strains.

d. Increased synthesis of inhibited enzymes or formation of resistant enzyme.

e. Development of alternate metabolic pathway.

Immunology

SECTION 3

Immunology

SECTION-3

SECTIONS

Immunity

INTRODUCTION

Immunology is the study of specific resistance to further infection by a particular microorganism or its products. Immunology is the science which deals with the body's response to antigenic challenge. It is a very broad scientific discipline whose relevance to most fields of medicine has become apparent in recent years. Immunological mechanisms are involved in the protection of the body against infectious agents but periodically they can also cause damage. Immunological tests are now routinely used in clinical practice, and in some cases they are indispensable for diagnosis of disease and subsequent care of patients. The introduction of a new technology, developed only a few years ago and called hybridoma technology, is revolutionizing immunology. This technique permits the production of antibodies against single antigenic determinants (epitopes). By this technique it is now possible to obtain unlimited amounts of very homogeneous and specific antibodies. Already we can use such antibodies for diagnosis and possibly in the future they will be used to treat the patient. Currently immunology concerns itself with all reactions, processes regardless whether they are less or more vigorous than original. These reactions may be harmful or protective and in some cases they may be both at the same time. In short immunology has broad biological role involving concept of recognition, specificity and memory. In this section on immunology discussion is restricted to the most relevant topics in the field of medicine.

HISTORICAL EVENTS IN IMMUNOLOGY

Practice of variolation was in progress in India and China from time immemorial. Here protection against smallpox was obtained by inoculating live organisms from the disease pustule. Jenner (1878) used nonvirulent cowpox vaccine against smallpox infection. Later, Pasteur tried a vaccine successfully using attenuated organisms against anthrax.

Metchnikoff (1883) suggested the role of phagocytes in immunity. Von Behring (1890) recognized antibodies in serum against diphtheria toxin. Denys and Leclef (1895) suggested that phagocytosis is enhanced by immunization. Ehrlich (1897) put forward side chain receptor theory of antibody synthesis. Bordet (1899) found that lysis of cells by antibody requires cooperation of serum factor now collectively known as complement.

Landsteiner (1900) declared human ABO groups and natural isohemagglutinin. Richest and Portier (1902) proposed the term anaphylaxis which is opposite of prophylaxis. Wright (1903) put forward opsonic activity to phagocytosis. Von Pirquet and Schick (1905) described serum sickness after injection of foreign serum. Von Pirquet (1906) correlated immunity and hypersensitivity. Fleming (1922) found lysozyme. Zinsser (1925) suggested the contrast between immediate and delayed type of hypersensitivity. Heidelberger and Kendall (1930-35) put forward quantitative precipitation studies on antigen-antibody reaction.

Coons (1942) introduced fluorescence antibody techniques. Medwar (1958) discovered acquired immunologic tolerance. Portar and Edelman (1972) determined structure of immunoglobulin. Rosalyn Yalow introduced radioimmunoassay in 1977 and Georges Koehler *et al.* reported monoclonal antibody (1984).

APPLICATION OF IMMUNOLOGY

1. It helps us to understand etiology and pathogenesis of diseases, e.g., rheumatic fever, asthma, acute glomerulonephritis, etc.
2. Diagnosis of disease is possible using ELISA, etc.
3. Development of vaccines.
4. Treatment using antibodies.
5. Transplantation and blood transfusion.
6. Surveillance, i.e. immune surveillance.
7. It helps to find out possible future susceptibility of a person to diseases with the help of HLA typing system.

IMMUNITY

The resistance offered by the host to the harmful effect of pathogenic microbial infection is called immunity. Immunity against infectious diseases is of different types (**Fig. 11.1**).

INNATE IMMUNITY

This is basic immunity which may be genetically passed on from one generation to other generation. It does not depend on prior contacts with microorganisms. It may be nonspecific when it indicates a degree of resistance to all infection, e.g., plant pathogens,

rinderpest, distemper. It is specific when it shows resistance to particular pathogens.

Innate immunity can be divided into following types:

Species immunity: Individuals of same species show uniform pattern of susceptibility to different bacterial infection. The mechanism of species immunity may be due to physiological and biochemical differences between tissue of host species which determine whether or not pathogen can multiply in them, e.g., poliomyelitis, measles, syphilis, leprosy, gonorrhea occur only in man. Many a time same species of bacteria produce different types of infection in different animals, e.g., *Salmonella typhi* produces typhoid fever in man whereas mice is resistant.

Racial immunity: Within a species different races show differences in susceptibility to infection, e.g., Negroes are resistant to yellow fever and malaria and high resistance of Algerian sheep to anthrax. Such racial differences are known to be genetic in origin principally induced by persistent environmental stimulus.

Individual immunity: Individual in population shows variation in their response to microbial infection, e.g., homozygous twins exhibit similar degree of resistance or susceptibility to lepromatous leprosy and tuberculosis. Such correlation is not seen in heterozygous twins.

Factors influencing level of innate immunity in an individual are:

1. *Age:* Two extremes of life carry high susceptibility to infectious diseases. The susceptibility of fetus to infection is related to immaturity of its immune apparatus, e.g., Coxsackie viruses cause fatal infection in sucking mice but not in adults.

    Old persons are highly susceptible to infection due to gradual waning of their immune responses.

    Many age differences in specific infections can be related to physiologic factors. Thus bacterial meningitis during first month of life is often caused by coliform

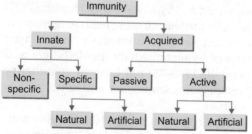

Fig. 11.1: Classification of immunity.

bacteria because bacterial antibodies to these bacteria are IgM and thus fail to cross the placenta. Other such examples are gonococcal vaginitis in small girls, rickettsial infection more severe in advancing age, rubella infection damages the fetus severely but otherwise produces only mild disease.

2. *Hormonal influence:* Endocrine disorders, e.g., diabetes mellitus is related to susceptibility to infection because of increased carbohydrate levels in tissue. Corticosteroids depress host's resistance by anti-inflammatory, antiphagocytic effect and by suppression of antibody formation and hypersensitivity. The elevated steroid levels during pregnancy may have relation to increased susceptibility of pregnant women to many infections.

3. *Nutrition:* Defective nutrition depresses all types of immune response and thus increasing the risk of infection.

Mechanism of Innate Immunity

The defence mechanisms of body are related to body coverings as under:

1. *Epithelial surfaces:* The intact skin and mucous membrane covering the body confers on it considerable protection against bacteria. They provide mechanical barrier. They also provide bactericidal secretions. Their bactericidal activity is related to the presence of lactic acid, saturated and unsaturated fatty acid in sweat and sebaceous secretion. The mucous membrane of gastrointestinal tract provides protection by bactericidal enzymes secreted in lumen. The anaerobic colony bacteria produce fatty acids with antibacterial activity. The term "colonization resistance" refers to resistance offered by the predominant normal flora to infection, e.g., the intestinal anaerobic microflora prevents superinfection by coliform during antibiotic therapy. Saliva is bacteriocidal. High acidity of stomach inhibits bacterial multiplication. The normal body flora play indirect role in defence of body, e.g.,

intestinal flora by producing bacteriocines which are destructive to other bacteria.

2. *Tissue defenses:* If barrier of body is overcome by the organisms, a number of factors in normal tissue and body fluid, play their role. Tissue factors may be divided into:
   a. Humoral factors.
   b. Cellular factors.

Humoral Factors

a. *Lysozyme:* It is a bacteriocidal enzyme found in nasal and intestinal secretion, seminal fluid and lacrimal secretion.

b. *Properdin:* It is euglobulin present in normal serum. It causes lysis of Gram-negative bacteria with the help of Mg^{++} and complement. It constitutes 0.02% of serum protein. It is not an antibody and its level remains constant in newborn and elderly individuals in both sexes. Its molecular weight is over one million.

c. *Beta lysin:* It is a relatively thermostable substance active against anthrax bacillus. It is liberated from platelets during clotting.

d. *Basic polypeptides:* They are bacteriocidal substances active at high pH (7 to 8). They act upon cell wall causing cell disintegration, e.g., lukins from leukocytes and plakin from platelets.

e. *C-reactive proteins (CRP):* The sera of patient with pneumococcal and other diseases give a precipitate when mixed with somatic polysaccharide C of *pneumococcus* in presence of calcium ions. These nonspecific substances (C-reactive protein) appear in blood of a person with tissue necrosis and inflammation. C-reactive protein does play an important role in the resolution of inflammatory process. It binds to many materials like bacterial polysaccharides and may then activate classical pathway, bringing complement components into play to potentiate bacterial killing. Recently, it is suggested that the functions of CRP is primarily to act as a binding mechanism, say for pneumococcal "C" polysaccharide which is most effectively precipitated on agglutination. The binding of such legands render them accessible to phagocytosis and as a result to clearance and metabolic breakdown. Characters of C-reactive protein are:

1. Calcium is essential for the reaction.
2. Reactive substance globulin is not detectable in normal serum. It is demonstrated in sera, pleural, peritoneal and joint fluids of patient.

The demonstration of C-reactive protein is useful in the diseases like rheumatic fever, and rheumatoid arthritis, etc.

f. *Bactericidin:* It is nonspecific serum factor active against *Neisseria, Streptococcus hemolyticus,* etc.

g. *Complement:* It is thermolabile substance present in serum and tissue fluid. It enhances phagocytosis and kills most of Gram-negative bacteria sensitized by specific antibodies.

h. *Nonspecific hyaluronidase inhibitors:* In tissue damage nonspecific inhibitor hyaluronidase appears in blood. It is heat labile and requires magnesium ion for its activity.

Production of antibodies against antigens of microorganisms may induce resistance because they:

1. Neutralize toxin or cellular products.
2. Have direct bacteriocidal or lytic effect with complement.
3. Block the infective ability of micro-organisms.
4. Agglutinate microorganisms thus subjecting them to phagocytosis.
5. Opsonize microorganisms.

Cellular Factors

1. *Phagocytosis:* Natural defence against invasion of blood and tissue by bacteria or others foreign particles is mediated by phagocytic cell which ingest and destroy them. The process of phagocytosis consists of:

i. The first phase involves the approach of the phagocyte to the microbe by means of positive chemotaxis. Under the influence of the products of life activities of microbes excitation of the phagocytes occurs, which leads to a change in the surface tension of the cytoplasm and gives the phagocytes amoeboid motility.

ii. In the second phase absorption of the microorganism on the surface of the phagocyte takes place. This process is completed under the influence of an electrolyte which alters the electrical potential of the phagocytized object (microbe).

iii. The third phase is characterized by submergence of the microbe into the cytoplasm of the phagocyte, which seizes minute objects quite rapidly and large ones (some protozoa, actinomycetes, etc.) are engulfed in pieces.

iv. In the fourth phase intracellular digestion of the engulfed microbes by the phagocytes takes place.

In the process of phagocytosis various changes in the microbes can be observed, e.g., the production of granules in *Vibrio cholerae*, swelling of *Salmonella*, fragmentation of *Corynebacterium diphtheriae*, destruction of anthrax bacilli and swelling of cocci. Ultimately the phagocytosed microorganisms become completely disintegrated.

Factors which speed up phagocytosis include calcium and magnesium salts, antibodies, etc. Phagocytosis proceeds more vigorously in immunes than in nonimmunes. Toxin of bacteria, leukocidin, capsular material of bacteria, cholesterol, quinine, alkaloids, and also a blockade of reticuloendothelial system inhibit phagocytosis.

Phagocytic cells may be:

a. Microphages, e.g., polymorphonuclear leukocytes.

b. Macrophages includes:
1. Histiocytes (wandering amoeboid cells in tissue).
2. Fixed reticuloendothelial cells.
3. Monocytes.

2. *Inflammation:* Tissue injury or irritation initiated by entry of bacteria or of other irritant leads to inflammation. It is important nonspecific mechanism of defense. Initially constriction and then dilatation of blood vessels of affected site is followed by escape of polymorphonuclear cells into tissue. Microorganisms are phagocytosed and destroyed. Out pouring of plasma helps to dilute the toxic products. A fibrin barrier is laid, serving to wall off the site of infection.

3. *Fever:* It is a natural defence mechanism. It may actually destroy the infecting organism. Fever stimulates the production of interferon and helps in recovery from virus infections. The substances which may cause fever are endotoxins and interleukin-1.

Acute phase proteins: Because of trauma or infection there may be abrupt rise of plasma concentration of some proteins (acute phase proteins). Some of the examples of acute phase proteins are 'C' reactive proteins, mannose binding proteins, alpha-1 acid glycoproteins, etc. They may increase host resistance, help in the healing of inflammatory lesions, prevent tissue damage, activate alternative pathways ('C' reactive proteins).

Outcome of infection: Following are some possible results of infection:
1. Elimination of pathogen without any clinical lesion when immune status of host is normal.
2. Localization of pathogen with production of local lesion when there is no impairment of the patient's general health and as a rule infection is soon eradicated, e.g., small staphylococcal pustule of the skin.
3. Localization of the pathogen with production of distant lesion as happens in diphtheria and tetanus because of exotoxin.
4. Local extension of infection to surrounding tissue as in case of hyaluronidase producing *Streptococcus pyogenes.* Other examples are tuberculosis and actinomycosis.
5. General dissemination as in case of septicemia and then involves various organs of the body.

ACQUIRED IMMUNITY

The immunity acquired during the lifetime of an individual is known as acquired immunity. Acquired immunity differs from innate immunity in the following respects:
1. It is not inherent in the body but is acquired during life.
2. It is specific for a single type of microorganism.

Acquired immunity may be:
1. Active.
2. Passive.

Active Immunity: It is the resistance developed by an immunity as a result of antigenic stimulus. Active immunity may be:

Natural active immunity: This is acquired after one infection or recovery from disease or subclinical infection after repeated exposure to small doses of the infecting organism.

Artificial active immunity: It may be acquired artificially by inoculation of bacteria, viruses or their products as below:
a. Living organisms: After proper attenuation, e.g., smallpox, BCG. Attenuation may be obtained as below:
   i. Subjecting the organism to drying, e.g., rabies virus vaccine.
   ii. Growing the organism at temperature higher than optimum, e.g., Pasteur's anthrax vaccine is prepared by cultivating the organism at 42°C.
   iii. By passage through animals of different species, e.g., variola virus through rabbit and calf.
   iv. By continued cultivation in presence of antagonistic substance, e.g., BCG vaccine is prepared by prolonged cultivation of tubercle bacillus (bacillus,

calmette and guerin) in medium containing bile.

    v. By repeated subculture in artificial media, e.g., streptococci.

b. Organisms are killed by heat or phenol without changing the antigenic structure of bacteria, e.g., typhoid vaccine, cholera vaccine.

c. Autovaccine.

d. Nonspecific protein therapy: Local cellular elements concerned with defensive mechanism respond to injection of nonspecific protein substance like milk injection. They cause increased proliferation resulting in more antibody release.

e. Toxoid: Bacterial inactivated toxin (not toxigenic but retains antigenicity) is injected repeatedly in increasing doses, e.g., diphtheria and tetanus toxoid.

Passive Immunity: Here subject is immunized by prepared antibodies and body cells do not take any active part in the production of immunity. It is of the following types:

Natural passive immunity: During intrauterine life transmission of antibodies from the mother to fetus can occur through placenta. It may be by way of colostrum of mother and milk during first few months of life. Breastfed infants resist establishment of enteroviruses in alimentary tract. These antibodies last for few weeks and protect infants from diphtheria, tetanus, measles, mumps, smallpox, etc.

Artificial passive immunity: Immunization in this case is passive and produced by injection of serum of animals that have been immunized actively. Antibodies remain in effective quantity for 10 days only. Following serum may be used:

a. *Antitoxic serum:* It is produced by injection of toxoid into horse in increasing doses till the blood is rich in circulating antibodies. The animal is bled and serum is separated. This serum contains prepared antibodies. Examples of antitoxic sera are diphtheria, tetanus, etc.

b. *Antibacterial serum:* Antibodies are produced by injection of bacteria into animals and serum is collected, e.g., pneumococcal, meningococcal, anthrax, dysentery, etc.

c. *Convalescent serum*: It is obtained from convalescent patient. It is also called convalescent serum. Such serum is used in the treatment of measles, poliomyelitis, infective hepatitis, etc.

Differences between active immunity and passive immunity are summed up as per **Table 11.1**.

Table 11.1: Differences between active and passive immunity.

Active immunity	Passive immunity
• Produced actively by host's immune system	• Received passively by the host. No participation by host's immune system
• Induced by infection or by contacts with immunogen	• Conferred by introduction of vaccines, e.g., readymade antibody
• Afford durable and effective protein	• Temporary and less effective protection
• Immunity effective after lag phase	• Immunity effective immediately
• Immunological memory present, i.e. subsequent challenge more effective	• No immunological memory
• Negative phase may occur	• No negative phase
• Not applicable to immunodeficient hosts	• Application to immunodeficient hosts
• Used as prophylaxis to increase resistance of body	• Used for treatment of acute infection
• Both cell mediated and humoral immunity take part	• Exclusively humoral immunity is involved
• No inheritance of immunity	• May be acquired from mother

Local Immunity: It has importance in infections which are either localized or where it is operative in combating infection at the site of primary entry of pathogen, e.g., influenza immunization with killed vaccine elicit humoral antibody response but antibody titer in respiratory secretion is not high enough to prevent infection. Natural infection or live virus vaccine administered intranasaly provide local immunity. A special class of immunoglobulin (IgA) forms major component of local immunity.

Herd Immunity: There is overall level of immunity in a community. It is relevant in the control of epidemic diseases. When herd immunity is low, epidemics are likely to occur on introduction of suitable pathogens. The term herd immunity means large proportion of individuals in a community are immune to pathogen.

VACCINATION

It is worthwhile to discuss it with the history of development of vaccine. Along with it other aspects are also taken up:

History of Development of Immunization

1721 — Variolation by Lady Montague
1793 — Smallpox immunization
1881 — Development of Pasteur's antirabies vaccine and also demonstration of efficacy of anthrax vaccine
1891 — Development of diphtheria antitoxin
1896 — Vaccine against typhoid fever
1904 — Production of tetanus antitoxin
1920 — Diphtheria antitoxin floccules
1930 — Diphtheria toxoid
1951 — Yellow fever live vaccine
1955 — Polio killed vaccine (SALK)
1960 — Polio live vaccine (SABIN)
1970 — Live vaccine of rubella and mumps. Also measles vaccine (killed as well as live).

Vaccines: Live attenuated or dead organisms when introduced into the body, artificial active immunization is produced. Killed vaccines produce relatively less immunity. The live vaccines contain major immunizing antigen and hence, more and longer antigenic stimulation resulting in prolonged immunity as compared to killed vaccine. Live vaccine is quite cheap and dose given is also small. The vaccines are classified as under **(Table 11.2)**.

A. Live attenuated vaccines are smallpox, yellow fever, polio, BCG, plague, brucellosis, mumps, rubella and measles. Attenuation is achieved by aging of culture, culture at high temperature, passage through another host species, drying (rabies) and selection of mutant (temperature sensitive).

B. Killed vaccines, e.g., whooping cough, TAB, cholera, polio (SALK), antirabic and measles. For this purpose organisms are killed by heat, formalin, phenol, alcohol, ultraviolet light and photodynamic inactivation. Killed vaccines may be preserved in phenol, alcohol or merthiolate.

C. Toxoid are exotoxin which are treated with formalin to destroy their toxicity but retaining their immunogenicity, e.g., formal toxoid of diphtheria and tetanus.

D. Subunit vaccines: They consist of only relevant immunogenic material such as the capsid proteins of non-enveloped icosahedral viruses or the peplomers (glycoprotein) of enveloped proteins.

Hazards of vaccination: Local sepsis, serum hepatitis, fever, malaise, soreness at injection site, arthralgia after rubella vaccine, convulsions in pertussis vaccine and allergic reaction may occur as untoward side effect after vaccination.

The problem with live vaccine is its stability of attenuation. The other problem with live vaccine is drastic consequences if given to immuno-deficient child. Antibodies in mother's milk may cause poor take if vaccinated infant is breastfed. Potency of vaccine may be maintained by lyophilization. The other problem is intestinal infections at subclinical levels and hence poor take of live vaccine as enteroviruses may prevent multiplication of the attenuated vaccine.

Table 11.2: Classification of vaccines available against microorganisms.

Vaccines	Vaccines against bacteria	Vaccines against viruses	Vaccines against parasites
Live vaccine	• *Mycobacterium tuberculosis* • *Vibrio cholerae* • *Salmonella* • *Escherichia coli*	• Polio • Mumps • Measles • Rubella • Vaccinia • Adeno • Rabies • Herpes zoster • Cytomegalovirus • Influenza • Yellow fever • Rotavirus	
Inactivated vaccine	• *Corynebacterium diphtheriae* • Pertussis • *Clostridium tetani* • *Vibrio cholerae* • Meningococcus (ACYW) • Pneumococcus • *Haemophilus influenzae* • *E. coli*	• Rabies • Polio • Influenza • Hepatitis B • Measles	• *Plasmodium falciparum* • *Trypanosomes cruzi* • *Schistosoma mansoni*

National Immunization Schedule (Table 11.3)

Table 11.3: National immunization schedule.

Vaccine	Administration	Dose	Route	Site
Infants				
Bacille Calmette–Guérin vaccine	At birth	0.05–1 mL	Intradermal	Upper arm
Diphtheria, tetanus, pertusis, *Haemophilus influenzae* and hepatitis B	6 weeks 10 weeks 14 weeks	0.5 mL	Intramuscular	Mid-thigh (lateral side)
Oral polio vaccine	6 weeks 10 weeks 14 weeks	2 drops	Oral	Oral
Intramuscular killed polio vaccine				
Measles vaccine	9 months	0.5 mL	Subcutaneous	Right upper arm
Japanese encephalitis	12 months			
Vitamin A	6-59 months	1 mL	Oral	Oral`
Children				
Diphtheria, tetanus, pertusis (booster)	16–24 months	0.5 mL	Intramuscular	Mid thigh (lateral side)
Measles, mumps, and rubella	1–14 months	0.5 mL	Subcutaneous	Right upper arm
Oral polio vaccine	16–24 months	2 drops	Oral	Oral
Measles (2nd dose)	16–24 months	0.5 mL	Subcutaneous	Right upper arm
Diphtheria, Tetanus, Pertusis (booster)	5-6 years	0.5 mL	Intramuscular	Mid-thigh (lateral side)
Tetanus toxoid	10 years-16 years	0.5 mL	Intramuscular	Right upper arm
Pregnant women				
Tetanus toxoid	Early pregnancy	0.5 mL	Intramuscular	Right upper arm
Tetanus toxoid	4 weeks after the 1st dose	0.5 mL	Intramuscular	Right upper arm

■ NEWER VACCINES

Nowadays, antigen identification and preparation of vaccine is achieved by recombinant DNA production of proteins and polypeptides, production of synthetic oligopeptides and epitopes by hybridoma technology, and directed mutation, selection and stabilization. Now it is possible to develop vaccines against agents that cannot even be grown.

In recombinant DNA genetic, the genes that code for immunologically important polypeptide antigens of viruses or bacteria are inserted into infectious nucleic acid vectors permitting the production of these proteins and polypeptides in new and unnatural hosts like bacterial, yeast or animal cells.

Hybridoma technology consists of the fusion of antibody producing lymphocytes with cancer cells to yield hybrid cells that can be propagated indefinitely and secrete only a single immunologic determinant a whole antigen. Monoclonal antibodies are highly specific tools for analysis of microbial antigens and allow selection of those that are of relevance to immunity. The other importance lies in their ability to define very short lengths of polypeptides that relate to specific immunity. This has opened the doors to chemical synthesis of vaccines.

Advantages of Newer Vaccines

1. Give specific immune response.
2. Rare reversion to virulence.
3. Fewer chances of contamination.

Disadvantages of Newer Vaccines

1. Limited immunogenicity of very simplified antigen.
2. Weak and inadequate immune responses.

■ APPLICATION OF VACCINE

❖ Prophylactic use for general population, e.g., BCG, polio
❖ Prophylactic use for selective group of persons, e.g., Hepatitis B vaccine for doctors, nurses, infant born to HBs antigen positive mothers, etc.
❖ New directions in vaccine development has slowly evolved from Jenner to recombinant genetics. It has provided a possible basis for prophylactic control of essentially all the infectious diseases.

Chapter 12

Antigen

INTRODUCTION

Antigen is a substance which, when introduced parenterally into the body, stimulates the production of an antibody with which it reacts specifically in an observable manner. Antigenic determinant is that portion of antigen molecule that determines the specificity of antigen-antibody reaction. It is also called epitope. An epitope corresponds to an area about 6 to 10 amino acids, or of 5 to 6 doses. Antibody recognizes epitope present on the surface of native antigen in solution, which may be proteins or polysaccharides, whereas T cell receptors bind to peptide fragment processed by antigen presenting cells. In these cells, the antigen undergoes proteolytic degradation, generating peptides which are then presented in association with class I or class II proteins of the major histocompatibility complex (HLA).

Antigenic Determinant

❖ Also called epitope
❖ It is smallest unit of antigenicity represented by small area on antigen molecule, which determines specific immune response and reacts specifically with antibody
❖ An antigen possesses several epitopes and each epitope induces specific antibody formation
❖ Size of epitope is 25 to 35 Å
❖ Molecular weight varies between 400 and 1000
❖ The determinant groups are:

a. Protein antigen (Penta of hexasaccharide)
b. Polysaccharide antigen (Hexasaccharide)
❖ A determinant is around 5 amino acid in size.
❖ The site on antibody molecule, which combines with corresponding epitope is known as paratope.

PROPERTIES OF ANTIGEN

A number of properties have been identified which make a substance antigenic.

1. **Foreignness**: Only antigens which are foreign to the individual induce an immune response. An individual does not normally give rise to immune response against his own constituent antigen.

   Antigenicity of substance is related to the degree of foreignness. Injection of sheep RBC or rat kidney tissue extract in rabbit will cause production of antibodies. But injection of rabbit RBC or kidney tissue extract into the same rabbit will not stimulate antibody production.

2. **Size**: Antigenicity bears a relation to molecular size. Very large molecules such as hemocyanin (molecular weight 6.75 millions) are highly antigenic. Usually antigens have a molecular weight of 10,000 or more.

   Substances of less than 10,000 dalton molecular weight, e.g., insulin (5700) are either non-antigenic or weakly antigenic.

However, substances with low molecular weight may be rendered antigenic by adsorbing the same on large inert particles like kaolin or bentonite.

Depending on the size of antigen and capacity to induce antibody production antigens can be divided into:

a. Complete antigen
b. Partial antigen.

a. *Complete antigen:* It is able to induce antibody formation and produce a specific and observable reaction with the antibody so produced, e.g., proteins, polysaccharide, etc.

b. *Partial antigen* (also called hapten): Haptens are substances which are unable to induce antibody production by themselves, but are able to react specifically with antibodies, e.g., lipids, nucleic acid, sulfonamide, penicillin, etc. Clinically they are important because a number of hypersensitivity reactions may develop as a complication of drug therapy. Haptens may be of two types:
   i. Complex hapten
   ii. Simple hapten

   i. **Complex hapten**: They are relatively higher molecular compounds which can precipitate with specific antibodies, e.g., Wassermann antigen (cardiolipin), polysaccharides (C substance of streptococci) and nucleic acid.

   ii. **Simple hapten**: They are low molecular weight compounds and are non-precipitating with specific antibodies, e.g., picric chloride, tartaric acid, para-aminobenzoic acid. Such substances when applied to skin, inhaled or injected can form compounds with proteins of skin and plasma proteins thereby producing foreign hapten group and sensitization.

3. **Chemical nature**: Most naturally occurring antigens are proteins and polysaccharides. Proteins are more effective in stimulating antibody production than polysaccharides except gelatin histone and protamines (non-antigenic protein) due to their low tyrosine contents (aromatic radicals). Not all proteins are antigenic. Gelatin is a well-known exception. Aromatic radical is a must for antigenicity. Gelatin is non-antigenic because of absence of aromatic radical.

4. **Susceptibility to tissue enzymes**: Only substances which are metabolized and are susceptible to the action of tissue enzymes behave like antigen. Substances insusceptible to tissue enzymes are not antigenic, e.g., polystyrene latex, D amino acids which are not metabolized in the body are not antigenic. Polypeptides composed of L amino acid are antigenic.

5. **Antigenic specificity**: Active sites are present at certain places in antigen molecules. These active sites are called antigenic determinants. The remaining portion of antigen molecule is antigenically inert. In antigen antibody reaction, antigen molecule reacts specifically at determinant site with complementary combining on antibody molecule, e.g., the antigenic specificity of the Lancefield group A *Streptococcus pyogenes* depends on N acetylglucosamine present in the side chain or rhamnose backbone. Antigenic specificity is of following types:

   a. *Species specificity*: Tissues of all individuals in species contain species specific antigen. It has been useful in:
      i. Tracing of evolutionary relationship.
      ii. Forensic application in identification of species of blood and seminal stains.

   b. *Isospecificity:* Isoantigens are antigens found in some but not all member of a species, e.g.:
      i. Human erythrocytes antigen on which individuals can be classified into group (blood group).
      ii. Histocompatibility antigen: HL-A (human leukocyte associated antigen system). It has its application in organ

transplantation from one individual to other.

c. *Auto-specificity:* A number of tissue antigen may act as autoantigen, e.g.lens protein, thyroglobulin, etc. These tissues under certain circumstances such as injury, infection or drug therapy alter the molecule so that they become foreign to one's own body and provoke autoantibody formation.

d. *Organ specificity:* They are restricted to particular organ or tissue of species. When they are restricted exclusively to an organ they are called organ specific, e.g., thyroglobulin, lens protein, brain, spinal cord and adrenal of one species share specificity with another species.

e. *Heterogenetic (Heterophile) specificity* (**Table 12.1**): This is found in a number of unrelated animals and microorganisms. The examples are:

  i. Forssman antigen found (**Table 12.2**) in the tissue of guinea pigs, cat, horse, sheep, bacteria, e.g., rickettsiae. It was first described by Forssman in 1911.

  ii. Weil-Felix reaction in typhus fever.

  iii. Paul-Bunnell reaction in infectious mononucleosis.

  iv. Cold agglutinin test in primary atypical pneumonia.

SUPERANTIGEN

Certain proteins that are capable of activating a large number of T-lymphocytes irrespective of their antigenic specificities are named as super antigen. They actually bind directly to the

Table 12.1: Cross-reacting antigens shown by heterophile reactions.

Antigen	Sharing antigen
• Blood group B substance	*Escherichia coli*
• Blood group A substance	Pneumococcus type 14 (cap polys)
• Blood group PI antigen	Hydatid fluid
• Blood group A substance	Streptococcal extract
• Rickettsiae causing typhus	Proteus OX_{19}, OXK_2, OXk
• Epstein-Barr virus	Sheep and Ox RBC

Table 12.2: Distribution of Forssman antigen.

RBC and other tissues	Kidney	Bacteria cells
Horse	Guinea pig	*Streptococcus pneumoniae*
Cat		*Shigella dysenteriae*
Mouse		*Pasteurella*
Chicken		*Clostridium perfringens*

lateral aspect of V regions of TCR beta chain. Superantigen may activate 20% of circulatory T-lymphocytes where as conventional antigenic stimuli can activate not more than 0.0001% of circulating T-lymphocytes. This excessive T-lymphocyte activation may result a huge outpouring of T-lymphocyte cytokines leading to multisystem problems. The examples are staphylococcal toxic shock syndrome and staphylococcal enterotoxin.

Antibodies—Immunoglobulins

Antibody is defined as humoral substance (γ-globulin) produced in response to an antigenic stimulus. It serves as protective agent against organisms. Antibodies are found in serum, lymph and other body fluids. Sera having high antibody levels following infection or immunization is called immune sera. Antibodies are:

1. Protein in nature.
2. Formed in response to antigenic stimulation.
3. React with corresponding antigen in a specific and observable manner.

The antibody molecule is chemically indistinguishable from normal gammaglobulin. Globulin is a very complex mixture of molecules consisting of closely related proteins. Now the term immunoglobulin is used to describe these closely related proteins.

▣ IMMUNOGLOBULINS

They are defined as proteins of animals origin endowed with known antibody activity and for some other proteins related to them by chemical structure.

Immunoglobulins are synthesized by plasma cells and also by lymphocytes. Immunoglobulins make 20 to 25% of the total serum proteins. The term immunoglobulins is the structural and chemical concept while antibody is biological and functional concept. All antibodies are immunoglobulins but all immunoglobulins may not be antibodies.

Based on their size, carbohydrate contents and amino acid analysis, five groups of immuno-globulins have been distinguished: IgG, IgA, lgM, IgD and IgE.

Structure of Immunoglobulin

Porter, Edelman and Nisonoff (1959-64) developed technique for fragmentation of immunoglobulin molecule by papain digestion which has led to the discovery of 5 main classes of immunoglobulin.

Papain Digestion (Fig. 13.1)

Enzymatic digestion: Porter and colleagues split rabbit IgG molecule to egg albumin by papain digestion in presence of cystein into two identical Fab (Fragment antigen binding) fragments and one Fc (Fragment crystallizable) fragment.

Papain acts on the exposed hinge region of molecule.

1. **Fab fragments:** Each fragment of 3.5S contains a single antigen binding site. The portion of the heavy chain in the Fab fragment is called Fd region. Each Fab fragment contains a light chain.
2. **Fc fragment:** It lacks the ability to bind antigen and appears to be identical in all rabbit IgG molecules. Each Fc fragment contains parts of both H chains. As this fragment is easily crystallizable, it is so named.

Pepsin Digestion (Fig. 13.2)

Pepsin strikes at a different point of the IgG molecule and cleaves the Fc from the remainders of the molecule leaving a large SS fragment, composed essentially of 2 Fab fragments. It is divalent and still precipitates with antigen. This fragment is formulated as $(Fab)_2$.

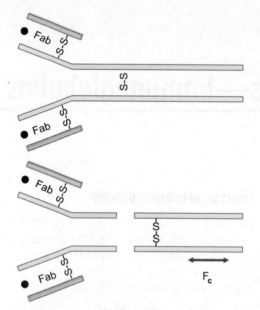

Fig. 13.1: Basic structure of an immunoglobulin molecule and papain digestion Fab and Fc fragments.

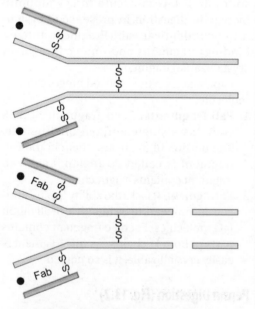

Fig. 13.2: Basic structure of an immunoglobulin molecule and pepsin digestion (Fab)₂.

Immunoglobulins are glycoproteins. Each molecule consisting of two pairs of polypeptide chains of different sizes held together by disulfide bonds (S—S) **(Fig. 13.3)**. The smaller

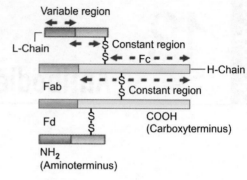

Fig. 13.3: Structure of immunoglobulin.

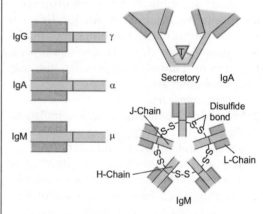

Fig. 13.4: Structure of IgG, IgA and IgM.

chains are called light (L) chain and larger ones heavy (H) chains. L chain has molecular weight 25,000 and H chain 50,000. The L chain is attached to the H chain by disulfide bond. The two H chains are joined together by one to five S—S bonds depending upon class of immunoglobulins. The H chains are structurally and antigenetically distinct for each class and designated by Greek letter as follows **(Fig. 13.4):**

IgG	γ	(gamma)
IgA	α	(alpha)
IgM	μ	(mu)
IgD	δ	(delta)
IgE	ε	(epsilon)

The L chains are similar in all classes of immunoglobulins. They may be either kappa or lambda in a molecule of immunoglobulins.

L chain: The antigen combining site of molecule is at its aminoterminus (N). Carboxyterminal portion is also called constant region. Of 214 amino acid residues that make up L chains, 107 constitute carboxyterminal half occur only in constant sequence and hence this part of chain is called constant region. Amino acid sequence in aminoterminal (N) half of chains is highly variable and so called variable region. This variability determines immunological specificity of antibody molecule. Like L chain, H chain also has constant and variable region.

The infinite range of antibody specificity of immunoglobulins depends on the variability of amino acid sequences at variable region of H chain and L chains which form antigen combining site.

Fc fragment: It is composed of carboxyterminal portion of H chain. It determines biological properties of immunoglobulins molecules like complement fixation, placental transfer, skin fixation, attachment to phagocytic cells, degranulation of mast cells and catabolic rate. It is crystallizable and contains carbohydrate.

Fd fragment: The portion of H chain present in Fab fragment is called Fd piece. Its function is not known.

Fab: It is aminoterminal half of heavy chain and one light chain. It does not crystallize. It does not contain carbohydrate and acts as antigen binding fragment.

Function of Immunoglobulins

The important functions of immunoglobulins are:

1. Complement activation causing lysis
2. Opsonization resulting in phagocytosis
3. Prevention of attachment of microbe to host cells
4. Neutralize toxins
5. Motility of microorganisms is restricted
6. Ultimately may result in agglutination of microbes.

Immunoglobulin Classes (Table 13.1)

1. **IgG:** It is the major serum immunoglobulin **(Fig. 13.5)**. It has molecular weight of

Table 13.1: Some properties of immunoglobulin classes.

	IgG	IgA	IgM	IgD	IgE
• Sedimentation coefficient	7	7	19	7	8
• Molecular weight	1,50,000	1,60,000	9,00,000	1,80,000	1,90,000
• Serum concentration (mg/mL)	12	2	1.2	0.03	0.00004
• Half-life (days)	23	6	5	2.8	2.3
• Daily production (mg/kg)	34	24	3.3	0.4	0.0023
• Intravascular distribution (%)	45	42	80	75	50
• Complement fixation	+		+		
• Placental transport	+		+		
• Present in milk	+		+		
• Secretion by seromucous glands	–		+		
• Heat stability (56°C).	+	+	+	+	–
• Examples antibodies	Many antibodies to toxin, bacteria and viruses	Secretory antibody in mucous membrane	Antipolysaccharide antibody and cold agglutination	Mainly IgD on surface of beta lymphocytes in newborn	Antiallergic antiparasitic antibodies

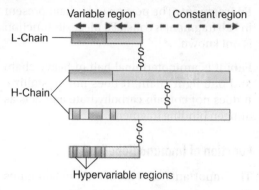

Fig. 13.5: IgG molecule.

1,50,000 and sedimentation constant is 7S. It is distributed equally between intravascular and extravascular compartments. It has half-life of 23 days. It appears to be spindle shaped 250 to 300 Å long 40 Å wide. The normal serum concentration of IgG is 5 to 16 mg/mL. It passes through placenta and provide natural passive immunity to newborn. It produces passive cutaneous anaphylaxis and participates in immunological reactions like precipitation, complement fixation, neutralization of toxin and viruses.

Four classes of IgG have been recognized, i.e., IgG1 IgG2, IgG3, IgG4. Each is having distinct type of gamma chain identifiable with specific antisera. Their properties are enumerated in **Table 13.2**.

2. **IgA:** It is the fast moving alpha globulin. It constitutes 10% of total serum globulin. Normal serum level is 0.6 to 4.2 mg per mL. It has half-life of 6 to 8 days and molecular weight is 1,60,000 with sedimentation constant of 7S. It is found in high concentration in colostrum, tear, bile, saliva, intestinal and nasal secretions. Its amount is greatly increased in cases of multiple myeloma. It does not pass through placenta. IgA does not fix complement but activates alternate complement pathway. It promotes phagocytosis and intracellular killing of organisms.

IgA exists in serum as monomer H_2L_2. Two subclasses of IgA are known, i.e., IgA_1 and IgA_2. IgA_2 in dominant form (60%) in the secretion and form only small component

Table 13.2: Properties of subclasses of immunoglobulin G.

Properties	IgG1	IgG2	IgG3	IgG4
• Fixation of complement	+	+	+	+
• Binding of macrophages	+	+	+	+
• Binding the heterogenous tissue	+	–	+	+
• Blocking of IgE binding	–	–	–	+
• Crossing of placenta	+	+	–	+
• Percentage of total IgG in normal serum	65	23	8	4
• Electrophoretic mobility	Slow	Slow	Slow	Fast
• Spontaneous aggregation	–	–	+++	–
• Combination with Staphylococcal A protein	+++	+++	–	+++
• Sedimentation of coefficient	7	7	7	7
• Molecular weight	150	150	150	150
• Heavy chains	γ1	γ2	γ3	γ4
• K/l ratio	2.4	1.1	1.4	8.0
• Half-life (days)	23	23	8	23
• Heavy chain allotype	6 gm	6 gm	6 gm	6 gm

of serum IgA. IgA$_2$ lacks interchain disulfide bonds between H and L chains.

IgA found in secretions contain additional structure unit called transport (T) or secretory (S) piece. T piece is synthesized in epithelial cells of gland, intestines and respiratory tract. It is attached to IgA molecule during transport across the cells. T piece links together two IgA molecule at Fc portion. J chain is also found in IgA. J chain is synthesized by lymphoid cell.

3. **IgM:** It is also called macroglobulin (**Fig. 13.6**). It constitutes 5 to 10% serum globulin (0.5 to 2 mg/mL). It has half-life of 5 days. It has molecular weight of 9,00,000 to 10,00,000 with sedimentation constant of 19S. Mostly it is intravascular. Polymeric form with J chains (one J chain per 10 L chains of IgM molecule) are frequently found and help in polymerization and stabilization of IgM molecule. It appears to be of spherical shape. IgM appears in the surface (membrane) of unstimulated β-lymphocytes and acts as recognition receptors for antigens. Two subclasses of IgM are identified, i.e., IgM-1 and IgM-2. IgM appears earlier in primary response and IgG is produced later. Its half-life is 5 days and it fixes complement. It does not pass through placenta. It is more efficient in agglutination, cytolytic and cytotoxic reaction. IgM deficiency is often associated with septicemia.

It was first detected by Rose and Fahey in 1965.

4. **IgD:** It is present in concentration of 0.03 mg per mL. It is mostly intravascular. It has half-life of 3 days. It is present on the surface of unstimulated B

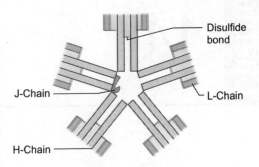

Fig. 13.6: IgM molecule.

lymphocytes blood. It acts as recognition receptors for antigens cell membrane bound IgD combination with matching antigen causes specific stimulation of these B lymphocytes. It results in either activation and cloning to form antibody or suppression. IgD has two subclass IgD$_1$ and IgD$_2$. Very little is known about its function. It seems likely that IgD may function as mutually interacting antigen receptor for the control of lymphocyte activation and suppression.

5. **IgE:** It is reaginic antibody responsible for immediate hypersensitive reactions. It has molecular weight of 1,90,000 with sedimentation coefficient of 8S. Its half-life is 2 days. It is inactivated by heat at 56°C for 1 hour. It has affinity for surface of tissue cells (particularly mast cells) of the same species. It mediates Prausnitz-Küstner reaction. It does not pass through placenta or fix complement. It is mostly intravascular in distribution. Normally it is found in traces in serum. Elevated levels are seen in atopic condition like asthma, hay fever and eczema. Children having parasitic infection in intestine show elevated levels of IgE.

Antigen and Antibody Reactions

Antigen-antibody reactions are useful in laboratory diagnosis of various diseases and in the identification of infectious agents in epidemiological survey. Antigen-antibody reactions *in vitro* are called serological reactions, e.g., precipitation, agglutination, complement fixation reactions **(Table 14.1)**.

Features of Antigens-Antibody Reactions

1. The reaction is highly specific.
2. Entire molecules react and not fragment.
3. There is no denaturation of antigen or antibody during reactions.
4. Combination occurs at surface and hence surface antigens are immunologically relevant.
5. The combination is firm but reversible. It is influenced by affinity or avidity. *Affinity* is intensity of attraction between antigen and antibody molecules. *Avidity* is strength of the bond after the formation of antigen antibody complex.
6. Both antigen and antibody participate in the formation of the agglutinates or precipitates.

Table 14.1: Comparative efficiency of immunoglobulins classes in different serological reactions.

Reactions	IgG	IgM	IgA
Precipitation	Strong	Weak	Variable
Agglutination	Weak	Strong	Moderate
Complement fixation	Weak	Strong	Negative
Lysis	Weak	Strong	Negative

7. Antigen and antibody may combine in varying proportions.

PRECIPITATION

When a soluble antigen combines with its antibody in presence of electrolytes (NaCl) at a suitable temperature and pH the antigen antibody complex forms insoluble precipitate.

Uses of Precipitation Reaction

1. Identification of bacteria, e.g., detection of group specific polysaccharides substance in streptococci in Lancefield grouping, etc.
2. Identification of antigenic component of bacteria in infected animal tissue, e.g., *Bacillus anthracis* (Ascoli test).
3. Standardization of toxin and antitoxins.
4. Demonstration of antibody in serum, e.g., Kahn's test for the diagnosis of syphilis.
5. Medicolegal serology for detection of blood, semen, etc.

Mechanism of precipitation: Lattice hypothesis explains it.

LATTICE HYPOTHESIS (FIG. 14.1)

Multivalent antigens combine with bivalent antibody in varying proportions, depending on antigen-antibody ratio in reacting mixture. Precipitation results when large lattice is formed consisting of alternating antigen and antibody molecules. This is possible only in the zone of equivalence. In zone of antigen and antibody excess lattice does not enlarge as valency of antigen and antibody is fully satisfied.

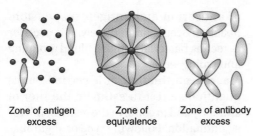

Zone of antigen excess   Zone of equivalence   Zone of antibody excess

Fig. 14.1: Lattice formation.

Techniques of Precipitation Reaction

1. **Ring test**: The test is very simple for detection of antigen. The antigen is layered over serum in a narrow tube. The reaction is visible as a white zone at the junction of two clear fluid. Examples are C-reactive protein test, Ascoli test, grouping of streptococci by Lancefield technique.
2. **Slide test**: When a drop of antigen and antiserum is placed on a slide and mixed by shaking, floccules appear, e.g., VDRL test for syphilis.
3. **Tube test**: The Kahn test for syphilis is an example of tube flocculation test.
4. **Gel diffusion**: The main advantages of this method are:
   a. The precipitate is relatively fixed by agar medium and is easily visible.
   b. If antigen or antiserum contains more than one factor then each factor produces separate precipitin line.
   c. Antigen and antibodies can be compared for common antigenic determinants.

Examples of Gel Diffusion (Fig. 14.2)

1. **Single diffusion in one dimension**: The antibody is incorporated in agar gel in a test tube and antigen solution is layered over it. The antigen diffuses downwards through the agar gel forming line of precipitation that appears to move downwards. Number of bands indicate number of different antigens present.
2. **Double diffusion in one dimension**: The antibody is incorporated in gel. Above it is placed a column of agar. Antigen is layered

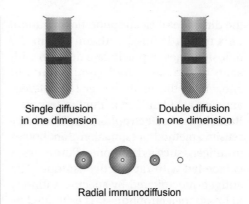

Single diffusion in one dimension   Double diffusion in one dimension

Radial immunodiffusion

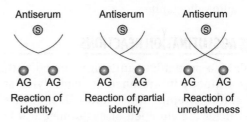

Reaction of identity   Reaction of partial identity   Reaction of unrelatedness

Fig. 14.2: Types of gel diffusion precipitations. (AG: Antigen)

over agar. The antigen and antibody move towards each other through intervening agar and form a band of precipitate where they meet at optimum proportion.

3. **Single diffusion in two dimension (radial immunodiffusion)**: Antiserum is incorporated in agar gel poured on slide. The antigen is added to well cut on the surface of gel. Ring shaped bands of precipitate are formed around wells. The diameter of ring gives an estimate of concentration of antigen.
4. **Double diffusion in two dimension**: Agar gel is poured on slide and wells are cut using template. Antiserum is placed on central well and different antigen in the surrounding wells. If two adjacent antigen are identical the line of precipitate will be formed by them. This method is a routine technique in the diagnosis of smallpox, Elek's test for the diagnosis of diphtheria, etc.
5. **Immunoelectrophoresis**: This is done in 2 steps. The first step is done in agar electrophoresis of the antigen. Rectangular trough is cut in agar on either side, parallel to

the direction of electrophoretic migration. This trough is filled with antiserum. By diffusion lines of precipitate develop with each of the separated components of antigen. By this method over 100 different antigens are identified in human serum.

6. **Radioimmunoelectrophoresis:** This is very sensitive method for estimation of antibodies to antigens such as hormones. Pure antigen is labelled with radioactive isotope. The antigen precipitated by specific antibody in immunoelectrophoresis is estimated by autoradiograph.

AGGLUTINATION REACTIONS

When a particulate antigen is mixed with its antibody in presence of electrolytes at a suitable temperature and pH, then the particles are clumped or agglutinated. It is more sensitive than precipitation for the detection of antibodies.

Uses

1. Identification of bacteria, e.g., serotyping of *Salmonella* and *Shigella* with known antisera.
2. Serological diagnosis of infection, e.g., Widal test for typhoid, etc.
3. Hemagglutination test, e.g., Rose-Waaler, Paul-Bunnell.

TECHNIQUE OF AGGLUTINATION TEST

Direct Agglutination Test

1. **Microagglutination (Fig. 14.3):** It is carried on a clean slide by mixing a drop each

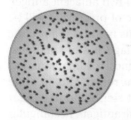 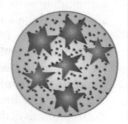

Fig. 14.3: Microagglutination test.

of antiserum and antigen suspension. Reaction occurs immediately. It is used for detecting bacterial antigen, blood grouping and typing, etc.

2. **Macroagglutination:** It is carried out as quantitative test to estimate the titer of antibody and to confirm the result of micro-agglutination. Following type of agglutination are observed with bacterial antigen:

a. Flagellar antigen or 'H' type of agglutination is seen when a formalized suspension of motile bacteria is treated with antiserum. It forms floccular, snowy flakes like deposit. Agglutination appears 2 to 4 hours after incubation at 52°C.

b. Somatic 'O' type of agglutination occurs when heat killed or alcohol treated suspension of bacteria is treated with homologous antiserum. The agglutination is compact with fine granulation. The reaction appears 18 to 24 hours after incubation at 37°C.

c. Vi agglutination is similar to O agglutination and occurs slowly at 37°C.

Coagglutination: Here the Fc fragment of any antibody gets attached to protein A of staphylococci (Cowan strain). Thus, staphylococci with a known attached antibody are agglutinated when mixed with the specific antigen **(Fig. 14.4)**.

Indirect or Passive Agglutination Test

Recently inert particles, e.g., latex, bentonite or red blood cells have been used as carrier of antigen. It is more sensitive test. Latex particles are used for the demonstration of rheumatoid factor, CRP, etc. A special type of passive hemagglutination test is the Rose-Waaler test. In rheumatoid arthritis patient's autoantibody (RA factor) appears in serum which acts as antibody to gammaglobulin. The RA factor is able to agglutinate red cell coated with globulins. The antigen used for test is a suspension of sheep erythrocytes sensitized with subagglutinating dose of rabbit anti-sheep erythrocytes (amboceptor).

Coombs' test (Fig. 14.5): It is used for the detection of incomplete antibodies (nonagglutinating anti-Rh antibody), *Brucella, Shigella* and *Salmonella* antigen. Coombs' test may be direct or indirect **(Table 14.2)**.

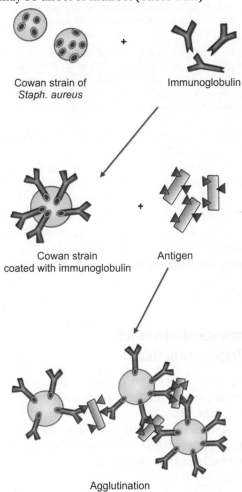

Cowan strain of
Staph. aureus

Immunoglobulin

+

Cowan strain
coated with immunoglobulin

Antigen

+

Agglutination

Fig. 14.4: Agglutination and coagglutination.

Sera containing incomplete anti-Rh antibodies is mixed with Rh positive red cells. Antibody globulin coats the surface of erythrocytes. Such erythrocytes coated with antibody globulin are washed free of all unattached proteins and treated with rabbit anti-serum against human gammaglobulin (Coombs' serum). The cells are agglutinated. This is the principle of Coombs' test.

Complement fixation test (CFT): This is a very sensitive test and is capable of detecting 0.04 mg of antibody nitrogen and 0.1 mg of antigen. It is used for serological diagnosis of diseases:

1. Bacterial diseases, e.g., gonorrhea, brucellosis.
2. Spirochetal disease, e.g., syphilis (Wassermann reaction), etc.
3. Rickettsial diseases, e.g., typhus fever.
4. Viral diseases like lymphogranuloma venereum.
5. Parasitic diseases, e.g., kala-azar, hydatid cyst, amoebiasis.

Principle: The ability of antigen antibody complex to fix complement.

Technique: Heat the patient's serum at 56°C for 30 minutes to destroy its own complement. Patient serum, complement (guineapig serum) and antigen are incubated at 37°C for 1 hour. Now sensitized sheep RBC are added as indicator system. The whole mixture is incubated at 37°C for 1 hour.

Interpretation: If complement has been used up, there would not be hemolysis. It means antigen antibody reaction has taken place. Test is reported as positive.

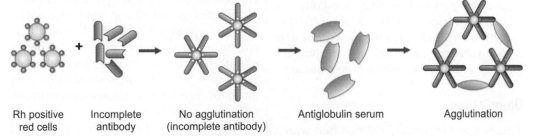

Rh positive
red cells

Incomplete
antibody

No agglutination
(incomplete antibody)

Antiglobulin serum

Agglutination

Fig. 14.5: Steps of Coombs' test.

Table 14.2: Differences between direct and indirect Coombs' test.

Direct	Indirect
• Detects the presence of incomplete antibodies adsorbed onto erythrocyte	• Detects incomplete antibody present in serum
• Indicated in autoimmune hemolytic anemia, erythroblastosis fetalis	• Indicated for detection of anti-Rh antibody in serum of Rh negative women of Rh positive husband
• Test is done by washing RBC in saline (3 times). Washed RBC are mixed with AHG in presence of bovine albumin. In positive test clumping of RBC occurs	• Serum of patient is mixed with saline washed Rh positive red cells (group O) and incubated at 37°C for 30 minutes. Wash red cell in saline and mix with Coombs' serum. • Agglutination occurs in positive cases

If sensitized RBC are lysed it means complement has not been fixed and test is reported as negative.

Neutralization Test

Specific antibodies are able to neutralize the biological effects of viruses, toxins and enzymes.

a. **Virus neutralization:** Viruses when mixed with immune serum lose their capacity to infect fresh host, e.g., vaccinia, influenza and poliomyelitis. Neutralization may be quantified on:
   i. Chorioallantoic membrane of chick embryo (pocks formation).
   ii. By enumeration of plaques on monolayer tissue culture.

b. **Toxin neutralization:** The toxicity of endotoxin is not neutralized by antiserum. On the other hand bacterial exotoxins are good antigens. They induce the formation of antibodies, i.e., antitoxin. These antibodies protect from diseases like diphtheria and tetanus. Schick test is based on the ability of circulating antitoxin to neutralize diphtheria toxin. Anti-streptolysin "O" test (ASO) in which antitoxin present in patient sera neutralize the hemolytic activity. Nagler's reaction is another example of neutralization.

Opsonization

This is another serological reaction which sensitizes bacteria for phagocytosis. The substances in serum which promote phagocytosis are called opsonins.

The opsonic index is defined as ratio of phagocytic activity of patient's blood having bacterium, to the phagocytic activity of blood from normal individual. It is measured by incubating fresh citrated blood with bacterial suspensions at 37°C for 15 minutes. Now estimate the average number of phagocytozed bacteria per leukocyte from stained blood.

Immune Adherence Test (Treponema pallidum)

When a suspension of living spirochete is treated with specific antibody and complement, the spirochetes becomes sticky. The test is used in the identification of spirochaetes. Adherence reaction is also shown by protozoa, microfilaria and bacteria.

Immunofluorescence

Fluorescence is the property of absorbing light rays of one wavelength and emitting rays with different wavelengths. Serological reactions employing tagged antisera are used to detect minute amounts of weakly active antigen or antibodies. The method is suitable for only qualitative reactions. The fluorescent antibody technique is used for:

1. Rapid serological diagnosis of number of bacteria.

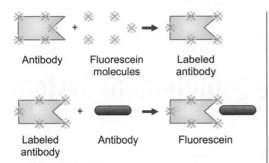

Fig. 14.6: Direct immunofluorescent technique.

2. Detection of antitoxoplasma antibody.
3. Demonstration of leptospira in human and animal muscles.
4. Detection of viruses in cells.

The various modifications of fluorescent antibody methods are as under:

a. *Direct method* **(Fig. 14.6):** It is commonly used for the detection of antigen by using of a single layer of fluorescent labelled antibody.

b. *Indirect method* (double layer technique): It is used by treating a slide smear of the antigen with specific unlabelled serum. The preparation is thoroughly washed and is treated with fluorescence labelled gamma-globulin against the human serum.

c. Sandwich technique is used for detection of antibody in tissue. Tissue section is treated with dilute solution of antigen. After washing (remove excess of antigen) section is exposed to fluorescein labelled antibodies.

Immunoelectron Microscopic Test

Immunoelectron microscopy: This is useful in the study of some viruses, e.g., Hepatitis B virus and viruses causing diarrhea. Viral particles are mixed with specific antisera are seen under electron microscope. Clumped virus particles are seen and studied.

Immunoferritin test: Ferritin is conjugated with antibody and such labelled antibody reacting with antigen can be visualized under electron microscope. Ferritin is electron dense substance obtained from horse spleen.

Immunoenzyme system: Some stable enzyme like peroxidase can be conjugated with antibody. Tissue section carrying corresponding antigen is treated with peroxidase labelled antisera. The peroxidase bound to the antigen can be visualized under the electron microscope by microhistochemical method. Some other enzymes such as glucose oxidase, phosphatase and tyrosinase may also be used in immunoenzyme test.

The Complement System

The bacteriocidal property of serum as well as of whole blood, has been recognized since 1888. These antibacterial substances were found to be inactivated by heating to 56°C for 30 minutes and function as bactericides only in the presence of specific antibody. Ehrlich discovered that antibody was also required for other activities, such as lysis of red blood cells (hemolysis) by this thermolabile (heat sensitive) component of serum which he named complement. Complement is well-known for its ability to react with a wide variety of antigen antibody combination to produce important physiological results. Included in this group of reaction are:

1. The destruction of erythrocytes as well as other tissue cells.
2. The initiation of inflammatory changes.
3. The lysis of bacterial cells.
4. Enhancement of phagocytosis involving some opsonized particles.

The complement refers to a series of factors occurring in normal serum that are activated characteristically by antigen-antibody interaction, and subsequently mediate a number of biologically significant consequences. Some genes controlling the production of complement components are located on human chromosome 6 in proximity to human leukocyte antigen (HLA) locus. Some components have enzymatic activity; others are enhancers or inhibitors. Complement is heat labile. The activity of complement is lost in 30 minutes at 37°C and in a few days at 4°C. This activity is also lost by bacterial contamination. It can be preserved at –25°C, lyophilization or after addition of high concentration of sodium chloride.

The concentration of complement in the serum is fairly constant for each species of animal. It constitutes 10 percent of human serum globulin. Its concentration is not increased by active immunization but is increased in abnormal conditions like carcinomatosis, coronary occlusion and rheumatic fever. Its concentration is decreased in acute glomerulo-nephritis, nephrosis, serum sickness, malaria, etc. Guineapigs possess higher levels of complements than any other laboratory animals. Therefore, guinea pigs serve as main source of complement in complement fixation test.

Components of Complement

At present, complement is known to have nine distinct components, one of which has three protein subunits making a total of 11 proteins.

C'_1: Heat labile (destroyed at 56°C for ½ hour) found in euglobulin fraction of serum.

C'_2: Heat labile, found in alpha and gamma-globulin fractions.

C'_3: Heat stable, inactivated by zymosan. It is found in euglobulin fraction of serum.

C'_4: Heat stable, inactivated by ammonia or hydrazine.

C_1 of human complement has the properties of proenzyme known as proesterase. C_1 component is composed of three fractions called C'_1q, C'_1r, C'_1s (held together by calcium ions). C'_1r is responsible for esterase activity, C'_1q attaches the whole C_1 component to antibody molecule.

The remaining components $C_{5,6,7,8,9}$ participate in cell lysis.

Genetics of Complement System

C-2, C-4 and factor B are present on chromosome-6. Some control proteins are coded for by a cluster of genes on chromosome-1, called RCA (regulation of complement activation) locus.

Regulation of Complement Activation

The lysis or damage of normal cells by excessive activity of complement is prevented by complementary regulatory proteins: plasma proteins and regulatory protein in cell membrane.

Biological Functions of Complement (Table 15.1)

1. Immune adherence and opsonization.
2. Chemotaxis, e.g., C_5a and $C_{5,6,7}$.
3. Anaphylatoxin, e.g., C_3a, C_4a, and C_5a.
4. Cytolysis, e.g., $C_{5,6,7,8,9}$.
5. Hypersensitive reaction of type II (blood transfusion) and type III (Arthus reaction and serum sickness).
6. Endotoxic shock, e.g., C_3 activation cause tissue damage by disseminated intravascular reaction. In endotoxic shock with Gram-negative septicemia of damage

Table 15.1: Biological activities of complement.

Complement	Activity
C_2b	Increased vasodilatation
C_4b	Anaphylotoxin histamine release
C_3a	Anaphylotoxin
C_5a	Anaphylotoxin chemotactic factor
C_4b	Immune-adherence opsonization
C_3b	Immune-adherence opsonization
$C_{5,6,7}$	Weak chemotactic factor
$C_5b—C_9$	Membrane disruption
C_4b, C_2	Virus neutralization

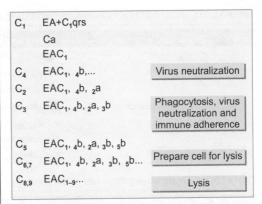

Fig. 15.1: The classical pathway of complement.

hemorrhagic fever, endotoxins become coated with C-3b and stick to platelets by immune adherence. $C_{5,6,7}$ generated in cascade reaction causes lysis of platelets with release of clotting factors.

Activities of Complement

The chain of events in which complement (C′) components react in specific sequence following activation of antigen antibody complexes and culminating in immune cytolysis is known as *classical C pathway* **(Fig. 15.1)**. The components of complement are fixed to sensitized cells in the order, $C_{1,4,2,3,5,6,7,8,9}$. Immune cytolysis is initiated by binding of C_1 to EA (erythrocyte antibody). C_1 occurs in serum as calcium chelation. With ethylenediaminetetra acetate acid (EDTA), it yields three component units C_1q, C_1r and C_1s. C_1q reacts with Fc piece of appropriate immunoglobulin (IgG, IgM) bound with antigen. This activates C_1r and C_1s and activated C_1 acquires enzymatic activity.

C_1 esterases act on C_4 and C_2. C_4 is splitted into C_4a and C_4b and C_2 into C_2a and C_2b. The $C_{4,2}$ splits C_3 into fragment C_3a and C_3b. At this stage, reaction is expressed as $EAC_1, {}_4b, {}_2a, {}_3b$, where E is erythrocyte, A is antihemolysin. $C_{1,4,2,3}$ acts on C_5 spitting it into C_5a and C_5b. C_6 and C_7 are then added. They are joined by C_8 and C_9 ($EAC_1, {}_4b, {}_2a, {}_3b, {}_5b, {}_{6,7,8,9}$) causing lysis of cell. The mechanism of lysis is by production of hole of 100 Å in diameter in cell membrane.

Table 15.2: Clinical conditions associated with deficiencies of complement components.

S. No	Deficiency	Clinical condition associated
1.	C_1 inhibitor	Hereditary angioneurotic edema
2.	C_1, C_2, C_4	• Systemic lupus erythematosus • Some collagen vascular diseases
3.	C_3, C_3b inactivator	Severe recurrent pyogenic infections
4.	C_5, C_6, C_7, C_8	• Bacteremia (mainly due to Gram-negative diplococci) • Toxoplasmosis
5.	Properdin	Severe meningococcal disease

Table 15.3: Comparative properties of alternative and classic pathways of complement activation.

Criteria	Alternative pathway	Classic pathway
1. Activating agents inulin, zymosan	Aggregated proteins LPS	IgM, IgG_1, IgG_2, IgG_3
2. Activation site	Unknown	Fc segment of Ig
3. Participation of C_1q, C_4b and C_2a	No	Essential
4. Participation of C_3 and C_5 through C_9	Yes	Yes
5. Divalent cation requirement	Mg^{++}	Ca^{++}, Mg^{++}
6. Non-immunologic initiation	Yes	No
7. Amplification mechanism	Yes	Yes

This disrupts osmotic integrity of membrane causing release of the contents of cell **(Table 15.2)**.

Deficiency of complement components may be associated with diseases **(Table 15.3)**.

Alternate Pathways of Complement

Activation of C_3 is without prior participation of $C_{1,4,2}$ is called alternate pathway and can be brought out by the following methods **(Fig. 15.2)**:

a. Zymosan with properdin (a glycine-rich beta-glycoprotein) forms complex in presence of Mg^{++} which activates C_3.
b. Cobra venom with cofactor (glycine-rich beta-glycoprotein) present in serum acts directly on C_3.
c. IgA and IgE are capable of activating alternate pathway.

The properdin system can enhance resistance to Gram-negative infections; it is involved in the lysis of erythrocytes from patients with paroxysmal nocturnal hematuria. The properdine system can also participate in the mediation of immunologic injury (e.g.,

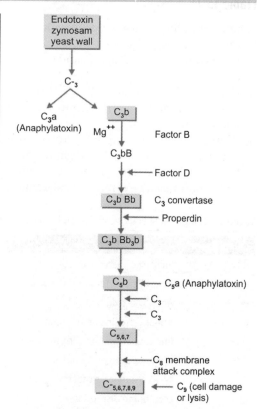

Fig. 15.2: Alternate complement pathway.

nephritis) and may be defective in sickle cell anemia.

Low serum complement levels: Low serum complements levels particularly C_3 are found in antigen-antibody complex diseases, e.g., lupus erythematosus, acute glomerulonephritis and in cryoglobulinemia.

By the way, alternative complement pathway differs from classical complement pathway as shown in **Table 15.3**.

Biosynthesis of Complement

❖ C_1 is synthesized in intestinal epithelium.
❖ $C_{2,4}$ is synthesized in macrophages.
❖ $C_{5,8}$ is synthesized in spleen.
❖ $C_{3,6,9}$ is synthesized in liver.
❖ The site of synthesis of C_7 is not known.

❖ Factor B macrophages, lymphocytes and hepatocytes.

Complement-dependent Serological Tests

1. Immune adherence test, i.e., some bacteria react with specific antibody in the presence of complement, particulate material, e.g., erythrocytes, platelets, and bacteria are aggregated and adhere to the cells, e.g., *Vibrio cholerae, Treponema pallidum.*
2. Complement fixation test.
3. Conglutinating complement absorption.
4. Immobilization test, e.g., *Treponema pallidum.*
5. Cytolytic or cytocidal test, e.g., *Vibrio cholerae.*
6. Opsonization.

Hypersensitivity

HISTORY

Immune response was thought to be protective. It may be activated by milk protein. Later on, Portier and Richet (1902) showed that immune responses possess harmful effects by administering sea anemones to dogs. The first dose did not produce any harmful effect but the second dose made the dog ill and died in a few minutes. Theobald Smith in 1904 observed same response in guinea pig using non-toxic antigen. With horse antisera and rabbit antisera used in human diseases, harmful effects of immune response became obvious. Von Pirquet (1906) suggested the term allergy which is an altered response of tissue to repeated contacts with antigenic agents. Allergy was thought to include:

a. Hypersensitivity (increased susceptibility).
b. Immunity (increased resistance).

HYPERSENSITIVITY

Hypersensitivity is defined as altered state induced by an antigen in which pathological reaction can be subsequently elicited by that antigen or by structurally similar substance.

In hypersensitivity, focus of attention is what happens to host as a result of immune reaction. In immunity, focus of attention is antigen (killing, neutralization of toxin).

Mechanism

The reactions that appear within minutes are mediated by freely diffusible antibody molecules (immediate type).

The other type is slow-evolving responses that are mediated by sensitized "T" lymphocytes. This is cell-mediated hypersensitivity (CMI, i.e., delayed type).

Classification

A. On the basis of time required for sensitized host to develop clinical reaction upon reexposure to the antigen, Chase classified them as:

   i. Immediate reaction.
   ii. Delayed reaction.

   The differences between immediate and delayed reactions are listed in **Table 16.1**.

B. *Coombs' and Gell classification (1969):* They have classified hypersensitivity reaction into five types on the basis of different mechanisms of pathogenesis **(Table 16.2)**. It is widely used:

   ■ **Type I:** Anaphylactic, reagin dependent, e.g., anaphylaxis, atopy, etc. IgG, IgE and histamine participate in this type of reaction.

   ■ **Type II:** Cytotoxic, e.g., thrombocytopenia, hemolytic anemia, IgG, IgM and complement take part in this reaction.

   ■ **Type III:** Immune complex or toxic complex, e.g., Arthus reaction, serum sickness, etc. In this reaction, IgG, IgM and complement take part.

   ■ **Type IV:** It is delayed type of hypersensitivity in which T cells, lymphokines and macro-phages take part, e.g., tuberculin type and contact dermatitis. The antigen activates specifically sensitized CD4 and

Table 16.1: Differences between immediate hypersensitivity reaction and delayed hypersensitivity reaction.

Immediate reaction	Delayed reaction
• Appears and recedes rapidly	• Appears slowly and lasts longer
• Induced by antigen or hapten by any route	• Induced by infection, injection of antigen with Freund's adjuvant or by skin contact
• Circulating antibodies present and responsible for reaction (antibody-mediated reaction)	• Cell-mediated reaction and not antibody mediated
• Passive transfer possible with serum	• Transfer possible by lymphocytes or transfer factor
• Desensitization easy but short lived	• It is difficult but long lasting
• Lesions are acute exudation and fat necrosis	• Mononuclear cell collection around blood vessels
• Wheal and flare with maximum diameter in 6 hours	• Erythema and induration with maximum diameter in 24 to 48 hours

Table 16.2: Hypersensitivity reactions.

Characters	I	II	III	IV	V
Reacting factor	Ab	Ab	Ab	Lymphocytes	Ab
Ig class and complement	Ig, E, G, C	Ig, G, M, C	Ig G, M, C	—	IgG
Cell	Mast cells		Leukocyte	T cells	T cells
Cutaneous response to Ag:					
i. Peak reaction	15 to 30 months		3 to 4 hours	24 to 48 hours	—
ii. Macroscopic	• Wheal and flare		• Erythema and edema	• Erythema and induration	—
iii. Microscopic	• Mast cells • Eosinophil • Edema		• Inflammation • Polymorph	• Lymphocytes • Macrophages Polymorph	— —
Transfer factor	Ab	Ab	Ab	T cell	Ab and T cell
Examples	• Anaphylaxis • Hay fever	• Thrombocyto-penia • Agranulocytosis	• Arthus reaction • Serum sickness	• Tuberculosis • Graft rejection	• Orchitis (guinea pig)
	Asthma	• Hemolytic anemia • Blood reaction	Farmer's lung Glomerular nephritis		• Thyro-toxicosis
Detection	PK reaction	—	—	• Lymphocytic transformation • MIF	

CD8. T cells resulting in secretion of lymphokines.

■ **Type V:** It is antibody-dependent cell-mediated and cytotoxic type of reaction, e.g., autoimmune orchitis in guinea pigs.

C. *Sell's classification (1972):* This classification is on the basis of pathogenesis (**Flowchart 16.1**).

We shall follow Coomb's and Gell (1969) classification for further discussion:

Flowchart 16.1: Sell's classification of hypersensitivity.

TYPE I REACTIONS

In type I reactions, antibodies are fixed on the surface of tissue cells (mast cells and basophils) in sensitized individual. Antigen combines with cell-fixed antibodies leading to release of pharmacological substance which produce the following clinical reactions:

Anaphylaxis

Anaphylaxis is a classical immediate hypersensitivity reaction. It is a shock-like condition resulting from the action of histamine-like substances released as a result of antigen-antibody union on a cell.

Antigen as well as hapten can induce anaphylaxis. There should be an interval, of at least 2 to 3 weeks between sensitizing dose and shocking dose. Once sensitized, the person remains so for a long time. The shocking antigen should be identical or immunologically closely related to sensitizing antigen. The organs involved in anaphylactic reaction are known as shock organs.

There exists a considerable species variation in susceptibility to anaphylaxis. In guinea pigs a small dose of egg albumin is injected intraperitoneally. After the interval of 2 to 3 weeks, a little larger dose of same antigen intravenously will bring out manifestation of anaphylaxis, i.e., guinea pigs become irritable, sneeze, cough, develop convulsion and die. At autopsy, lungs show congestion. Here the shock organ is lungs. Death may be due to constriction of smooth muscle of bronchioles.

In rabbits, death in anaphylactic shock is due to constriction of pulmonary arteries. Thus causing dilation of right side of heart. In man, fatal anaphylaxis is rare. There is itching of scalp and tongue, flushing of skin of body and difficulty in breathing due to bronchial spasm. It is followed by hypotension, loss of consciousness and death. Human anaphylaxis is associated with serum therapy, antibiotic injection and insect stings.

Cutaneous Anaphylaxis

Cutaneous anaphylaxis is a local anaphylactic reaction. It can be elicited by scratch or intradermal injection of antigen into the skin in man or guinea pig. At the site of injection of antigen, there will be erythema, itching, wheal, pseudopods and spreading flare. The reaction becomes maximum in 10 to 30 minutes and fades away in a few hours. Cutaneous anaphylaxis (skin test) is useful for testing hypersensitivity and in identifying the allergen responsible for atopic diseases.

Passive Cutaneous Anaphylaxis

Passive cutaneous anaphylaxis (PCT) can be produced by injecting antibody into local area of skin and antigen intravenously. The capillary dilatation takes place rapidly and can be made visible by incorporating Evans blue dye in the serum. The reaction (PCA) is one of the convenient methods for detecting small amounts of human IgG and IgE antibody.

Schütz-Dale Phenomenon

Isolated tissue, e.g., intestinal or uterine muscle strips from sensitized guinea pigs are kept in Ringer's solution in a bath. On addition of specific antigen to the bath, it will contract vigorously. This is called Schütz-Dale phenomenon. It is a specific reaction.

Mechanism of Anaphylaxis

The mast cells and circulating basophils are the key cells in the allergic response. Bridging of cell-bound IgE molecules, anaphylotoxins, and non-specific stimuli all precipitate in the release of mediators from some population of these cells. In case of IgE bridging, a protease in the cell membrane is activated and cyclic AMP produced. Membrane phospholipids become methylated, forming phosphatidylcholine, leading to opening of the calcium channel and further conversion to arachidonic acid which is converted to

prostaglandin by the lipoxygenase pathway. Mast cell granules that contain preformed histamine, eosinophilic chemotactic factors, neutrophil chemotactic factor, bradykinin and serotonin are broken down and move to periphery of the cell, and the granule and cell membranes fuse, causing a pore to form through which the granule contents are extruded.

In addition to the factors described, there are lymphocyte chemotactic factors, prostaglandin generating factor, inflammatory factors of anaphylaxis, and the basophil kallikrein, prekallikrein activator and Hageman factor activator involved. However, current research focuses on platelet-activating factor as a possible key mediator in anaphylactic and septic shock, and asthma.

By injection of serum, anaphylactic hypersensitivity can be transferred from sensitive person to normal person. IgG and IgE are responsible for anaphylaxis. In man, IgE is responsible entirely.

The mediators of anaphylactic response are pharmacological active substances. They are released by degranulation of mast cell (in tissue) and basophil (in circulation). Their release is by two mechanisms:
a. Shocking dose of antigen combines with circulating IgG antibody.
b. Shocking dose of antigen combines with IgE fixed to mast cell. Alternatively, antigen combines with circulating IgE forming soluble antigen-antibody complex. This gets fixed to mast cell by Fc fragment of IgE. Desensitization can be done either by repeated small injection of antigens or by a single non-fatal shocking dose.

Pharmacological Mediators of Anaphylaxis (Table 16.3)

Histamine: It is the most active amine. When released into skin, it stimulates sensory nerves producing burning and itching sensation. It causes vasodilatation and hyperemia by axon reflex and edema by increasing capillary

Table 16.3: Mediators of anaphylaxis.

Mediator	Source	Function
Histamine	Preformed in mast cell/basophil	—Elevates cycle AMP levels
		—Feedback regulation
		—Increases vascular permeability
	—Smooth muscle contraction	
		—Generates prostaglandins
		—Pulmonary vasoconstriction
		—Increases gastric secretion
		—Stimulates suppressor lymphocytes
		—Cardiac effect
Heparin	-do-	Anticoagulant
Tryptase	-do-	Activates C_3
B-glucosaminidase	-do-	Splits of glucosamine
NCF	-do-	Neutrophil chemotaxis
Serotonin	Preformed in mast cell	Increases vascular permeability
Eosinophilic chemotactic factor	Preformed in mast cells	—Attract and deactivate eosinophils
		—Increase eosinophilic complement receptors
Platelets-activating factor	Generated in mast cells	—Aggregate platelets
	—Macrophages	—Release amines and thromboxane
	—Neutrophils	—Increase vascular permeability
	—Eosinophils	—Bronchoconstriction
		—Myocardial depressions
		—Vasoconstriction
		—Sequesters platelets
Prostaglandins	Generated in mast cells	—Increase cAMP
		—Smooth muscle constriction
		—Increase vascular permeability
Thromboxane		Aggregation and vasodilation
Leukotrienes	Generated in mast cells	—Smooth muscle constriction
	—Macrophages	—Increase vascular permeability
	—Neutrophils	—Decrease peripheral blood flow
	—Eosinophils	—Generate prostaglandins
		—Cardiac depression
		—Coronary vasoconstriction
		—Decrease lymphocyte response
Neutrophil chemotactic factor	Preformed in mast cells	Attract and deactivate lymphocytes

permeability. It also stimulates smooth muscle contraction and secretions. Histamine is present in platelets, mast cells, basophil, etc.

Serotonin (5-hydroxy tryptamine): It is found in intestinal mucosa, brain tissue and platelets. It causes smooth muscle contraction, increased capillary permeability and vaso-constriction. It is important in anaphylaxis of rat and mice. Its role in man is not known.

Kinins: They cause smooth muscle contraction, increased vascular permeability, vasodilatation and pain. The best known kinin is bradykinin. Its role in human anaphylaxis is not established.

Many other pharmacological active substances are also released during anaphylaxis, e.g., heparin, acetyle choline, prostaglandin E and F and eosinophilic chemotactic factor of anaphylaxis (ECF-A).

Anaphylactoid reactions: It is non-specific reaction involving the activation of complement and release of anaphylotoxins. It has no immunological base. Intravenous injection of peptone, trypsine, etc. provokes clinical reaction resembling anaphylactic shock. This is anaphylactoid reaction.

ATOPY: It is naturally occurring familial hypersensitivity of man manifested by hay fever and asthma. The substances which are more frequently responsible for these manifestations are pollen, feather, animal dander, dust, milk and wheat husk. It is difficult to induce atopy artificially.

Predisposition to atopy is genetically determined and so it runs in families. IgE is known to be an atopic reagin, it is characterized by the following properties:

1. IgE can be detected by sensitive technique like passive hemagglutination, etc.
2. Reagin is believed to be synthesized in man. It is now possible to induce atopic sensitivity to guinea pigs though with difficulty.
3. Reaginic antibody has an affinity for skin. This is the basis of Prausnitz-Kustner (PK) reaction. When serum collected from Kustner (having atopic hypersensitivity to certain species of cooked fish) was injected intracutaneously into Prausnitz followed 24 hours later by an intracutaneously injection of a small quantity of cooked fish antigen into the same site, within few minutes wheal and flare reaction occurred. Since IgE is homocytotropic, test has to be carried out in man only.
4. They are heat sensitive antibodies and are inactivated at 56°C in one hour. Heating destroys Fc fragment of IgE molecule.
5. It does not pass through placenta.

Atopic sensitivity is due to an over production of IgE. The symptoms are caused by release of pharmacological active substances following combination of antigen and cell-fixed reagin. Exposure of antigen to eyes, respiratory tract, intestine and skin may cause conjunctivitis, rhinitis, gastrointestinal symptoms and dermatitis. Sometimes, it may cause urticaria even after ingestion of allergen.

Demonstration of atopic antigens:
a. *In vivo:* PK reaction.
b. *In vitro:* Schültz-Dale test and degranulation of sensitized mast cells.

TYPE II REACTIONS

Cytotoxic and Cytolytic

This type of reaction is initiated by antibodies that react with either antigenic determinant of cell or tissue element. Cell damage occurs in the presence of complement or mononuclear cells.

In sedormid purpura, sedormid (allyl isopropyl acetyluria) is administered. It combines with platelets altering their surface antigenecity. Antibodies are formed against sedormid-coated platelet antigen. In subsequent administration of drug, antibodies cause complement-dependent lysis of platelet leading to thrombocytopenic purpura.

Cytolytic reactions are responsible for transfusion reaction, hemolytic diseases of newborn and autoimmune anemia.

TYPE III REACTIONS

Immune Complex Diseases

Here the damage is caused by antigen-antibody complex. This may precipitate on or around blood vessels causing damage to cells secondarily or on membrane interfering with their function. In antigen excess, soluble circulating complex may be formed with antibodies. These may be deposited on blood vessel walls or on basement membrane, causing local inflammation and massive complement ($C_{5,6,7}$) activation.

Arthus Reaction

When rabbits were injected subcutaneously with normal serum, initial injections were without any local effect; but with later injections, there occurred local reaction consisting of edema, induration and hemorrhagic necrosis. This is a local manifestation of generalized hypersensitivity and is called Arthus reaction. The tissue damage in this case is due to formation of antigen-antibody precipitations which are deposited in blood vessels. This leads to increased vascular permeability and infiltration of site with neutrophils. Leukocyte platelets thrombi reduce blood supply causing tissue necrosis. Leukocytes release lysosomal enzymes causing vasculitis of blood vessels wall. Arthus reaction can be passively transferred with sera containing IgG in high titer.

Serum Sickness

Serum sickness is a systemic form of type III hypersensitivity. It appears 7 to 12 days following single injection of high concentration of foreign serum like diphtheria antitoxin. Clinical manifestations are fever, lymphadenopathy, splenomegaly, arthritis, glomerulonephritis, endocarditis, vasculitis, urticarial rash, abdominal pain, nausea and vomiting. The pathogenesis is the formation of immune complex (foreign serum and antibodies to

it that reaches high titer by 7 to 12 days). It gets deposited on endothelial lining of blood vessels in various parts of body causing inflammatory infiltrations. The plasma concentration of complement falls due to massive activation and fixation by antigen-antibody complex. The disease is self-limited. When all foreign antigens are eliminated and free antibody appears, symptoms clear without any sequelae. It differs from other types of hypersensitivity reaction; in that single injection can serve both sensitizing and shocking dose.

Other immediate hypersensitivity diseases are:
1. Cot death.
2. Food hypersensitivity.
3. Atopic dermatitis.
4. Goodpasture disease.
5. Myasthenia gravis.

DELAYED HYPERSENSITIVITY (TYPE IV REACTION)

Delayed or cell-mediated hypersensitivity is one aspect of cell-mediated immunity. The antigen activates specifically macrophages and sensitized T lymphocytes leading to secretion of lymphokines. Locally, the reaction is manifested by infiltration with mononuclear cells.

Characters: These reactions have the following characters:
1. Antigenic stimulus is necessary.
2. In sensitive subjects, reaction occurs on exposure to specific antigen, e.g., tuberculin reaction.
3. Induction period is 7 to 10 days.
4. Delayed hypersensitivity is transferred by cells from lymphoid tissue, peritoneal exudate or blood lymphocytes.

Manifestations

1. **General toxemia:** A total of 0.1 mL tuberculin in tuberculous patient produces severe reaction which is manifested as malaise, cough, dyspnea, limb pain, vomiting, rigors and lymphopenia.

2. **Focal reaction:** If antigen in a large quantity is introduced in a fresh sensitized tissue, allergic reaction with necrosis of tissue occurs, e.g., tubercular bronchopneumonia.

3. **Local reactions:** It is a typical cutaneous response. If 0.1 ml of 1 : 1000 dilution of old tuberculin is injected intradermally, there will be slowly developing inflammatory response which will be maximum in 48 hours. It subsides in 7 days.

Types: Delayed hypersensitive reactions are of two types:

    a. Classical or tuberculin type.

    b. Granulomatous reactions.

CLASSICAL TYPE

Classical type plays a part in clinical conditions:

1. **Infective disease (bacterial, viral, fungal and parasitic):**

    a. Bacteria hypersensitivity, e.g., Koch's phenomena (tuberculosis), psittacosis, trachoma, lymphogranuloma venerum, leprosy, syphilis, brucellosis, etc.

    b. Viral hypersensitivity, e.g., mumps and revaccination with vaccinia virus.

    c. Fungal hypersensitivity, e.g., coccidioides, sporotrichosis, blastomycosis and aspergillosis.

    d. Parasitic hypersensitivity, e.g., hydatid cyst, filariasis, schistosomiasis, etc.

2. **Contact sensitivity:** Plant substances like poison oak, poison ivy, poison simac, laundry ink (dhobi's itch on the back or neck), cottonseed, penicillin ointment, nickel, mercuric chloride, quinine, formaldehyde, sulfonamides, etc. may cause skin dermatitis by forming papules, vesicles which ooze and desquamate.

GRANULOMATOUS REACTIONS

Granulomatous reactions is characterized by granuloma formation consisting of altered mononuclear cells, histiocytes, epithelioid cells and foreign body type of giant cells. It takes longer time than delayed hypersensitivity and need poorly soluble substances. It occurs in tuberculosis, tuberculoid leprosy, etc.

Mechanism of delayed hypersensitivity: Wax D of *Mycobacterium tuberculosis*, complete Freund's adjuvant, etc. induces delayed hypersensitivity. There are two suggestions regarding nature of agent causing delayed hypersensitivity reactions:

1. Cytophilic antibodies in low concentration may bind effectively with macrophages.

2. Sensitized cells with antigen liberate substances altering vascular permeability.

Type V or Stimulation Hypersensitivity

Stimulation hypersensitivity is an antibody-mediated hypersensitivity. In this case, antibody reacts with key surface component like hormone receptor. It may switch on or stimulate the cell, e.g., thyroid overactivity due to thyroid-stimulating antibody which develops into Grave's disease.

Thyroid-stimulating hormone (TSH) from pituitary gland gets attached to thyroid cell receptors thus activating adenyl cyclase in the membrane. It converts ATP to AMP. AMP stimulates activity of thyroid cell and hence secretion of thyroxine. The thyroid-stimulating antibody in sera of thyrotoxic patient is actually an antibody directed against receptors of TSH. This antibody may bind to these receptors and bring about the same results as that of TSH.

SCHWARTZMAN REACTION

Schwartzman reaction is not an immune reaction but rather an alteration in factors affecting intravascular coagulation.

Culture filtrate of *Salmonella typhi* if injected intradermally in a rabbit followed 24 hours later by same filtrate intravenously, a hemorrhagic necrotic lesion develops at the site of intradermal injection. The intradermal and intravenous injections need not be of same or even related endotoxin. The absence of specificity and short interval of time between the two doses exclude any immunological basis for reaction.

The initial dose is characteristically of an endotoxin. The intravenous injection can be of a variety of substances, e.g., bacterial endotoxin, starch, serum, kaolin, etc. The preparatory injection causes accumulation of leukocytes which condition the site by release of lysosomal enzymes damaging capillary wall. Following the intravenous dose, there occurs intravascular clotting. The thrombi leads to necrosis of vessel walls and hemorrhage.

If both the injections are given intravenously, the animal dies in 12 to 24 hours after the second dose. It is suggested that mechanism like Schwartzman reaction may operate in conditions like purpuric rash of meningococcal septicemia and acute hemorrhagic adrenal necrosis found in overwhelming infection.

Immunohematology

INTRODUCTION

Blood has been considered in diseases of man right from dawn of time. Blood also was believed to restore youth and vitality of old persons. Blood transfusion became successful only after the discovery of blood groups by Landsteiner. Currently, more than 400 red cell antigens are known. Most of them are poorly immunogenic, ABO and Rh blood groups bear significant importance in blood transfusion, medicine, transplantation, etc.

Blood Groups

Various blood group systems are available, e.g.
1. ABO   2. Rh   3. MN   4. Lutheran
5. Lewis   6. Duffy   7. Kidd.

ABO and Rh systems are the important one and are called major blood group antigens.

ABO Antigens and Isoantibodies

The ABO blood group system was described first of all by Landsteiner in 1900. It contains four major blood groups on the basis of antigen A and antigen B present on the membrane of red cells (**Table 17.1**). Their presence or absence is under genetic control. Red cells of group A have antigen A, cells of group B antigen B and cells of group AB carry both A and B antigens while group O cells have neither A nor B antigen. **Table 17.2** shows ABO distribution in India.

Group A is divided into A-1 and A-2 thus increasing blood groups in ABO system to 6, i.e.,

Table 17.1: Major ABO group antigens.

Group	Genotypes	Antigen in red blood cells	Isoantibodies in plasma
O	OO	—	Anti-A, Anti-B
A	AA, AO	A	Anti-B
B	BB, BO	B	Anti-A
AB	AB	AB	None

Table 17.2: ABO distribution in India.

Group	Frequency
A	22%
B	33%
AB	5%
O	40%

A-1, A-2, B, A1B, A-2B and O. Other subgroups of group A are, 3, A4 A5. About 80% of group A and group AB belong to subgroup A-1 and A-1B while the remainders belong to the subgroups A-2 and A-2B, respectively. Since A-2 cells are sensitive to very high titer anti-A serum, confusion may be there in blood grouping. Hence, A-2 group can be interpreted as group O and A-2B as B. So it is obligatory to use anti-A serum carefully and selected appropriately that it agglutinates A2 and A-2B cells satisfactorily. Both anti-A and anti-B are natural antibodies of IgM type. These antibodies appear in blood of infants. A and B agglutinogens are not well developed at birth but by the age of one, they reach full strength.

H-Substance

Red cells of all ABO groups have a common antigen, which is a precursor for formation of A and B antigens. The amount of the H substance is related to ABO group of the cells. Group O cells have the maximum quantity of H-substance while group A-2B the least amount. Since it is universally distributed, the H-substance is generally not important in blood grouping or transfusion. Sometimes, A and B antigens as well as H antigens are absent from red cells. This is called Bombay or OH blood. Such persons carry anti-A, anti-B and anti-H antibodies. So, the sera of such persons is incompatible with all red cells except of those with same rare blood group.

A, B and H substances are glycoproteins. In addition to red cells A, B and H substances are present in most of the tissue and body fluids. Blood group antigens are also present in secretions such as saliva, gastric juice and sweat but not cerebrospinal fluid (CSF) of certain individuals and they are called secretors. The secretion of ABH antigen is under control of two allelic genes—Se and se. Individuals inheriting Se are secretors and those with Se-se are not secretors.

Blood group antigens are encountered in animals (stomach of horse and dogs) and plants anti-A agglutinin extracted from *Dolichos biflorus* and anti-H from *Ulex europacus*). The blood group agglutinine of plant origin is called lectins.

It is worth to understand that ABO locus is on chromosome number 9. By the way, Rh locus is on chromosome-1.

The Rh System

Levine and Steksib (1957) detected an antibody in the serum of woman who recently delivered a baby with Rh refers to a factor present in human red cells which was discovered in 1940 by Landsteiner and Wiener through the use of sera prepared by the injections of red corpuscles of Rhesus monkeys into rabbits and guinea pigs. It was found that the red cells of 80% of white persons were agglutinated by anti-Rhesus (anti-Rh) serum and the remainders failed to react this way. The former were referred as Rh positive and the latter Rh-negative.

The chemical nature of Rh substance is by and large unknown. There are different theories and nomenclature for the genes and antigens of Rh system. Fisher's hypothesis was that Rh antigens of Rh system were controlled by three pairs of closely linked allelomorphic genes, Cc, Dd and Ee. Every person carries one member of each pair of these genes derived from each parent. Each gene is responsible for production of a specific antigen. The antigen controlled by D locus in the strongest immunogene called Rh-D antigen. The six genes give rise to eight allelomorphs and eight antigenic patterns. The six sera corresponding to the antigens are denoted by the terms Anti-C, Anti-c, Anti-D, Anti-d and so on. Five of the six antisera have been detected in human but no serum containing anti-d has been found. May be the counterpart of D is not antigenic or the gene is amorphic.

As per Wiener view, Rh antigens are controlled by any one of several allelic genes present in a single locus on chromosome. The concerned gene determines the production of appropriate antigen.

The genotype is expressed by two letters R, R2 in Wiener's system; whereas in Fisher system, it is by two sets of letters CDe/cDE. However, in practice, Rh positive or Rh negative blood depends on the presence of D antigen on the surface of red cells, which may be detected by testing with anti-D (anti-Rh serum). About 6 to 7% Indians are Rh negative.

Utilization of Blood Groups in Clinical Practice

1. Blood Transfusion

ABO and Rh antigens are considered for routine blood transfusion. The other blood group antigens are quite weak in this regard. In selecting appropriate donors, the following facts bear some importance:

❖ Serum or plasma of recipient should be free from antibody capable of damaging donor's erythrocytes.

❖ Donor should not carry any antibody that may lyse the recipient's erythrocytes.

❖ Donor's red cells should not possess any antigen which is deficient in the recipient.

Nowadays, it is preferred that recipient and donor both have same blood group. O group used to be transfused to the recipient of any group and was called universal donor. Likewise, AB group person was designated as universal recipient.

Rh compatibility is important when recipient is Rh negative. If Rh negative person receives Rh positive blood, antibodies against Rh antigen are formed and subsequent transfusions with Rh positive blood may cause hemolytic reactions. In case of childbearing age women, hemolytic disease of newborn occurs additionally.

2. Blood Group and Diseases

❖ Blood group antigens may become weak in leukemia.

❖ *Pseudomonas aeruginosa*, become agglutinable by all blood group sera and also by normal human sera. This is called Thomsen-Friedenreich phenomenon and it may be due to unmasking of hidden antigen normally present on all human red cells. This hidden antigen is known as T antigen and anti-T agglutinins are normally present in the sera of all human beings.

❖ Duodenal ulcer is found mostly in individuals of blood group O.

❖ Patients of cancer stomach usually belong to blood group A.

Blood transfusion can be hazardous even after matching blood group and tests from various viral infections are performed. Blood from disaster could be avoided if blood banks irradiate all blood with gamma rays. Bones from cadavers could replace metal implants if they were subjected to gamma rays. These recommendations of irradiation were made known and emphasized by Professor Mammen Chandy at international conference on the application of radioisotopes and radiation held at Mumbai in February 1988.

IMMUNE DEFICIENCY SYNDROME

When there lies defect in persons to produce immune response or to express immune response into effective function, then there is failure in the development and function of lymphoreticular system **(Table 18.1)**. It is associated with diminished resistance to infection.

The following are types of immune deficiency in man:
1. Reticular dysgenesis means failure of stem cell development.
2. Di George syndrome in which there is defective development of thymus.
3. Agammaglobulinemia where there is deficient production of immunoglobulins, e.g., ataxia telangiectasia.

Table 18.1: Clinical immunodeficiency diseases.

Disorder	Postulated B cell	Cell defect T cell	Observed immunologic defect
• Congenital X-linked agammaglobulinemia (Biuton's)	+	–	Absent plasma cells, all classes of immunoglobulins extremely deficient, cellular immunity normal
• Transient hypogammaglobu-linemia of infancy	+	–	Usually self-limited
• Selective immunoglobulin deficiency (IgA, IgM, IgG subclass)	+	–	IgA, IgM, IgG producing plasma cells absent, respective immunoglobulin absent, cellular immunity normal
• Thymic hypoplasia (Di George's syndrome)	–	+	Immunoglobulins normal but some antibody responses deficient. Cellular immunity defective
• Chronic mucocutaneous	–	+	
• Immunodeficiency with ataxia telangiectasia	+	+	Variable deficiency in immunoglobulins and antibodies. Cellular immunity defective for some antigens
• Immunodeficiency with thrombocytopenia and eczema (Wiskott-Aldrich syndrome)	+	+	Variable deficiency of enzymes, immunoglobulins and antibodies. Cellular immunity defective for some antigens
• Immunodeficiency (e.g. thymoma); with short-limbed dwarfism, autosomal recessive, combined, X linked	+	+	Extremely deficient antibodies and cellular immunity defective for all antigens

4. Tumors that affect antibody-producing cell and there is excessive production of plasma cells. They form single immunoglobulin. Such tumors are called myelomas.
5. Agranulocytosis means defect in granulocyte production.
6. Chédiak-Higashi disease in which there is neutrophil lysosomal abnormality. The other example is lazy leukocyte syndrome in which there is defective mobilization of leukocytes at sites of infection. In chronic granulomatous disease, there is defect in granulocyte function.

ACQUIRED IMMUNE DEFICIENCY SYNDROME

Acquired immune deficiency syndrome (AIDS) is characterized by opportunistic infections, defective cellular immunity, autoimmune phenomenon and unusual malignancies, e.g., Kaposi's sarcoma. It may remain symptomless; but sometimes, certain symptoms may appear, e.g., weight loss, pyrexia and generalized adenopathy which is not responding to therapy, chronic diarrhea, involvement of brain and deep sores around mouth and anus. The four "H" type groups at high risk of contacting AIDS have been identified as: (a) Homosexuals, (b) Heroin addicts, (c) Hemophiliacs, and (d) Haitians.

Dr Robert C Gallo discovered HTLV-III (Human T cell lymphotropic virus) in 1983. Now it is called HIV (human immunodeficiency virus). It has been incriminated for AIDS. Some scientists believe that AIDS may be a result of virus mutation. This is considered to be the first such mutation in medical history to have caused a virulent new disease.

It is suggested that all tissues, body fluids particularly blood, semen, saliva, other secretions and excreta must be assumed infective. So utmost care should be taken to avoid needle injury, or contamination of wound, skin lesions or mucosal surfaces. Clinical and laboratory workers should have six monthly serum samples tested for HIV.

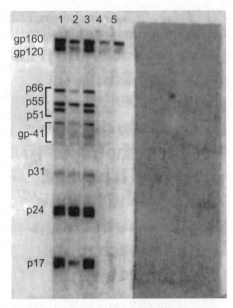

Fig. 18.1: Western blot test number 1, 2 and 3 are showing positive bands.

They must wear gowns, gloves and plastic aprons. They must protect eyes appropriately. AIDS patients should be nursed properly.

For the diagnosis of AIDS, the following procedures may be helpful:
a. ELISA
b. Western blot technique (**Fig. 18.1**) in which viral antigens are separated electrophoretically and transferred onto a nitrocellulose paper. These spots are exposed to the test specimen. If specific antibodies are present, they react with corresponding antigen.

AUTOIMMUNE DISEASES

Normally, body does not produce antibodies against its own constituents. In certain situations, body produces autoantibodies against its own constituents.

Mechanism of Autoimmune Disease

1. Hidden antigen may not be recognized as self-antigen and hence production of antibodies against hidden antigen, e.g., thyroid, lens of eye, testis, etc.

2. In some cases, new antigen is formed by infection or physical or chemical processes, e.g. drugs. This mechanism may have role in rheumatoid arthritis where there is denaturation of gammaglobulin.
3. Immunization with foreign antigen results in the production of antibodies. These antibodies may crossreact with some host components, e.g., antibodies against *Streptococcus pyogenes* may cross-react with human heart muscle in rheumatic heart disease.
4. There may be breakdown of general mechanism of immune tolerance through genetic mutation. Breakdown of immunological homeostasis may lead to cessation of tolerance and production of forbidden clones, e.g., systemic lupus erythematosus (SLE). **Table 18.2** shows classification of autoimmune diseases.

Table 18.2: Classification of autoimmune diseases.

Disease	Antigen involved
Diseases associated with inaccessible antigens	
• Hashimoto's disease of thyroid	
• Sjogren's disease	
• Sympathetic ophthalmia	Organ specific antigens are not present normally in circulation
• Multiple sclerosis	
• Peripheral neuritis	
• Male sterility	
Diseases associated with common body antigen	
• Rheumatoid arthritis	
• Acquired hemolytic anemia	Denatured γ globulin, red cell antigen, platelets antigen, nuclear (DNA) and cytoplasmic constituents
• Idiopathic thrombocytopenic purpura	
• Systemic lupus erythematosus constituents	
• Scleroderma	
• Polyarteritis nodosa	

Features Observed in Autoimmune Diseases

1. Immunoglobulin levels are elevated.
2. Autoantibodies demonstration.
3. Deposition of immunoglobulins at the place of lesion, e.g., renal glomeruli.
4. Lymphocytes and plasma cells are collected at lesion site.
5. Corticosteroids and immunosuppressive agents are invariably useful.
6. Usually more than one autoimmune conditions encountered in a patient.
7. Genetic predisposition.
8. It is irreversible.
9. Females are mostly susceptible to autoimmune disorders.

IMMUNOLOGY OF TRANSPLANTATION

Transplantation is one of mankind's old dreams. In case of irreparable damage to organ because of disease or injury or when the organ is congenitally defective or absent, grafting or transplantation becomes inevitable for restoration of function. The individual from whom organ is obtained is the donor, the individual on whom it is applied is recipient and organ transplanted is graft or transplant.

Classification of transplant: Transplants are classified in the following ways:
1. Based on the organ transplanted they are classified as heart, kidney, skin transplant.
2. On the basis of anatomical site of origin and site of placement of transplant, e.g., orthotopic, when grafts are applied in anatomical normal sites (e.g., skin graft), whereas heterophic grafts are placed in anatomically abnormal sites, e.g., when thyroid tissue is transplanted in subcutaneous pocket.
3. Transplants could be fresh organs or stored ones.
4. Transplants may be living (kidney, heart) or dead (bone, artery), former is called vital graft whereas latter one is structural graft.
5. Transplants may be classified on the basis of genetic relationship between the donor and recipient **(Table 18.3)**. Transplant

Table 18.3: Terminology of antigen, antibodies and tissue graft.

Relationship between donor and recipient	Genetic terminology	Antibody antigen	Transplantation terminology
• Same animal	—	Auto-antibody Auto-antigen	Autograft
• Identical twins and inbred strain	Synergic (isogeneric)	—	Isograft
• Same outbred species or different inbred strains	Allogenic iso-antigen	Iso-antibody (homograft)	Allograft
• Different species	Heterogenic Xenogenic	Hetero-antibody Hetero-antigen	Xenograft (Heterograft)

may be autograft (taken from individual and placed on himself), isograft (placed on another individual of same genetic constitution, e.g., graft made between identical twins), and allograft (placed in genetically non-identical member of same species). Autograft and isograft are compatible with host tissue genetically and antigenically and hence are successful. On the other hand allograft and xenograft are incompatible genetically and antigenically and hence are rejected.

Allograft rejection: If skin graft from rabbit is applied on genetically unrelated animal of the same species, initially graft appears to be accepted up to two or three days. By fourth day, graft is invaded by lymphocytes and macrophages, blood vessels get occluded with thrombi, vascularity decreases, graft undergoes ischemic necrosis and in ten days' time the graft sloughs off. This sequence of events is called first set response. In this animal, which has rejected a graft by the first set response, another graft from same donor is applied, it will be rejected in an accelerated way. Initially, vascularization does occur but is interrupted by inflammatory response with necrosis and graft sloughs off by sixth day. This is called second set response.

Mechanism of allograft rejection (Fig. 18.2): The first set of response is brought about by T lymphocytes. Hence, it is predominantly cell mediated. Humoral antibodies are also produced during allograft rejection and may be detected by hemagglutination, lymphocyte toxicity, complement fixation and immunofluorescence. Antibodies are formed more rapidly and abundantly during second set response, of course, along with cell-mediated response.

Humoral antibodies may act in opposition to cell mediated response by inhibiting graft rejection. This phenomenon is called *immunological enhancement.* If the recipient is pretreated with one or more injections of killed donor tissue and transplant applied subsequently, this transplant may survive quite longer than in control animals. It should be remembered that allograft immunity is a generalized response directed against all the antigens of donor.

Factors favoring allograft survival: (i) Immunosuppression, e.g., neonatal thymectomy, irradiation, corticosteroids and antilymphocytic serum (ALS), (ii) Blood cross-matching and tissue typing for various HLA antigens. There are certain privileged sites where allografts are permitted to survive, e.g., intrauterine allograft, cartilage, brain, testis and cornea.

IMMUNOLOGICAL SURVEILLANCE

Immunological surveillance means destruction of malignant cell that may arise by somatic mutation. Such malignant mutation does occur frequently in living body and can develop into tumor if constant vigilance of immune system is defective. Increased incidence of cancer is there because of

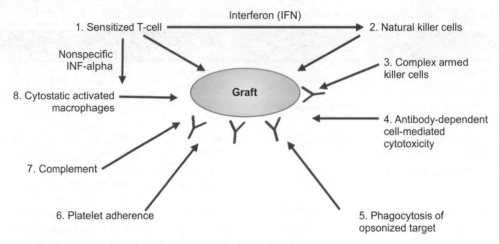

Fig. 18.2: Mechanism of graft rejection.

inefficiency of surveillance mechanism on account of aging, congenital or otherwise immunodeficiency disorders. In other words, cancer should not occur if surveillance is effective enough.

Escape from immunological surveillance may result in development of tumor. The possibilities of escape are: (i) very fast proliferation of malignant cells to an extent which may be beyond the control of immunological attack, (ii) circulating tumor antigen may coat lymphoid cells and thus preventing them from acting on malignant or tumor cells, and (iii) tumor antigen on malignant cells may not be accessible to sensitized cells.

Tumor antigens: The following are tumor surface antigens:

a. Virally controlled antigens may be produced in cell infected with oncogenic virus. These antigens are of two types, the first is 'V' antigen which is identical with an antigen on the isolated virion. The second is 'T' which may be present only on infected cells.

b. Embryonic antigens are L-fetoproteins in hepatic carcinoma and carcinoma embryonic antigen (CEA) in cancer of intestine.

c. Idiotypic antigen: Tumors induced by benzopyrene possess specific

transplantation antigen. Even when carcinogen produces two different primary tumors in same animals still each tumor produced by given chemical has its own idiotypic antigen. They may not exhibit the same antigenic specificities and do not confer cross-resistance by immunization.

IMMUNOLOGICAL TOLERANCE

Immunological tolerance is a kind of immunological unresponsiveness involving antibody production as well as cell-mediated response. This non-reactivity may be specific to the particular antigen only, whereas immune reaction to other antigens remains unaffected. Tolerance can be induced for any of the substances that induce antibody production. It may be induced by exposure to antigen in fetal life or by exposure to a large amount of antigens in adult life.

When antigen comes in contact with lymphocytes, they may respond positively (stimulation) or negatively (tolerance). Factors responsible for positive or negative response of lymphocytes are concentration of antigen, degree to which these recognized antigens fit the combining site of antigen, the way these antigens are presented whether on molecules or cell surfaces and the presence or absence of other lymphocytes which may help to suppress immune response. Tolerance may occur when lymphocytes are confronted with high concentration of antigen. This is called high zone of immunological tolerance. Constant of small concentration of antigen below threshold is required for stimulation results in low zone immunological tolerance.

Tolerance can be overcome spontaneously to injection of cross-reacting immunogens. Tolerance to living agent is more lasting than that to non-living substances. Natural occurring tolerance is found in some viral infections, e.g., rubella and cytomegalovirus in which there is constant viremia with decreased ability for production of neutralizing antibodies.

Mechanism of immunological tolerance: The mechanism is not clear. Inactivation of antigen sensitive cells may be the mechanism of tolerance production. Contact of antigen with antigen sensitive cell without being processed through macrophages or T cells may result in inhibition of antigen sensitive cells. Initiation of tolerance by this method may be further maintained by reintroduction of antigen in a suitable manner which cause inhibition of newly emerging antigen sensitive cells.

The other possible mechanism of tolerance is by alteration of regulation mechanism of immune system. Strong activity of suppressor "T" cell can give rise to state of tolerance.

LIMULUS AMEBOCYTE LYSATE TEST (LAL TEST)

Principle: Limulus amebocyte lysate (extract of blood cells from horseshoe crab) forms a firm clot when incubated with endotoxin at 37°C.

This test is less expensive and rapid semiquantitative which may be useful as under:
1. Detection of lipopolysaccharide (LPS) in toxemia or septicemia.
2. Detection of purity of fluid used for intravenous therapy.
3. Detection of water pollution with Gram-negative bacilli.
4. Detection of Gram-negative bacilli in food.

5. Diagnosis of meningitis due to Gram-negative organisms.

RADIOIMMUNOASSAY METHOD

Radioimmunoassay method is useful for accurate quantitative estimation of polypeptide hormones. It is specific, precise and simple method available.

Principle: Radioiodine-labeled hormones compete with non-labeled hormones of a sample under test for antihormone antibodies. The more of the hormone in test sample, the less chance the labeled hormone has of combining with the limited number of antibody molecules. Thus by measuring the quantity of labeled hormone combined with antibody, a measure in the test sample can be obtained.

This method is useful for an assay of IgE levels in serum and for detection of Australia antigen in human serum.

Immunoblotting

Here mixture of antigen is electrophoretically separated in a polyacrylamide gel. The separated antigens are passed on or blotted electrophoretically from gel to nitrocellulose paper and incubated with antibody No. A (against antigen). Antibody No. A is then revealed by another antibody (antibody No. B). Nitrocellulose sheet with transferred DNA is called Southern blot and when same technique is applied to analyze transferred RNA, it is called Northern blot. Nitrocellulose sheet with transferred proteins (Antibodies to HIV) is called Western blot.

ENZYME-LINKED IMMUNOSORBENT ASSAY

Enzyme-linked immunosorbent assay (ELISA) is especially useful for detection of rotavirus and Hepatitis-A virus (stool samples). This method is widely accepted as reagents are stable and cheap. Procedure is easy to understand and perform. Simplicity and sensitivity are the highlights of ELISA.

Principle: Antigen is coated on plastic plate or tube. To it is added serum which is supposed to contain antibodies. Addition of antiglobulin linked with enzymes (alkaline phosphatase or peroxidase) is done. This will attach with antigen-antibody complex. Now add enzyme substrate (p-nitrophenyl phosphate). There will be color reaction indicating the presence of antibodies.

Procedure: Absorb antigen, (e.g. in malaria schizont may be used as an antigen) to the surface of plastic plates or tubes. Excess of antigen is removed by washing. Test material is then added, say patient serum. Unbound antibody is removed by washing. Now enzyme (alkaline phosphatase) linked anti-human gamma globulin (known) is added. Again excess is removed by washing. This mixture is incubated at 37°C. Finally, corresponding enzyme substrate, (p-nitrophenyl phosphate) is added which may be hydrolized by enzyme yielding yellow product. The optical density of this yellow product is measured in a spectrophotometer **(Figs. 18.3A to C)**. The optical density is directly proportional to the amount of enzyme deposited on plates or tubes which in turn is related to the amount of antibodies in a test sample. Likewise, we may detect antigen from specimen by coating antibody on the surface of plates or tubes and adding enzyme linked known antigen. Rest of the procedure is same.

ELISA is useful for assay of hormones (estrogen, progesterone, HCG, T3, T4), onco-protein (alpha 2-hepatoglobulin), snake poisoning, virological infections (Hepatitis B antigen, Hepatitis A antigen, Herpes simplex, Rota, Rubella, EB, CMV, and antibodies to influenza and measle viruses). Besides these, it is often useful in bacteriological conditions (enteric infection, antibodies against M protein of streptococci, *E. coli* antibodies in urinary tract infection in urine specimen, *Mycobacterium tuberculosis*, leprosy, etc.), fungal diseases (candidiasis, aspergillosis), surveillance of disease in particular area and histochemical complex reactions.

■ MONOCLONAL ANTIBODIES

Hybridoma technology for the production of antibodies was introduced by Kohler and Milstein for which they have been awarded the Nobel prize in medicine in 1984. Now it is possible to successfully generate not only mouse hybridomas but also interspecies (ratmouse and human-mouse) hybridomas. Even human to human hybridomas have also been produced.

Monoclonal antibodies derived from one clone of cells are homogeneous, i.e., composed of same class of immunoglobulin with identical combining site (specificity), affinity and physiochemical properties. The advantages of monoclonal antibodies versus conventional antisera are summarized in the **Table 18.4**.

Hybrids are made from two types of cells: (i) antibody forming cells, i.e., "B" lymphocyte with limited lifespan, and (ii) myeloma cells with ability to multiply indefinitely **(Fig. 18.4)**. The hybrids secreting the desired antibody are cloned and may be maintained in culture or frozen or grown as solid tumor or as an ascitic tumor in mouse peritoneal cavity. The yield of the antibody is usually up to 100 mg/L tissue culture medium or up to 10 gm/L in serum or ascitic fluid tapped from peritoneal

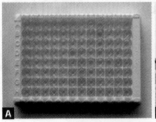
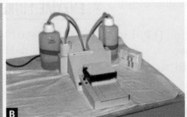
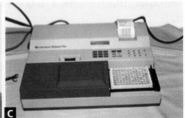

Figs. 18.3A to C: (A) ELISA plates; (B) ELISA plate reader; (C) ELISA plate washer.

Table 18.4: Properties of monoclonal and conventional antibodies.

Property	Conventional antibody	Monoclonal antibody
• Useful antibody contents	Low	High
• Composition	—Heterogeneous	—Homogeneous
	—Multiple (variable from animal to animal)	—Defined and consistent
• Cross-reaction with other antigen	Partial with antigen bearing common antigenic determinant	Usually absent
• Class and subclass of immunoglobulin	Mixture of many classes	Only one
• Supply	Limited	Abundant

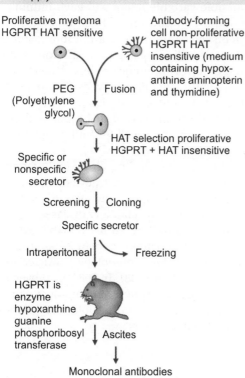

Proliferative myeloma HGPRT HAT sensitive

Antibody-forming cell non-proliferative HGPRT HAT insensitive (medium containing hypoxanthine aminopterin and thymidine)

PEG (Polyethylene glycol)

Fusion

HAT selection proliferative HGPRT + HAT insensitive

Specific or nonspecific secretor

Screening | Cloning

Specific secretor

Intraperitoneal | Freezing

HGPRT is enzyme hypoxanthine guanine phosphoribosyl transferase

Ascites

Monoclonal antibodies

Fig. 18.4: Formation of monoclonal antibodies.

Table 18.5: Mouse/human monoclonal antibodies of clinical interest.

Normal tissue	Hemopoietic cell antigen, thymocytes, kidney, liver, heart, limbic system neurons and trophoblast antigen.
Bacteria	*Streptococcus group B, Escherichia coli, Pneumococcus, Neisseria meningitis, Neisseria gonococci, Mycobaterium leprae and Mycoplasma.*
Viruses	Measles, Hepatitis "B" surface antigen, influenza virus, and Epstein-Barr virus.
Parasites	*Plasmodium falciparum and Toxoplasma gondii.*
Hormones	hCG, progesterone, vasopressin, growth hormone, estradiol 17B.
Tumor associated	Leukemia, lymphoma, carcinoma, sarcoma and neuroblastoma.
Miscellaneous	HLA—A/B/C/DR, microglobulin, transferrin receptor, acid phosphatase, digoxin, tetanus toxoid. Clq, H-Y antigen, etc.

cavity of tumor-bearing mice for producing human monoclonal antibodies. Lymphocytes from peripheral blood film, spleen, lymph nodes of immunized volunteers are used as fusion partners **(Fig. 18.4)**.

Hybridoma technique has been widely adapted to generate monoclonal antibodies against a wide variety of antigen as shown in **Table 18.5**.

The relative eclipse of interest in the *in vivo* use of antibacterial antibodies that followed the introduction of chemotherapy and antibiotics has now been reversed by introduction of monoclonal antibodies and can be produced in unlimited quantities of specific immunoglobulin.

Monoclonal antibodies have numerous application in the diagnosis, treatment and prophylaxis of various clinical disorders **(Table 18.5)**. They provide powerful means for the study of pathogenesis of many diseases especially those related to autoimmune and immune deficiency. Formation of monoclonal antibodies is illustrated in **Figure 18.4**.

NOBEL PRIZE IN MEDICINE IN 1987

Generation of Immunoglobulin Diversity

The Nobel Assembly of Karolinska Institute in Stockholm awarded the Nobel prize in medicine in 1987 to Susumu Tonegawa, a Japanese scientist, for his discovery of the genetic principle for the generation of antibody diversity.

We are aware that no immunoglobulin can be produced by a cell unless it has a blueprint for it in its genes. Since, the human genome contains only about 100,000 genes, it seems unreasonable that they could allow the production of a billion of different antibodies. This was the dilemma unsolved for four to five decades.

Tonegawa, in an important series of experiment reported in 1976, showed for the first time that different genes coding for the proteins that make up an immunoglobulin had physically moved closer on chromosome, thus making it possible to combine at random different proteins that make up these antibodies. He used genetic engineering techniques to compare the arrangement of genes in embryonic and adult mouse B cells. When the embryonic cells mature into adult cells, as they develop, they shuffle the genes, so that some genes end up closer together on the chromosomes.

Tonegawa's experiment showed that during development of a mammal, one each of these different genes (in humans there are 200 different 'V' genes, 20 'D' genes and 4 'J' genes on variable part of heavy chain of immunoglobulin molecule) come together at random producing thousands of different possible variable regions. Since, there are four possible variable regions to each immunoglobulin, and on top of this, the genes are themselves inherited in a random fashion, there are billions of possible variations in the final group of immunoglobulins. It means that the blueprint for different types of proteins are already existent. The foreign protein particle on identification has only to be matched with a corresponding B-cell for immunoglobulin production to start.

This pioneer finding along with genetic engineering which is fast developing today, will, of course, open new avenues for the treatment of many refractory diseases.

Tonegawa performed his valuable experiments during the time he spent working at the Basel Institute for Immunology in Switzerland between 1971 and 1981. In 1981, he moved to Massa-chusetts Institute of Technology where he has concentrated on the molecular genetics of the T cell receptors.

Systemic Bacteriology

SECTION OUTLINE

SECTION 4

Staphylococcus

MICROCOCCACEAE

The family Micrococcaceae has three genera:
a. Micrococci are found on skin or mucous membrane. They are usually not associated with infection.
b. Planococci are motile cocci and are not pathogenic in man. They are arranged in tetrads and produce a yellow-brown pigment on nutrient agar, e.g., *Planococcus citreus* and *Planococcus halophilus*.
c. *Staphylococcus* genus possesses 30 species. Fourteen species are associated with man and animals. Quite a number of central nervous system (CNS) infections are caused by *Staphylococcus epidermidis* (70%) followed by *Staphylococcus saprophyticus*, *Staphylococcus hominis*, *Staphylococcus simulans*, *Staphylococcus hemolyticus*, etc.

Staphylococci were first seen in pus by Koch in 1878. Pasteur cultivated them for the first time in 1880. They were named by Sir Alexander Ogston in 1881.

General characters: They are Gram-positive cocci, ovoid or spheroidal, non-motile arranged in groups. On nutrient agar, they form colonies, white, yellow or golden yellow in color. Their hemolytic capacity is variable. Pathogenic strains produce coagulase, ferment sugar (glucose, lactose, mannitol) with acid production, liquefy gelatin and produce pus in lesion. Under the influence of certain chemicals (e.g., penicillin), they are lysed or changed into L forms. They are not affected by bile salts or optochin.

Classification

A. On the basis of pigment production, three types of staphylococci are identified.
   1. *Staphyloccus aureus* produces golden yellow colonies and are pathogenic.
   2. *Staphylococcus albus* produces white colonies and may be nonpathogenic.
   3. *Staphylococcus citreus* produces lemon yellow colonies and are nonpathogenic.
B. On the basis of pathogenicity:
   1. Pathogenic species — *Staphylococcus aureus*.
   2. Nonpathogen species—*Staphylococcus epidermidis*.
C. Baird-Parker classification.

STAPHYLOCOCCUS AUREUS (STAPHYLOCOCCUS PYOGENES)

Morphology: It is ovoid or spherical, (0.8 to 0.9 μ), non-motile, rarely capsulated, non-sporing strain with ordinary aniline dye and is Gram-positive. It is arranged in clusters (grape-like) **(Figs. 19.1 and 19.2)**. Cluster formation is due to cell division occurring in three planes with daughter cells tending to remain in close proximity.

Cultural characteristics: *Staphylococcus aureus* is aerobic and grows readily on simple media at optimum temperature 37°C and pH 7.4.

Fluid media: It produces uniform turbidity. No pigment is produced.

Nutrient agar: After 24 hours' incubation, colony is pigmented, golden yellow, 2 to 4

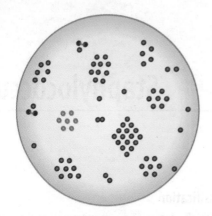

Fig. 19.1: Colonies of *Staphylococcus aureus.*

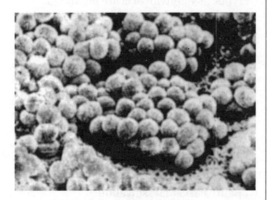

Fig. 19.2: Colonies of *Staphylococcus aureus*
(electron microscope)

mm (pinhead size), circular, convex, smooth, shiny, opaque, with entire edge and emulsifies easily. Pigment production occurs optimally at 22°C and only in aerobic culture. Pigment production is enhanced when 1% glycerol monoacetate or milk is incorporated in medium. Pigment is lipoprotein.

Blood agar: A wide zone of beta hemolysis (clear zone) is produced around colonies. Hemolysis is marked on rabbit or sheep blood and weak on horse blood agar.

Egg yolk medium: The organism produces opacity on glucose egg yolk medium through lipolytic enzyme which acts on lipoprotein of yolk (lipovitellin).

MacConkey medium: Colonies are small and pink in color (lactose fermenter).

Selective Media

1. Media containing 8 to 10% NaCl (salt milk agar, salt broth).
2. Lithium chloride.
3. Tellurite.
4. Polymyxin.
5. Mannitol salt agar **(Fig. 19.3)**.

Factors Influencing Pigment Production

1. **Temperature:** Maximum pigment production is at room temperature 20 to 25°C.
2. **Oxygen:** Pigment is produced under aerobic condition.
3. **Medium:** Pigment is produced on solid medium. Milk agar and glycerol monoacetate are useful in rapid identification of *Staphylococcus aureus* on the basis of pigment production.
4. **Light:** In the presence of light, pigmentation of colony is better.

Biochemical Reactions

It ferments a number of sugars producing acid and no gas (glucose, lactose, sucrose, maltose, mannitol). Fermentation of mannitol

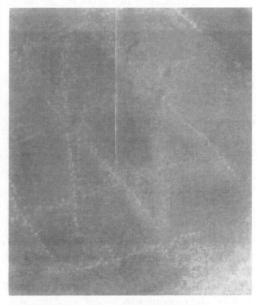

Fig. 19.3: Mannitol salt agar *Staphylococcus aureus.*

is important in *Staphylococcus aureus*. It is catalase positive and coagulase positive. It liquefies gelatin. It is lipolytic in media-containing egg yolk medium. Phosphatase is produced only by *Staphylococcus aureus*.

Characteristics of Pathogenic Strain

1. Coagulase positive.
2. Mannitol fermentation.
3. Beta hemolysis.
4. Golden yellow pigment.
5. Liquefies gelatin.
6. Phosphatase is produced.
7. Sensitivity to lysostaphin.
8. Hydrolyses urea.
9. Reduces nitrates to nitrites.
10. Tellurite reduction.
11. Deoxyribose nuclease enzyme production.

Resistance: It is among the more resistant of non-sporing organisms. It withstands 60°C for 30 minutes. It resists 1% phenol for 15 minutes.

Mercury perchloride (1%) kills it in 10 minutes. Crystal violet (1 in 500,000) and brilliant green (one in 10 million) is lethal for it. Staphylococcal resistance to penicillin is due to the production of an enzyme penicillinase (beta lactamase) which inactivate penicillins. Broadly, resistance falls into several classes:

a. Beta lactamase is under plasmid control.
b. Methicillin resistance.
c. Plasmids can carry genes for resistance to tetracycline erythromycin and amino glycosides.
d. "Tolerance" implies that staphylococci are inhibited by drug and not killed by it.

Antigenic structure: It has specific antigens in cell wall **(Fig. 19.4)**. It can be demonstrated by agglutination or precipitation. Pathogenic strains are more uniform and 15 types have been recognized.

Staphylococci contain both antigenic polysaccharides and proteins that permit grouping of strains to a limited extent. Peptidoglycan, a polysaccharide, plays an important role in the pathogenesis of staphylococcal infection. It elicits production of interleukin-1 and opsonic antibodies by monocytes. It can also be a chemoattractant for polymorphonuclear leukocyte. It produces a localized Schwartzman phenomenon and activates complement. Teichoic acids (polymers of glycerol or ribitol phosphate) linked to cell wall peptidoglycan can be antigenic. Antiteichoic antibodies may be particularly associated with active staphylococcal endocarditis. Surface protein may interfere with phagocytosis.

Protein A, a cell wall component of *Staphylococcus aureus* (Cowan 1 strain), happens to bind strongly to Fc portion of any IgG molecule. This makes the Fab portion of an antibody molecule to face outwards, so that it is free to combine with specific antigen. Staphylococcal protein A is involved in coagglutination. Moreover, protein A may interfere with phagocytosis and cause damage to platelets.

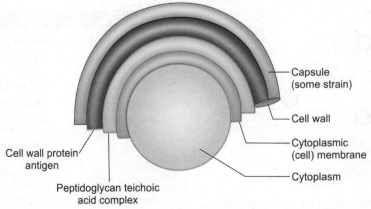

Fig. 19.4: Antigenic structure of staphylococci.

Antigenic structure is, however, of little use in the identification of *Staphylococcus*.

BIOTYPES

There are six biotypes (A, B, C, D, E, F and G). Biotype A strain is pathogenic to man. Biotype A is characterized by pigment production, fibrinolysis, coagulation test positive, hemolysin (a or b), telberite reduction, etc.

Bacteriophage typing: The phage typing is useful in the investigation of *Staphylococcus aureus* infection. An internationally accepted set of phages is used for typing. Staphylococcal phage typing is by pattern method **(Fig. 19.5)**.

A set of twenty-eight phage may be employed. The strains are divided into four groups. Human strains belong to phage group I, II or III. Hospital infections are usually due to strains belonging to group I or III.

Typing set of staphylococcal phages:

Group I.   29, 52, 52A, 79, 80.
Group II.   3A, 3B, 3C, 55, 71.
Group III.   6, 7, 42 E, 47, 53, 54, 75, 77, 83
                 A, 84, 85.
Not Allocated   42D, 81, 94, 95, 96.

Enzymes Produced

1. *Coagulase (free coagulase):* It is filterable and heat labile enzyme produced in lag and early log phase of bacterial growth. It is antigenic.

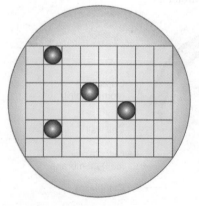

Fig. 19.5: Bacteriophage typing of staphylococci.

About seven distinct antigenic types have been described. Human strain produces A variety. It has antiphagocytic action.

Clotting of human or rabbit plasma is brought about by coagulase. Along with coagulase-reacting factor (CRF) present in plasma, it converts fibrinogen into fibrin.

Enzyme coagulase can be demonstrated by mixing 0.1 mL of an overnight broth culture of organism and 0.9 mL of 1 in 10 diluted rabbit plasma in a glass tube and incubated at 37°C. Result is noted after every 2 hours. The plasma forms clot if organism is coagulase positive.

2. *Clumping factor (bound coagulase):* It is heat stable protein. Antigenically, it is homogenous. It does not require coagulase-reacting factor (CRF) and fibrinogen is not converted into fibrin.

Clumping factor is a component of cell wall. It can be liberated upon autolysis of the cell.

When a drop of saline suspension of *Staphylococcus aureus* is mixed with rabbit plasma, the cocci are clumped or agglutinated. This clumping of *Staphylococcus* is due to combination of fibrinogen with receptor present on the surface of organism. It is not associated with pathogenicity of organisms.

Table 19.1 depicts differences between clumping and coagulase factors.

Table 19.1: Differences between clumping and coagulase factor.

Clumping factor	Coagulase factors
• It remains on the surface of the organism	It is secreted outside the body of the organism
• It is heat stable	It is heat labile
• One type of clumping factor is present serologically	Seven types of coagulase are differentiated. They are named as A, B, C, D, E, F and G. All human strains of Staphylococcus aureus produce "A" type of coagulase

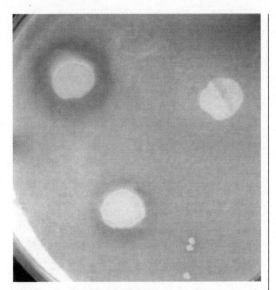

Fig. 19.6: DNase activity of *Staphylococcus aureus* observed on DNase test agar (M482) flooded with 1 N HCL.

3. *Phosphatase:* It is produced by coagulase positive strain of staphylococci. For its demonstration, organisms are cultured on agar medium containing phenolphthalein diphosphate. When such a mixture is exposed to ammonia vapor, colonies assume a bright pink color due to the presence of free phenolphthalein.
4. *Hyaluronidase:* Most strains of *Staphylococcus aureus* form hyaluronidase especially those producing impetigo contagiosa.
5. *Deoxyribonuclease (Fig. 19.6):* Coagulase positive *Staphylococcus* also produces this enzyme.
6. Colony-compacting factor.

TOXINS

1. **Hemolysin**: *Staphylococcus aureus* produces at least four types of hemolysin known as alpha, beta, gamma and delta. All hemolysins are antigenically distinct. Alpha hemolysin may cause hemolysis of rabbit and sheep red cell rapidly. Alpha hemolysis is produced by coagulase positive strain and is important in the pathogenesis of infection in man. It is leukocidal, cytotoxic, dermonecrotoxic and lethal. It is antigenic and is neutralized by antitoxin.

   Beta hemolysin is produced by *Staphylococcus* isolated from animals. It is hemolytic for sheep red cells. It is produced aerobically as well as anaerobically. It is less toxic to laboratory animals.

   Delta lysin is lytic for sheep RBC. It is less toxic to laboratory animals.

   The gamma lysin, the weakest of other hemolysins, acts on human, sheep, rabbit and monkey erythrocytes.
2. **Leukocidin**:
   i. The alpha lysin has leukocidal activity.
   ii. Panto valentine is an independent toxin which kills human and rabbit polymorph and macrophages without lysing them. It is heat and oxygen labile and consists of two antigenically distinct proteins F and S.
   iii. Leukolysin is closely associated with delta lysin. It is thermostable.
3. **Enterotoxin**: The toxin is responsible for manifestations of *Staphylococcus* poisoning—nausea, vomiting and diarrhea within 6 hours of taking contaminated food. It is heat stable. It is antigenic and is neutralized by antitoxin. It is a trypsin-resistant protein. Six antigenic type have been distinguished (A to F). Type A and B are most common. Ingestion of 25 µg of enterotoxin B results in vomiting and diarrhea in humans or monkeys.

   Strain producing this toxin belongs to bacteriophage group III (66/47). Its mode of action is not known. It is believed that it acts peripherally on sensory nerve endings of smooth muscle of intestine. It has emetic effect on cats perhaps by acting centrally.
4. **Fibrinolysin**: *Staphylococcus aureus* produces staphylokinase during the later stages of growth which causes lysis of fibrin. This fibrinolysin may dislodge the infected intravascular thrombi and then contribute to the development of *Staphylococcus* septicemia.

5. **Exfoliative toxin**: It consists of two proteins which may cause desquamation of staphylococcal scalded skin syndrome. Specific antibodies against it are protective.
6. **Toxic shock syndrome toxin**: Some strains of staphylococci may produce a toxin called toxic shock syndrome toxin-1 which resembles enterotoxin-F and exotoxin-C. In man it may cause fever, shock, skin rash, etc. It may involve many organs of man. In rabbit, it causes effects like toxic shock syndrome but lack skin rash with desquamation.

Other Toxins

1. Nucleases
2. Lipases
3. Proteases
4. Scarlatina toxin.

Numerous *Staphylococcus* strains are found in air, dust, clothing and fomites. They may be pathogenic to newborn babies when they come from fomites. These may be normally present on skin, nose and mouth. They may enter skin through hair follicles, sebaceous glands, sweat glands, cracks, abrasions or injury to the skin.

Virulence Factors

The virulence factors important in *Staphylococcus aureus* are:
1. Cell wall polysaccharide confers rigidity and integrity to bacterial cells. Besides, it activates complement and induces release of inflammatory cytokines.
2. Teichoic acid is an antigenic part of cell wall. It facilitates attachment of cocci to host cell surfaces. It also protects the cocci complement-mediated apsonization.
3. Capsule around the bacteria inhibits apsonization.
4. Protein A is chemotactic, antiphagocytic and anticomplementary. It induces platelet damage and hypersensitivity.

Protein A is also a 'B' cell mitogen. It has been used as ligands for isolation of IgG.
5. Clumping factor is the bound coagulase.
6. Coagulase.
7. Lipases help the organism in infecting skin and subcutaneous tissues.
8. Hyaluronidase.
9. Nuclease is heat stable in *Staphylococcus aureus*.
10. Protein receptors facilitate staphylococcal adhesion to host cell tissue, e.g., fibronectin, fibrinogen, IgG and C_1q.

Pathogenicity: *Staphylococcus* may cause the majority of acute pyogenic lesions in man. Staphylococcal lesions are characteristically localized. Staphylococcal disease may be classified as:
1. *Cutaneous lesions:* Furuncles, styes, boils, abscess, carbuncles, impetigo, pemphigus neonatorum.

    The majority of hospital cross-infections are of staphylococcal in origin.
2. *Deep infection:* Acute osteomyelitis, tonsillitis, pharyngitis, sinusitis, pneumonia, pulmonary abscess, breast abscess, meningitis, endocarditis and renal abscesses. Staphylococcal septicemia is a rare but serious disease. Staphylococci of phage group II cause bullous exfoliation— the "scalded skin" syndrome. Toxic shock syndrome usually begins within five days of onset of menses in young women who use tampons. There is an abrupt onset of high fever, vomiting, diarrhea, myalgias, scarlatiniform rash, hypotension with cardiac and renal failure. This syndrome may recur in successive menstrual periods and is tentatively attributed to staphylococcal toxin.
3. *Staphylococcal food poisoning:* It results when food contaminated with enterotoxin, produced by *Staphylococcus* is consumed, e.g., meat, fish, milk and milk products. Diarrhea and vomiting set in within 6 hours of taking contaminated food.

Laboratory Diagnosis

1. Hematological Investigations

a. *Total leukocyte counts:* There is leukocytosis and total leukocyte count is above 10,000 cells per cubic mm.

b. *Differential leukocyte count:* There is increase in neutrophil count. It is usually more than 80%.

2. Bacteriological Methods

Specimen like pus from suppurative lesion and sputum from respiratory infection is taken. In food poisoning, feces and remains of suspected food should be collected. For detection of carrier, usual specimen like nasal swab, swabs from perenium and umbilical stump is necessary. It is studied as follows:

a. *Smear examination:* A smear is prepared from the specimen obtained as above. It is stained with Gram method. Stained smear shows a large number of pus cells and Gram-positive cocci arranged in cluster or in small groups.

b. *Isolation of organism:* The specimen is plated on blood agar media. Staphylococcal colonies appear after overnight incubation at 37°C. They are golden yellow colonies, showing beta hemolysis. The colonies are tested for coagulase and phosphatase pro-duction. Antibiotic sensitivity test is done as a guideline to treatment. Bacteriophage typing may be done if the information is required for epidemiological purposes.

Swabs from carrier's feces and from food poisoning are inoculated on selective media like Ludlam's and salt agar media.

c. *Serological diagnosis:* It is helpful in the diagnosis of hidden deep infections. This includes demonstration of specific antibodies (e.g., antibodies to teichoic acid in staphylococcal endocarditis), and toxin or leukocidin in patient's blood.

d. Bacteriophage typing, antibiogram, plasmid, typing, ribotyping and DNA finger printing can be done.

METHICILLIN-RESISTANT STAPHYLOCOCCUS AUREUS

Methicillin-resistant *Staphylococcus aureus* (MRSA) was isolated in 1960. They are emerging increasingly because of indiscriminate use of antibiotics. Methicillin resistance is most accurately found by standard agar screen. Classic methicillin resistance is encoded by the methicillin resistance determinant (mec), a 30 to 50 Kb transposon-like segment of DNA that is present in methicillin-resistant *Staphylococcus aureus* strain. The mec A gene, which resides on mec encodes a variant penicillin-binding protein (PBP) called PBP2' or PBP2a. PBP2 has reduced affinity for β-lactam antibiotics and is able to substitute for the essential PBPs if they have been inactivated by β-lactam. They are resistant to most of antibiotics because they carry large conjugative plasmids bearing multiple resistance determinants. They are uniformly sensitive to vancomycin.

Methicillin-resistant *Staphylococcus aureus* (MRSA) is responsible for more than 50% nosocomial infections. The prevalence of MRSA is around 10 to 30% of all *Staphylococcus* infection. Multidrug resistance is a common feature of MRSA. Ciprofloxacin has been suggested the alternative for the treatment of MRSA infections. The dominant phage pattern of MRSA are 6/47/54/75/77.

Epidemiological markers useful in the identification of methicillin-resistant *Staphylo coccus aureus* includes antibiotype, phage type, plasmid profile, electrophenotypes and many other genotype typing methods.

Biotyping is simple, quick, reproducible and can be incorporated in bench routine. However, strain discrimination is limited.

Phage typing is standardized and reproducible, rapid to perform. It carries drawback as one has to maintain of stocks to check phages. Reverse phage typing may come up as valuable supplement to the routing phage typing. In this case, strain differentiation is limited.

Antibiotic susceptibility pattern has been used widely for typing purposes. It is not reproducible.

PREVENTION OF MRSA

❖ Maintain good hand and body hygiene.
❖ Keep cuts, scrapes and wounds clean and covered till healed
❖ Avoid sharing personal items like towels, razors, etc.
❖ Get early treatment using intravenous antibiotics of patients of infections with suspected MRSA.

STAPHYLOCOCCUS SAPROPHYTICUS

1. They are opportunistic microorganisms capable of causing:
   a. Urinary tract infection in young females
   b. In patients undergone cardiac surgery may develop septicemia endocarditis because of *Staphylococcus saprophyticus*.
2. They are resistant to novobiocin.
3. They are coagulase negative.

STAPHYLOCOCCUS ALBUS

Staphylococcus albus is coagulase negative *Staphylococcus* which is a part of skin flora.

Cultural Characters

Nutrient agar colony is pinhead size and white in color.

Blood agar colony is white and there is no hemolysis around them.

Pathogenicity: It is usually nonpathogenic. It may act as opportunist pathogens causing acne, pustules and stitch abscess. If resistance is poor, it may cause serious illness like septicemia. In persons with structural abnormalities of urinary tract, it may cause cystitis.

Differentiation Between *Staphylococcus aureus and Staphylococcus saprophyticus*

Properties	Staphylo-coccus aureus	Staphyloccus saprophyticus
• Coagulase test	+	–
• Mannitol fermentation	+	–
• DNAase production	+	–
• Phosphatase production	+	–
• Alfa lysine production	+	–
• Presence of Protein A in cell wall	+	–
• Resistance to novobiocin	–	+

STAPHYLOCOCCUS CITRUS

Staphylococcus citrus is found as saprophyte and is never pathogenic. On nutrient and blood agars, it forms lemon yellow pigmented colonies. On blood agar, it is never hemolytic. It does not ferment sugar and toxin or coagulase.

Differentiation Between *Staphylococcus aureus and Micrococcus*

Properties	Staphylococ-cus aureus	Micrococcus
• Gram staining	Gram positive, grape-like cluster exhibiting uniform staining	Gram positive in group of four or eight larger than *Staphylococcus*, not uniformly stained and darkly stained
• Colony character	Golden yellow colonies	White colored colonies
• Coagulase test	+	–
• Carbohydrate fermentation	Fermentatively	Oxidatively

MICROCOCCUS TETRAGEN (GAFFKYA TETRAGENA)

Micrococcus tetragen is a commensal of mucosa of upper respiratory tract. It is Gram-positive cocci slightly longer than staphylococci and occurs in tetrads. It is capsulated when in tissue.

Cultural Character

Fluid media: In broth, a thick deposit may develop. Supernatant fluid may remain clear.

Nutrient agar: The colony is white. It is emulsified with difficulty.

Blood agar: A zone of hemolysis may appear around colonies.

Biochemical reactions: It ferments lactose, glucose, sucrose and maltose with acid production only. Gelatin is not liquefied.

Pathogenicity: May be responsible for dental abscess, cervical adenitis, pulmonary abscess and rarely endocarditis.

SARCINA

Sarcina is similar to *Micrococcus* except that it forms pockets of 8. Some of them may be motile. It is mostly nonpathogenic.

Streptococcus

General characters: They are Gram-positive cocci arranged in chains, nonmotile and nonsporing. They require media enriched with blood, serum or ascitic fluid for their growth. They are important human pathogens causing pyogenic infection with a characteristic tendency to spread. They are also responsible for nonsuppurative lesions like acute rheumatic fever and glomerulonephritis.

Classification of *Streptococcus*: Several systems of classification have been employed:

1. **Morphological classification:** Attempt to classify streptococci into long chain (pathogenic strain) and short chain (nonpathogenic) forming cocci **(Fig. 20.1)** is not a satisfactory method of classification. Length of chain, however, depends upon the medium in which organism is grown and on several other factors.
2. **Classification based in cultural character:** Streptococci are divided into obligate anaerobe (Peptostreptococci) and aerobes or facultative anaerobes. The aerobic or facultative streptococci are further classified on the basis of hemolytic property on blood agar plate.
   a. *Alpha hemolytic:* Streptococci produce a zone of greenish discoloration around the colony. This zone of partial lysis is of 1.2 mm wide with irregular margin.
   b. *Beta hemolytic:* Streptococci produce sharply defined, clear, colorless zone of hemolysis 2 to 4 mm wide.
3. **Classification based on biochemical reactions:** Fermentation is used in differentiating different species of streptococci, e.g., mannitol is fermented by enterococci while *Streptococcus pyogenes* and *Streptococcus viridans* do not ferment mannitol.
4. **Classification based on antigenic structure:** The aerobic streptococci producing beta hemolysis are divisible into Lancefield group A, B, C, D, E, F, G, H, K, L, M, N, O, P, Q, R, S, T, U, V, on the basis of specificity of polysaccharide-C hapten antigen present on the cell wall. A majority of hemolytic streptococci that produce human infection belongs to group A. Hemolytic *Streptococcus* of group A is known as *Streptococcus pyogenes*. It may be further subdivided into types based on protein (M, T, R) present on cell surface (Griffith typing). More than 80 Griffith types of *Streptococcus pyogenes* have been recognized so far. **Table 20.1** shows diseases caused by streptococci of various groups.

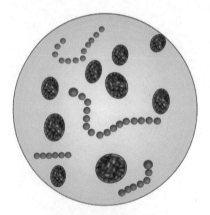

Fig. 20.1: *Streptococcus.*

Table 20.1: Diseases caused by streptococci of various groups.

Group disease caused	Habitat
A. Majority of human streptococcal diseases	Man
B. Mastitis in cows, post-natal infections in human and sepsis in newly born	Cow, human genital tract
C. Diseases in various animals. Mild respiratory infections in human.	Various animals and upper respiratory tract of humans.
D. Infections of urogenital tract in humans, endocarditis and wound infections.	Milk products, intestines of humans and animals
E. Diseases in pigs and cows	Pigs and cows
F. Respiratory infections in humans and endocarditis	Upper respiratory tract of humans
G. Mild respiratory infections in humans Genital tract infections in dogs	Upper respiratory tract of humans and dogs
H. Endocarditis	Upper respiratory tract of humans
K. Endocarditis	Upper respiratory tract of humans
L. Genital tract infections in dogs	Dogs
M. Genital tract infections in dogs	Dogs
N. Genital tract infections in dogs	Dogs
O. Endocarditis	Milk products
P. Not known	Chicken, pigs
Q. Not known	Human intestines
R. Not known	Human intestines
S. Not known	Human intestines
U. Not known	Animals
V. Not known	Animals

GROUP A

Streptococcus pyogenes

Morphology: It is 0.5 to 1 mm in diameter and arranged in chain. Chain formation is due to cocci dividing in one plane only and failure of daughter cell to separate completely. The length of a chain depends upon medium in which organism is grown. It is usually encapsulated, non-sporing and non-motile. When capsule is present it is composed of hyaluronic acid (Group A and Group C). *Streptococcus* Group B and Group C show polysaccharide capsule.

Cultural character: *Streptococcus pyogenes* is aerobic and facultative anaerobes with optimum temperature of growth being 37°C. Enriched media with whole blood, serum, ascitic fluid or glucose favors rapid growth.

1. *Fluid media:* Serum broth, 24 hours after culture shows granular growth with powdery deposits. There is no pellicle formation.
2. *Blood agar:* After 24 hours' incubation, colony is small, 0.5 to 1 mm (pin-point colonies), circular, transparent, low convex with area of hemolysis. Strains with capsules produce mucoid colonies. Virulent strains produce matted colonies (granular). A virulent strain produces glossy colonies **(Fig. 20.2)**.

Selective media: Blood agar medium having 1:5,0 0,000 crystal violet may be used as selective medium **(Fig. 20.3)**.

Biochemical reactions: It ferments lactose, glucose, salicin, sorbitol, maltose, dextrin, etc. producing acid but no gas. It is catalase negative. It does not liquefy gelatin and is not soluble in 10% bile. It hydrolysis pyrrolidonyl naphthylamide (PYR test), producing red colors. It does not ferment ribose.

Resistance: It is easily destroyed by heat at 56°C for 80 minutes. It can survive in dust for several weeks if protected from sunlight. It is resistant to crystal violet. It is susceptible to sulfonamide, etc. *Streptococcus pyogenes* is highly sensitive to bacitracin and this property is used in rapid identification of group A hemolytic streptococci.

Antigenic structure: Hemolytic streptococci possess a group specific polysaccharide C and three type specific protein antigen M, T, R and nucleoproteins **(Fig. 20.4)**.

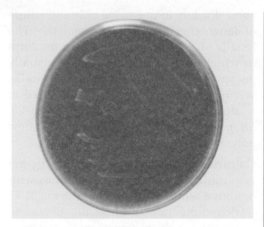

Fig. 20.2: *Streptococcus pyogenes* growth of blood agar medium.

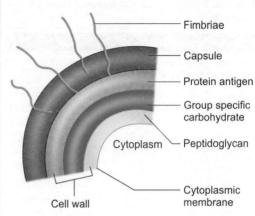

Fig. 20.4: Antigenic structure of *Streptococcus pyogenes*.

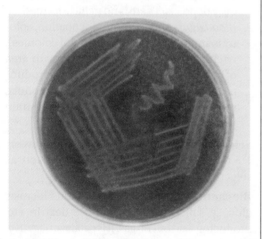

Fig. 20.3: Crystal violet blood agar plate—selective medium for *Streptococcus pyogenes*.

Polysaccharide C antigen: It confers serological specificity and hence it has 20 Lancefield groups. Human strain belongs to group A and bovine strain belongs to group B.

This antigen is an integral part of cell wall and so it has to be extracted for grouping by precipitation with specific antigen. Extraction can be done by:

1. Hydrochloric acid (Lancefield's acid extraction method).
2. Formamide (Fuller's method).
3. An enzyme produced by *Streptomyces albus* (Maxted method).
4. Autoclaving (Rantz and Randall's method).

M antigen: M protein besides determining type specificity also acts as virulence factor by inhibiting phagocytosis. Antibody to M protein is protective. M protein is alcohol soluble and is destroyed by trypsin. Over 65 protein types have been recognized in group A.

T antigen: It is acid and heat labile but trypsin resistant. It is demonstrated by agglutination with the specific antisera. Antibodies against the antigen are not protective.

It has no relationship to virulence of streptococci. It is obtained from streptococci by proteolytic digestion (otherwise rapidly destroy M proteins). It permits differentiation of certain types. Other types share the same T substance.

R antigen: *Streptococcus pyogenes* (serotypes 2, 3, 28, 48) and in some strain of group B and C, this R protein antigen is found. It has no relation to virulence.

Fimbriae are hair like consisting of M protein which are covered by lipotecoic acid and are present in streptococci group A important to attach streptococci to epithelium.

Nucleoproteins: Extraction of nucleoproteins of streptococci by treatment with weak alkali yields mixture of proteins and other substances called P substances which probably make up most of streptococcal cell body.

Other factors: M-associated protein (MAP) is identified. Some M types of *Streptococcus pyogenes* produce serum opacity factor.

Toxin Production

1. *Hemolysins:* It is filterable toxic substance. It is of two types:
   a. Streptolysin O demonstrable in deep colonies which is oxygen labile, heat labile, strongly antigenic, important in contributing to virulence (intravenous injection into animal has specific cardiotoxic activity) and it is inhibited by cholesterol.
   b. Streptolysin S is oxygen labile, non-antigenic, inhibited non-specifically by serum lipoprotein and may be nephrotoxic.
2. *Erythrogenic toxin* is filterable and heat stable toxin and is of three types: A, B and C. In small dose if injected intradermally causes erythema in susceptible persons. Administration of larger amount causes generalized rash, fever and malaise. It is erythrogenic toxin and is associated with pathogenesis of scarlet fever.
   The production of erythrogenic toxin A and C is dependent on lysogenization of streptococci with certain temperate bacteriophage. B type is chromosomal.
3. *Streptokinase (fibrinolysin)* is produced mostly by strain of group A, C and G. It is heat stable and antigenic. It promotes lysis of human fibrin clots by activating a plasma precursor. Fibrinolysin appears to play a part in streptococcal infection by breaking down fibrin barrier around lesion and spreading infection.
4. *Deoxyribonucleases (streptodornase)* causes depolymerization of DNA. It helps to liquefy thick pus. Four distinct streptodornase A, B, C and D have been recognized of which B is more antigenic in man.
5. *Diphosphopyricine nucleotidase (DPNase)* is antigenic and is specifically neutralized by antibody in convalescent sera. It is believed to be leukotoxic. It acts on the coenzyme DPN and liberates nicotinamide from the molecule.
6. *Hyaluronidase* is a spreading factor present in culture filtrate of *Streptococcus pyogenes.* It breaks down hyaluronic acid of the tissue. This favors spread of infection along intercellular space. Streptococci possess a hyaluronic acid capsule and also elaborate hyaluronidase, self-destructive process. But strains that produce hyaluronidase in large amounts (M type 4, 22) are non-capsulated and hence no hyaluronic acid.
7. *Protease* is intracellular enzyme produced at acidic pH in cultures grown at 37°C. It destroys M type specific protein and also inhibits production of fibrinolysin and hyaluronidase. It is produced in areas of inflammation. The biological significance of this enzyme is not known.
   Amylase and esterase are also produced but it is not known whether they play any role in natural infection or not.

Pathogenicity: *Streptococcus pyogenes* is more invasive and produces septicemia readily. There is a tendency to spread locally along lymphatics and through bloodstream.

1. *Respiratory infection:* Throat is the primary site of invasion causing sore throat. It may be localized in tonsils (tonsillitis) or may involve pharynx (pharyngitis).
   Scarlet fever is caused by a strain-producing erythrogenic toxin. This accounts for characteristic erythematous rash. This is uncommon in the tropics and does not occur in India.
   From throat, streptococci may spread to the surrounding tissue causing otitis media, mastoiditis, Ludwig angina and suppurative adenitis. It may cause meningitis. Bronchopneumonia may occur when *Streptococcus pyogenes* acts as secondary invader, e.g., influenza. Sometimes empyema may result.
2. *Skin infection:* It may cause suppurative infection of skin, e.g., wound, burns, lymph-

angitis and cellulitis. Infection of abrasion may lead to fatal septicemia.

Apart from this, it may cause erysipelas and impetigo. Erysipelas is a diffuse infection involving superficial lymphatic. The involved skin becomes red, swollen and indurated. It is found in old patients. In impetigo, *Streptococcus pyogenes* of group A type 4, 25 are involved. It is seen in young children. Impetigo may lead to glomerulonephritis in children of tropics but do not often lead to rheumatic fever.

3. *Genital tract: Streptococcus pyogenes* is an important cause of puerperal sepsis. The source of infection is nasopharynx of doctors, nurses and attendants, etc.

4. Other infections like abscess of organs (brain, lungs, liver, kidneys) may occur. It may cause septicemia and pyemia.

5. *Non-suppurative complications:* They are:
   a. Acute rheumatic fever.
   b. Acute glomerulonephritis.

The pathogenesis of these conditions is not clearly understood. They require 1 to 3 weeks after acute infection. No organism is detected when sequelae sets in. Comparison of acute rheumatic fever and acute glomerulonephritis is shown in **Table 20.2**.

Acute rheumatic fever: It is a systemic non-suppurative inflammatory condition characterized by fever, pancarditis, migratory polyarthritis, sometimes chorea and subcutaneous nodules. Usually, disease is preceded by an attack of streptococcal sore throat, septic tonsillitis or respiratory tract infection.

The hypersensitivity to streptococci or its products is suggested in pathogenesis of rheumatic fever because of:
1. Absence of organism in the lesion.
2. Latent period between attack of sore throat and onset of rheumatic disease.
3. Similarity of disease produced experimentally in rabbit.

It is suggested that lesion of rheumatic fever may be the result of hypersensitivity to some streptococcal component produced by repeated attacks. Rheumatic fever has marked

Table 20.2: Comparison of rheumatic fever and glomerulonephritis.

	Acute rheumatic fever	Acute glomerulone-phritis
Site of infection	Throat	Throat or skin
Prior sensitization	Essential	Not necessary
Serotype of Streptococcus pyogenes	Any	Nephritogenic only (12, 49, 2, 52, 55, 57, 4)
Immune response	Marked	Moderate
Complement levels	Unaffected	Lowered
Hereditary tendency	Present	Not known
Repeated attack	Common	Absent
Penicillin prophylaxis	Essential	Not indicated
Course	Progressive	Spontaneous
Prognosis	Variable	Good

tendency to be reactivated by recurrent streptococcal infections, whereas nephritis does not have this characteristic. It has also been suggested that there may be an element of anti-immunity involved and antigenic cross-reaction between streptococci and heart tissue also has been demonstrated.

Acute glomerulonephritis: It is caused by only few nephritogenic strain of group A (4, 12, 49, 2, 52, 57), type 12 being the most common. The most important antigen is probably in streptococcal protoplast membrane. The immunity in streptococcal infection is type specific and so acute glomerulonephritis is non-recurring condition. Not only sore throat but pyoderma or impetigo may also lead to nephritis. It is self-limited episode that resolves without any permanent damage.

Pathogenesis may be due to antigenic cross-reaction, between glomerular antigens and some components of nephritogenic streptococci. More often, it may be immune complex disease.

Laboratory Diagnosis

1. **Hematological investigations:**
   a. Total leukocyte count may show considerable increase.

b. *Differential leukocyte* counts show increase in neutrophil count. Polymorph neutrophil may constitute more than 80%.

c. Erythrocyte sedimentation rate (ESR) is raised especially in rheumatic disease. It is done to estimate the activity of disease.

2. **Bacteriological method**: Most important specimens are throat swab, nasopharyngeal swab, pus swab, sputum, cerebrospinal fluid, blood, etc.

a. Smear from above material after Gram's straining, show Gram-positive cocci arranged in chains.

b. *Culture:* Specimen is cultured on blood agar or crystal violet blood agar media with loop. After overnight incubation at 37°C, colonies are studied. These are small (pin-point); raised colonies showing beta hemolysis. Hemolytic streptococci are grouped further by Lancefield technique. A rapid presumptive identification of group 'A' streptococci can be made by performing bacitracin sensitivity test **(Fig. 20.5)**. For rapid diagnosis, swab or pus specimens are cultured in broth; and after 2 to 3 hours, smears are stained with fluorescein labeled group A antiserum.

c. *Serological test:* The titer of antistreptolysin O in a patient serum in dilution above 1: 200 is an indication of streptococcal infection. It is also useful for detecting asymptomatic carriers of *Streptococcus pyogenes.* A titer above 286 of antistreptolysin O is suggestive of rheumatic activity. A use in antibody titer to other streptococcal antigens may be estimated, e.g., anti-DNase, anti- hyaluronidase (especially in skin infections), antistreptokinase, anti-M type specific antibodies, etc. Streptozyme test is useful in detection of antibodies to antigen and enzymes.

3. **Skin test** is known by the name Dick test.

Dick test: It is done to find out susceptibility of a person to scarlet fever. 0.2 mL erythrogenic toxin is injected intradermally on the forearm and same amount of heated inactivated toxin on the other forearm. A bright red rash appears within 6 hours and becomes maximum in 24 hours and thereafter this fades away. Control forearm does not show any reaction. A positive reaction means no immunity to scarlet fever. A negative reaction means immunity.

4. **Schultz-Charlton reaction**: Erythrogen antitoxin is injected intradermally in a patient with scarlatinal rash. There is local blanching of rash.

Treatment: *Streptococcus pyogenes* is sensitive to penicillin, sulfonamide and several other antibiotics. However, penicillin is the drug of choice. Antitoxic serum was used to be administered effectively in scarlet fever.

▌GROUP B

Streptococcus agalactiae is responsible for mastitis in cow. It may be present in human throat and vagina as commensal. It can be identified by CAMP (Christie-Atkins-Munch-Petersen) reaction.

On the basis of type specific capsular antigens, they are divided into four groups, ia, ib, ii and iii. All the strains of type ia and ib are from human source.

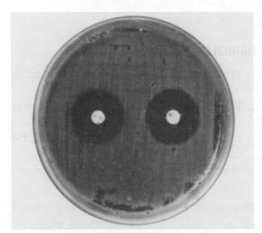

Fig. 20.5: *Streptococcus pyogenes* showing bacitracin and pencillin sensitivity.

DISEASES CAUSED BY GROUP 'B' STREPTOCOCCI

Newborn

❖ Pneumonia
❖ Meningitis
❖ Respiratory diseases
❖ Osteomyelitis.

Adult

❖ Endocarditis
❖ Septicemia
❖ Meningitis
❖ Arthritis
❖ Wound sepsis
❖ Pyoderma.

It is rarely pathogenic in man. Sometimes, they may cause puerperal infection, septicemia, meningitis and ulcerative endocarditis, etc.

GROUP C

Streptococcus equisimilis is isolated from horses and cows. It may produce streptolysin O and fibrinolysin. The organisms have been isolated from puerperal infection, cellulitis, wound and scarlet fever.

GROUP D

Group D streptococci can be divided into enterococci, e.g., *Enterococcus fecalis* (**Fig. 20.6**), *Enterococcus fecium, Enterococcus durans, Enterococcus avium* and so on. *Enterococcus fecalis* is the most common of all above. It ferments mannitol with gas production, VP positive with PYR test positive and can be grown on blood tellurite producing black colonies.

Enterococcus fecalis may cause urinary tract infection, wound infection, infective endocarditis, biliary tract infection, peritonitis, suppurative abdominal lesions and septicemia. Important characteristics of enterococci are:
❖ Normal flora of lower intestinal tract and vagina.
❖ Can grow in 6.5% sodium chloride, 40% bile and at 45°C.

Fig. 20.6: Slanetz and Bartley medium *Enterococcus fecalis*.

❖ On sheep blood agar may produce alpha, beta hemolysis or may be non-hemolytic too.
❖ Tiny, deep pink colonies appear on Mac-Conkey agar medium.
❖ Most strains are resistant to penicillin, sulfonamide and also to cephalosporin, gentamycin, streptomycin, etc.
❖ Survive heat up to 60°C for 30 minutes.
❖ Non-motile, Gram-positive cocci, non-capsulated and may be arranged in pairs or short chain.
❖ PYR test positive.

Cultural Characters

1. **Fluid media**: It shows uniform turbidity after 24 hour incubation at 37°C.
2. **Blood agar**: Colony is little bigger than *Streptococcus pyogenes,* circular, raised, low convex and emulsifies easily. Most of the strains are non-hemolytic.
3. **MacConkey agar medium**: Colonies are tiny, and deep pink in color.

Biochemical reactions: It ferments mannitol, sucrose, sorbitol, aesculin and grows on tellurite blood agar producing black colonies.

Resistance: It grows at pH 9.6 in the presence of 6.5% sodium chloride, and also in the presence of 40% bile. It survives at 60°C temperature for 30 minutes.

Pathogenicity: It invades tissues and may produce pyogenic lesions, e.g., cystitis, pyelitis, vaginitis, cervicitis, puerperal sepsis and subacute bacterial endocarditis.

Non-enterococci, e.g., *Streptococcus bovis, Streptococcus equinus, Streptococcus avium,* etc. may cause urinary tract infection, endocarditis, septicemia. They may be nonhemolytic and susceptible to penicillin.

Group F, G, H and O may occur as commensal in the throat.

ALPHA HEMOLYTIC STREPTOCOCCI

Some streptococci do not produce soluble hemolysin. It is characterized by production of alpha hemolytic colonies on blood agar. It includes:

a. *Streptococcus viridans.*
b. *Streptococcus salivarium.*
c. *Streptococcus mitis.*
d. *Streptococcus MG.*

Streptococcus viridans: It is present as a commensal on mucosa of mouth, nasopharynx and saliva of man. On the basis of biochemical reactions, it is classified into five species *(Streptococcus salivarium, mutans, sanguis, mitior, milleri).* On blood agar, it produces alpha hemolysis **(Fig. 20.7).**

It is normally nonpathogenic. Sometimes, it may cause subacute bacterial endocarditis and formation of plaque on teeth leading to dental caries, etc.

Diagnosis of subacute bacterial endocarditis is established by repeated blood culture. It is susceptible to penicillin.

Streptococcus salivarium: It is nonpathogenic found in mouth and intestine of man. *Streptococcus salivarium* can grow at 45°C and produce large mucoid colonies on agar containing 5 percent raffinose and salicin.

Streptococcus mitis: It does not grow at 45°C. Colonies are non-mucoid, smaller and surrounded by a wide zone of alpha hemolysis.

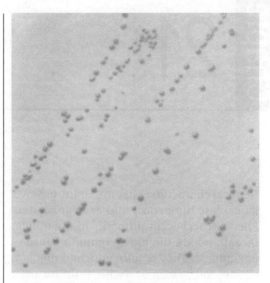

Fig. 20.7: Colonies of *Streptococcus viridans.*

Streptococcus MG: It belongs to group E. It is isolated from sputum of patient suffering from primary atypical pneumonia. It is capsulated. The organism is agglutinated by the serum of some patient suffering from atypical pneumonia.

ANAEROBIC STREPTOCOCCUS

Peptostreptococcus putridus: The natural habitat of anaerobic streptococci is female genital tract. The culture on blood agar medium is incubated anaerobically in McIntosh Fildes jar for 48 hours. The colony is 2 to 4 mm, circular, raised and translucent. There is no hemolysis.

It ferments glucose, maltose and fructose with abundant gas production. It produces puerperal sepsis, and puerperal septicemia, brain abscess and other suppurative and gangrenous lesions.

ANAEROBIC COCCI

Gram-positive	Gram-negative
Peptococcus	Veillonella
Streptococcus	Acidaminococcus
Peptostreptococcus	Megaphaera
Ruminococcus	
Caprococcus	

General characters: They are Gram-positive, lanceolate diplococci and are capsulated. Pneumococci occur primarily in the human throat and are the most common cause of pneumonia. They require enriched medium with blood, serum or ascitic fluid for their growth. On blood agar, they produce alpha hemolysis. Of late, they are reclassified as *Streptoccocus pneumoniae*.

Morphology: It is typically small (1 μ) slightly elongated with one end broad and other pointed (flame shaped). It occurs in pairs **(Fig. 21.1)**. It is capsulated, capsule enclosing each pair. It is non-motile and non-sporing. It is Gram-positive. In India, ink preparation capsule appears as a clear halo **(Fig. 21.2)**.

Cultural characters: It requires serum or whole blood for growth. It grows best at 37°C and at pH 7.6. It is aerobic and facultative anaerobic. Growth is improved by providing them 5 to 10% CO_2. Characters of growth on following media are:

1. Serum and glucose broth shows uniform turbidity after 24 hours growth. After 36 hours, autolysis occurs. There is no pellicle formation.
2. *Blood agar:* Colony is small (0.5 to 1 mm), dome shaped with area of greenish discoloration (alpha hemolysis) around them. On further incubation, the colonies become flat with raised edges and central umbonation (draughtsman appearance) **(Fig. 21.3)**. Type III pneumococci are longer and have mucoid appearance.

Biochemical reaction: It ferments many sugars, forming acid only. Inulin is fermented

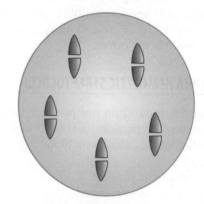

Fig. 21.1: *Pneumococcus.*

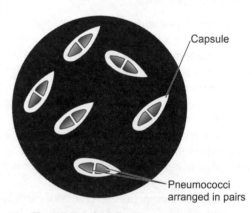

Capsule

Pneumococci arranged in pairs

Fig. 21.2: India ink preparation showing capsule of pneumococci.

by all Pneumococci. They are bile soluble (few drops of 10% sodium desoxycholate solution are added to 1 mL of overnight broth culture). The culture clears due to lysis of cocci. It is catalase and oxidase negative.

Resistance: It is readily destroyed by heat (52°C for 15 minutes), in one hour by

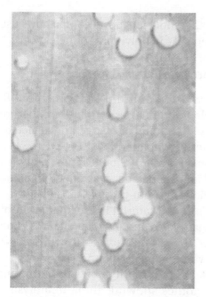

Fig. 21.3: Draughtsman colonies of *Pneumococcus.*

phenol, potassium permanganate and other antiseptics.

It is sensitive to sulfonamide. It is sensitive to optochin (ethyl hydrocuprein) in 1/80,000 and it is useful in differentiating them from streptococci.

Strain may be maintained on semisolid blood agar or by lyophilization.

Antigenic structures: Pneumococci possesses a number of antigens:

1. *Nucleoprotein:* It is neither species specific nor type specific. Antibody to this antigen is not protective.
2. *Species specific polysaccharides hapten:* It is situated at the cell surface and is not related with capsular antigen.
3. *Capsular polysaccharide:* It is found in capsulated form. It determines type specificity of organism and virulence. Pneumococci isolated from lobar pneumonia are classified into four types: I, II, III and heterogeneous group IV. Members of group IV are further classified into various types. Now about 90 types are known named 1, 2, 3, etc.

Typing may be carried out by:

1. Agglutination of cocci with type specific antiserum.
2. Precipitation of capsular polysaccharides with specific serum.
3. Capsular swelling reaction (Quellung reaction): Here suspension of Pneumococci is mixed with type specific antiserum. In the presence of homologous antiserum the capsule becomes apparently swollen, delineated and refractile.

Toxin and Other Virulence Factors

1. *Hemolysin: Pneumococcus* produces soluble hemolysin in young culture. It gives characteristic green coloration around colonies. It is oxygen labile and its role in the pathogenesis of Pneumococcal infection is not known.
2. *Capsular polysaccharide:* It is specific soluble substance which protects the organism from phagocytosis. It is acidic and has hydrophilic properties. Hence, this substance has association with virulence.
3. Pneumococci produce large amounts of enzyme resembling receptor destroying enzyme of influenza virus.
4. *Leucocidin:* It kills leukocytes.

Pathogenesis: Pneumococci get attached to nasopharyngeal cell through bacterial surface adhesion (pneumococcal surface antigen-A or choline-binding proteins) with epithelial cell receptors. Epithelial binding sites include glycoconjugates containing the disaccharide GlcHAcgb1-4 Gal or assialo-GM1 glycolipid.

Once nasopharynx is colonized, infection may result if pneumococci are carried to eustachian tubes or nasal sinuses, etc.

Pneumococci produce disease through their ability to multiply in the tissue. They produce no toxin of significance. The virulence of organism is a function of its capsule, which prevents or delays ingestion of encapsulated cells by phagocytes.

Pneumococcal infection causes an outpouring of fibrinous edema fluid into alveoli, followed by red cells and leukocytes, which results in consolidation of portion of lung. Many pneumococci are found throughout this exudate. Later mononuclear cells actively phagocytose the debris, and this liquid phase is gradually reabsorbed. The pneumococci are taken up by phagocytes and are digested intracellularly.

In man, 80% lobar pneumonia and 60% bronchopneumonia are caused by pneumococci. It also produces suppurative infection in various parts of body as under:

1. *Lobar pneumonia:* Airborne infection of respiratory tract is a frequent occurrence. The organism is generally eliminated by natural defence mechanism. If resistance is lowered, organism penetrates bronchial mucosa and spreads through lung along peribronchial tissue and lymphatics. Bacteremia is frequent during early stages. Toxemia is due to diffusion of capsular polysaccharide into blood and tissue. The fall of temperature by crisis and relief coincide with complete neutralization of capsular polysaccharide by anticapsular antibodies. Serotypes 1 to 8, 12, 14, are mostly the cause of pneumonia. Type 3 strain produces particularly severe infection.

2. *Bronchopneumonia:* It is always secondary infection following viral infection of respiratory tract. Bronchopneumonia may be caused by any serotype of pneumococci.

3. *Pneumococcal meningitis* is most serious pneumococcal infection. It occurs when pneumococcal pneumonia is persistant. Disease is common in children.

4. They may produce suppurative lesions like empyema, pericarditis, otitis media, sinusitis, conjunctivitis and peritonitis.

Laboratory Diagnosis

1. Hematological Investigations

a. Total leukocyte count usually shows leukocytosis. Count may be more than 15,000 per cu mm.

b. Differential leukocyte count shows usually increase in polymorphonuclear cells.

2. Bacteriological Investigations

a. *Material:* Sputum, cerebrospinal fluid, pleural fluid, pericardial fluid, peritoneal fluid and pus discharge are collected in a sterile container.

b. *Smear examination:* Gram staining shows flame-shaped cocci arranged in pairs and they are Gram-positive capsulated.

c. *Culture:* Material is inoculated on blood agar plates and incubated at 37°C under 5 to 10% carbon dioxide. Growth occurs after overnight incubation.
Blood culture: It shows flat, umbonated colonies showing alpha hemolysis. The colonies are treated for inulin fermentation, bile solubility and optochin sensitivity test to differentiate it from *Streptococcus viridans.*

d. *Immunologic methods:* The detection of pneumococcal capsular polysaccharides in sputum and other body fluids by immunologic methods such as counterimmunoelectro phoresis or latex agglutination provides an alternative to bacteriologic techniques for presumptive diagnosis of pneumococcal infection. Because of crossreactions between the polysaccharides of pneumococci and other bacterial species, immunologic diagnosis is less specific than bacteriologic diagnosis.

e. *Animal pathogenicity:* Mice are most susceptible to pneumococcal infection (except type 14). It is used for rapid diagnosis. Sputum is emulsified with saline. One mL is inoculated intraperitoneally into 2 mice. Animal usually dies within 24 hours. The encapsulated diplococci can be demonstrated in heart blood and peritoneal fluid.

Treatment: Sulfonamides and penicillins are quite effective drugs. Resistance may develop with antibiotics like sulfonamides and tetracycline. Rarely, penicillin-resistant

Table 21.1: Differentiation between *Pneumococcus* and *Streptococcus viridans*.

Pneumococcus	Streptococcus viridans
• Morphology	
– Capsulated	• Non-capsulated
– Flame-shaped diplococci	• Oval or round arranged in chain
• Quellung test positive	• Negative
• Colonies Initially dome shaped and later on draughtsman colonies	• Dome shaped
• Growth in liquid media shows uniform turbidity	• Granular turbidity and powdery deposits
• Bile solubility is positive	• Negative
• Inulin fermentation is positive	• Negative
• Optochin sensitivity is positive	• Negative
• Intraperitoneal inoculation in mice brings fatal infection	• Nonpathogenic

strains of pneumococci do occur. It is possible to immune persons with type specific polysaccharides. It provides 90% protection. A vaccine has also been developed, (include type 1, 2, 3, 4, 6, 8, 9, 12, 14, 19, 23, 25, 51 and 56) which may be useful for elderly, debilitated or immunosuppressed individuals. This vaccine was licensed in the USA in 1977. In 1983, an expanded polysaccharide vaccine containing 23 types was licensed in the USA. Currently, pneumococcal vaccines of capsular polysaccharides conjugated to proteins such as diphtheria toxoid are being developed.

However, pneumococci may be differentiated from *Streptococcus viridans* as shown in **Table 21.1**.

General characters: They are Gram-negative, aerobic, non-sporulating, non-motile, oxidase positive cocci arranged in pairs. The genus contains about 30 species. Two important pathogens are:
a. *N. meningitidis*
b. *N. gonorrhoeae*

NEISSERIA MENINGITIDIS

Morphology: It is Gram-negative, oval or spherical 0.8 μ to 0.6 μ, arranged in pairs with adjacent sides flattened **(Fig. 22.1)**. Its considerable variation in size, shape and staining property especially in old culture is due to autolysis. In smear from lesion, the cocci are more regular and are intracellular. Sometimes, microcapsule may be demonstrated by Quellung reaction.

Cultural characters: Growth occurs in media enriched with blood, serum or ascitic fluid. Growth is improved by adding 10% carbon dioxide. It is aerobic and grows at optimum temperature 37°C and pH 7.4.

Fluid media: The serum broth shows mild or moderate turbidity after 24 hours incubation at 37°C.

Blood agar: The colony is moist, elevated, smooth, translucent, round and convex. It is of 1 mm diameter with glistening surface and entire edge. The colony is butyrous in consistency and easily emulsifiable. There is no hemolysis.

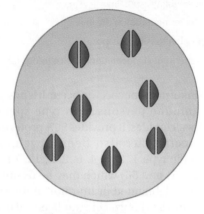

Fig. 22.1: *Meningococcus.*

Chocolate agar plate: Character of the colony is same as described above. Involution forms appear soon due to active autolysis.

Biochemical reaction: It is catalase and oxidase positive. Glucose and maltose are fermented producing acid and no gas.

Classification: At least 13 serogroups of meningococci have been identified (A, B, C, D, X, Y, Z, W-135, 29E, H, I, K and L) by immunologic specificity of capsular polysaccharides. This grouping is assuming practical importance due to the recent attempts to develop vaccine against protein which is group specific.

The nucleoproteins meningococci (P substance) have some toxic effect. Certain DNA extracts are capable of inducing streptomycin resistance in Meningococci.

Resistance: It is highly susceptible to heat, desiccation, alteration in pH and to disinfectants. It may acquire resistance to streptomycin readily.

Pathogenicity: Meningococci are strict human parasites. The route of infection is usually nasopharynx. They produce cerebrospinal meningitis and meningococcal septicemia. Bacteremia favored by absence of bactericidal antibody (IgG) or its inhibition by blocking IgA antibody or a complement deficiency (C5, C6, C7 or C8).

From nasopharynx, meningococci may spread along perineural sheath of olfactory nerve, through cribriform plate to subarachnoid space. Alternatively, spread may be through blood and conjunctiva. On reaching central nervous system, a suppurative lesion of meninges is set up involving surface of spinal cord, base and cortex of brain. The cocci are invariably demonstrated from cerebrospinal fluid lying free or intracellular in leukocytes.

Meningococcemia: It presents as acute fever with chills and malaise. Hemorrhagic manifestation is characteristic. In early disease, petechial rash may occur which is due to thrombosis of many small blood vessels in many organs, with perivascular infiltration and petechial hemorrhage. Meningococci may be isolated from petechial rash lesion. There may be metastatic involvement of joint, ear, lungs, myocardium and adrenals.

Toxin: Endotoxin is released by the autolysis of organism. There are hemorrhagic manifestations.

Laboratory Diagnosis

1. *Hematological investigations:*
   a. Total leukocyte count shows marked leukocytosis. Count may be more than 15,000.
   b. Differential leukocyte count shows increase in polymorphonuclear cells.

2. *Cerebrospinal fluid examination:*
   a. Macroscopically fluid is mild to moderately turbid. It is under pressure and contains many pus cells when examined microscopically.
   b. One portion of fluid is centrifuged and studied after Gram staining. Meningococci will be seen mainly inside polymorph and extracellularly also.
   c. Meningococci second portion is inoculated on blood agar or chocolate agar under 5 to 10% carbon dioxide. After 24 hours' incubation, we will identify Meningococci on the basis of morphology and biochemical reactions.
   d. Third portion of CSF is incubated overnight and then subcultured on chocolate agar. This method may succeed when direct method fails.

3. *Blood culture:* In meningococcal and in early cases of meningitis culture is positive.

4. *Nasopharyngeal swab:* It is useful in carriers.

5. *Petechial lesion:* Meningococci may be collected from petechial hemorrhage.

6. *Autopsy:* It is done on meninges, lateral ventricles, surface of brain and spinal cord. After smear and culture, organisms are identified. These must be tested within 12 hours of death of patient.

7. *Retrospective evidence:* It may be obtained by demonstrating complement fixing antibodies in convalescent sera. However, antibodies to meningopoly-saccharides can be measured by latex agglutination or hemagglutination test.

8. *Polymerase chain reaction (PCR):* DNA from cerebrospinal fluid or blood may be amplified and detected. Hence PCR may be used as rapid method.

Treatment: Sulfonamides or chloramphenicol are used in the treatment of meningitis. With sulfonamide drug resistant strain may emerge and hence in such situation penicillin G or chloramphenicol is used. Immunization with polysaccharide vaccine has given good protection and so may be used

prophylactically. The various preparations of capsular polysaccharides available are:
1. Monvalent, i.e. group A or C.
2. Bivalent, i.e. group A and C.
3. Quadrivalent, i.e. group A, C, Y and W 135. Dose is 50 mg subcutaneously. Children require two doses with interval of 3 months, whereas adults require single dose. Protective efficacy of this vaccine is claimed as 90 percent.

NEISSERIA GONORRHOEAE

Morphology: It is strictly a parasite of man. The coccus is Gram-negative, oval or spherical 0.8 to 0.6 μ with adjacent side concave (bean shaped) arranged in pair as compared with mieningococci (**Table 22.1** and **Fig. 22.2**). It is found predominantly within the polymorphs.

Cultural characters: It is aerobic. Growth occurs best at 37°C and at pH 7.4. Addition of 5 to 10 percent carbon dioxide is essential. An enriched media is required for its growth. The following media may be used:

Serum broth: Growth is poor at 37°C in 24 hours. Growth is mainly on the surface with no turbidity.

Chocolate agar: After 48 hours of incubation, colonies are round, convex, translucent, gray white, 0.5 to 1 mm in diameter with glistening surface and entire margin. Consistency is viscid and difficult to emulsify.

Thayer-Martin medium: It is a selective medium. It inhibits many contaminants including non-pathogenic *Neisseria*. This medium contains vancomycin, colistin and nystatin.

Chacko Nair egg enriched medium: It supports good growth.

Biochemical reaction: It ferments glucose with formation of acid only. Catalase and oxidase is positive.

Classification: On the basis of colony morphology, auto-agglutinability and virulence, there are four biotypes (T1, T2, T3 and T4). T1 and T2 are small, brown, autoagglutinable and virulent. T3 and T4 produce large non-pigmented colonies which are avirulent.

Antigenic structure: Gonococci are serologically heterogenous. Gonococci possess

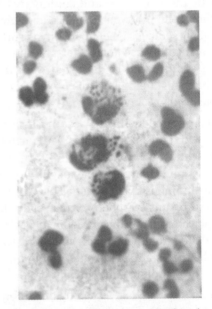

Fig. 22.2: Gonococci from smear of urethral discharge.

Table 22.1: Differences between *Gonococcus* and *Meningococcus*.

Neisseria meningitidis	Neisseria gonorrhoeae
• They occur as intracellular diplococci in smear of exudate	• S ame
• Adjacent sides are flat	• They are concave
• Colonies are butyrous easily emulsified	• Viscid colonies difficult to emulsify
• Produce acid in glucose and maltose	• Acid is produced in glucose only

polysaccharides and nucleoproteins. They also possess capsule demonstrated by negative staining. H8 is a surface exposed protein which is heat stable. The outer membrane is a macromolecular complex, an iron regulated protein are other antigenic constant proteins of Gonococci and all of them have poorly defined role in pathogenesis.

Resistance: It is killed by heat, drying and antiseptics. It is susceptible to sulfonamides, penicillin and other antibiotics.

Pathogenicity: The Gonococcus is a specific human parasite causing a venereal disease called gonorrhea. It produces lesions as follows:

Incubation period is 2 to 8 days. In male it starts as acute urethritis with mucopurulent discharge containing Gonococci. Infection may extend along urethra to prostate, seminal vesicle and epididymis. It may spread to periurethral tissue causing multiple discharging sinuses (watercan perineum).

In females, infection involves urethra and cervix uteri. Vagina is spared because of acidic pH. The infection may spread to Bartholin glands, endometrium and fallopian tubes. Salpingitis may lead to sterility.

Proctitis occurs in both sexes. Pharyngitis and conjunctivitis may occur. Blood invasion for primary infection may lead to lesions like arthritis, ulcerative endocarditis and rarely pyelonephritis, meningitis and pyemia. Ophthalmia neonatorum may occur in newborn as a result of infection from genital tract of mother.

Gonococci contain several plasmids. At least one such plasmid carries the gene for betalactamase production that makes the Gonococcus resistant to penicillin. Gonococci attach to surface epithelial cells with pili. Some *Gonococci* secrete proteases that can break down surface IgA antibodies.

In low concentration of free iron, Gonococci cannot grow. Gonococci only bind human transferrin and lactoferrin by producing iron repressible proteins (Fe RPs) that function in the removal of iron from transferrin and lactoferrin. This specificity has been used to explain why Gonococci are obligate human pathogens.

Attachment of Gonococci to mucosal cells is mediated in part by pili and by protein II. Pili also impede phagocytosis of Gonococci by neutrophils and antibody to pili is opsonic. An enzyme IgA protease which inactivates SIg Al interfere with IgA mediated antiadherence activity and hence increased attachment. Other factors which are important in pathogenesis are tumor necrosis factors (damage to fallopian tube), peptidoglycan fragments (toxic for fallopian tube mucosa), several proteases, peptidases and phospholipases.

Laboratory Diagnosis

1. *Hematological investigations:*
   a. Total leukocyte count shows leukocytosis.
   b. Differential leukocyte count shows increase in polymorphonuclear cells.

2. *Bacteriological examination:*
   Smear examination: Gram's staining of smear from purulent discharge (urethra, cervix, etc.) shows Gram-negative diplococci inside polymorphs. The use of fluorescent antibody technique is specific and sensitive method of identification. In male, meatus is cleaned with gauze soaked in saline and sample of discharge is collected with platinum loop for culture and smear. In female, besides urethral discharge, cervical swab should also be studied.

   In chronic infection, there may not be any urethral discharge. Here exudate may be obtained after prostatic massage.

Culture: It is done on soft blood agar not chocolate agar incubated in jar containing 10 percent CO_2. Material should be incubated immediately. In case of delay charcoal impregnated swab should be sent to laboratory in Stuart transport medium. In chronic cases, where mixed infection is usual, it is better to use selective medium like Thayer-Martin medium.

Serological test: Serum and genital fluid contain IgA and IgG antibodies against Gonococcal pili, outer membrane protein and lipopolysaccharide.

1. *Complement fixation test (CFT):* It is done with polyvalent antigen. It becomes positive 2 weeks after infection and remains positive for long time even after the cure of disease. It becomes positive even after meningococcal infection.
2. *Flocculation test:* It is simpler test than CFT. It has all disadvantages of CFT.

   Other serological techniques are radio-immunoassay, and ELISA. However, these tests lack specificity and reliability as diagnostic aids.

Nucleic acid probe: It may be used to detect Gonococci in urethral and cervical specimen.

Treatment: Sulfonamides and penicillin with probenecid is quite effective. Alternatively, tetracycline or erythromycin can be used. With the emergence of beta lactamase-producing Gonococci we require the use of spectinomycin, trimethoprim sulfamethoxazole or cefoxitin.

Following vaccines are being considered:

1. A Gonococcal pilus vaccine effective against only homologous strain (prevents attachment of Gonococci to mucosal surface).
2. Vaccines containing 3 or 5 serotypes of protein 1 (bacteriocidal effect).
3. Gonococcal lipopolysaccharide vaccine (under study).
4. Finally multicomponents vaccine may be prepared.

Commensal Neisseriae

They may inhabit normal respiratory tract. Their pathogenic significance is uncertain. *N. flavescens* and *N. catarrhalis* have been reported occasionally as having caused meningitis. Characteristic features of some of them are shown in **Table 22.2.**

Table 22.2: Characteristics of species of *Neisseria*.

Species	Colonies	Growth on nutrient agar	Growth at 27°C	Glucose	Fermentation Maltose	Sucrose	Serological
N. meningitidis	Round, smooth, glistening and creamy consistency	—	—	A	A	—	8 antigenic groups
N. gonorrhoeae	Same as above but small and opalescent	—	—	A	—	—	Antigens heterogeneous
N. flavescens	Same but pigmented	+	±	—	—	—	Antigenically distinct yellow homogeneous group
N. sicca	Small, dry, opaque, wrinkled, and brittle	+	+	A	A	A	Autoagglutinable
N. catarrhalis	Variable, small, trans-lucent, opaque and not emulsifiable	+	+	—	—	—	Autoagglutinable

Non-gonococcal Urethritis

Urethritis due to causes other than Gonococci is described as non-gonococcal or non-specific urethritis. Here Gonococci cannot be demonstrated from urethral lesions.

Etiology

1. Gonococci (L form).
2. Chlamydial infection (TRIC).
3. *Mycoplasma* (*Ureaplasma urealyticum, Mycoplasma hominis*).
4. *Haemophilus vaginalis (Gardnerella vaginalis).*
5. *Candida albicans.*
6. *Trichomonas vaginalis.*
7. *Mobiluncus* (recently classified genus).
8. *Acinetobacter iwoffi.*
9. Chemical and mechanical irritation.

   Since etiological diagnosis is difficult to make, hence management is also difficult.

Veillonella

They are small, anaerobic, Gram-negative cocci that are part of normal mouth flora. They ferment a few sugars and probably are not pathogenic.

General characters: They are Gram-positive, non-acid fast and non-motile bacilli occurring in palisade. They frequently show club-shaped swelling at the ends and irregular staining. *Corynebacterium diphtheriae* is the pathogenic member and it shows metachromatic granules in Albert-stained smear. It produces powerful exotoxin.

CORYNEBACTERIUM DIPHTHERIAE

Morphology: It is thin, slender, rod 3 to 6 μ × 0.6 to 0.8 μ showing clubbing at one or both ends. It is non-sporing, non-capsulated and non-motile. It is Gram-positive and shows pleomorphism. The presence of metachromatic granules (Babes-Ernst granules) serve to distinguish it from diphtheroid. The granules are colored dark purple with methylene blue, Albert or Neisser's differential stain. There may be one or more granule in a simple cell. The granules consist of polymerized metaphosphate.

The bacilli are arranged in characteristic fashion. It is seen in pairs or groups. Bacilli form various angles with each other like V or L. This is called Chinese letter arrangement **(Fig. 23.1)**. This is due to incomplete separation of daughter cells after binary fission.

Cultural character: Enrichment of media with blood, serum or egg is necessary for good growth. The optimum temperature is 37°C and pH 7.2. It is aerobic and facultative anaerobic.
1. *Serum broth:* Turbidity, pellicle formation, amount and nature of deposit is useful in

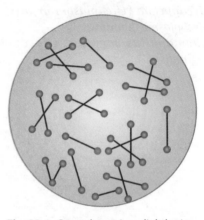

Fig. 23.1: *Corynebacterium diphtheriae.*

identification of types of *Corynebacterium diphtheriae.*
2. *Loeffler's slope culture* shows abundant growth after 6 to 8 hours incubation. The colony is small, granular, moist, creamy and glistening with irregular edges.
3. *Blood tellurite medium* (0.04%): It is useful in differentiation of *Corynebacterium diphtheriae* into gravis, mitis and intermedius types. It acts as selective media inhibiting the growth of other organisms. Diphtheria bacilli reduce tellurite to metallic tellurium giving gray to black color to colonies **(Fig. 23.2)**.

Biochemical Reactions

It ferments glucose and maltose with acid production only. Fermentation of starch, glycogen and dextrin is useful for recognition

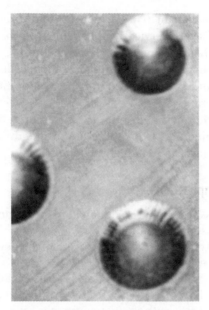

Fig. 23.2: Colonies of *Corynebacterium diphtheriae.*

of gravis, intermedius and mitis. Gravis ferments starch, glycogen and dextrin while intermedius and mitis have no action on starch and glycogen.

It is catalase positive, oxidase negative and do not liquefy gelatin. Urea is not hydrolyzed. It is indole negative and do not form phosphatase.

Resistance

It is readily destroyed by heat (58°C for 10 minutes). It is resistant to drying. It is sensitive to penicillin, erythromycin and broad spectrum antibiotics.

Antigenic Structure

Antigenically they are heterogeneous. Gravis has 13 types, intermedius 4 types and mitis 40 types.

Bacteriophage Typing

About 42 bacteriophages types are known. Type I and III are mitis, IV to VI intermedius, VII is avirulent gravis and remaining virulent gravis. A system of bacteriocin typing has also been described.

Toxin

Diphtheria bacilli produce very powerful exotoxin. The strain most universally used for toxin production is Park William 8 strain.

Toxin consists of two factors A and B. A is a lethal factor and B is a spreading factor. Fragment A inhibits polypeptide chain elongation in the presence of nicotinamide adenine dinucleotide, by inactivating the elongation of EF-2. So toxin fragment-A inactivates EF-2 by catalyzing a reactions that yields free nicotinamide plus an inactive adenosine diphosphate ribose EF-2 complex. It is presumed that abrupt arrest of protein synthesis is responsible for necrotizing and neurotoxic effects of diphtheria toxin. Diphtheria toxin is protein in nature (mol wt. 62,000). It is extremely potent. Lethal dose for 250 gm guinea pig is 0.0001 mg. It is labile.

It can be converted into toxoid (toxin that has lost toxicity but not antigenicity) by:
1. Prolonged storage at 37°C.
2. Incubation at 37°C for 4 to 6 weeks.
3. 0.2 to 4% formalin.

The toxigenicity of diphtheria bacilli depends upon the presence of a beta phage which acts as genetic determinant controlling toxin production. Toxigenicity remains as long as the bacillus is lysogenic. When bacillus is cured of phage, it looses toxigenicity.

Toxin production is also influenced by the concentration of iron in the medium. 0.1 mg of iron per ml is the optimum concentration in the medium for toxin production. 0.5 mg per ml of iron in the medium inhibits toxin production. Other factors influencing the toxin production are osmotic pressure, pH, and availability of suitable carbon and nitrogen. The mechanism of action of toxin is not well understood. It inhibits protein synthesis and rapidly kill susceptible cell. It has affinity for myocardium, adrenal tissue and nerve endings.

Mode of Action of Toxin

The bacilli remain confined to site of entry where they multiply and form toxin. This toxin produces area of necrosis. The resulting fibrinous exudate together with epithelial cells, leukocytes, erythrocytes and bacteria form pseudomembrane.

Diphtheria does not occur naturally in animal but infection can be produced experimentally, e.g., cat, dogs, chicks, pigeons, guinea pig, rabbits, etc. Subcutaneous injection in guinea pig, with culture of virulent diphtheria bacilli will cause death of animal in 1 to 4 days. At autopsy of guinea pig, we may find:

1. Gelatinous, hemorrhagic edema and necrosis at the site of inoculation.
2. Swollen and congested lymph nodes.
3. Peritoneal exudate which may be hemorrhagic.
4. Congested abdominal viscera.
5. Enlarged and hemorrhagic adrenals.
6. Blood-stained pleural exudate.
7. Pericardial effusion.

Pathogenicity

Incubation period is 3 to 4 days. Pathogenicity is because of toxin production. *Corynebacterium diphtheriae* does not actively invade deep tissues and never enters the bloodstream. The site of infection may be:

1. Faucial.
2. Laryngeal.
3. Nasal.
4. Otitic.
5. Genital, vulval, vaginal, etc.
6. Conjunctival.
7. Cutaneous around mouth and nose, etc.

Anyhow, faucial diphtheria is the most common.

On the basis of clinical severity, diphtheria may be classified:

1. Malignant in which there is severe toxemia. There is cervical lymphadenitis (bull neck). Death is due to circulatory failure.
2. Septic which leads to ulceration, cellulitis and gangrene around the pseudomembrane.
3. Hemorrhagic type is characterized by bleeding from the edge of membrane, epistaxis, conjunctival hemorrhage.

Complications

1. Asphyxia—a mechanical obstruction by pseudomembrane.
2. Acute circulatory failure which may be peripheral or central.
3. Post-diphtheritic paralysis, e.g., palatine, ciliary, occurring in 3rd or 4th week of disease with spontaneous recovery.
4. Septic, e.g., pneumonia and otitis media.

Laboratory Diagnosis

Hematological investigations
It is not significant.

Bacteriological Investigations

Laboratory confirmation of diphtheria is necessary for control measures and epidemiological purposes. Specific treatment should be given immediately without waiting for laboratory test report.

1. *Smear examination:* Gram-staining shows thin, Gram-positive bacilli showing Chinese letter arrangement. Albert staining is done for the demonstration of metachromatic granules **(Fig. 23.3)**.
2. *Culture:* The swab is inoculated on Loeffler's slope, blood tellurite media and blood agar plate. The serum slope shows growth in 6 to 8 hours. Smear is stained with Albert stain and we may find bacilli with metachromatic granules and typical arrangement. Blood tellurite plate may be incubated for at least 2

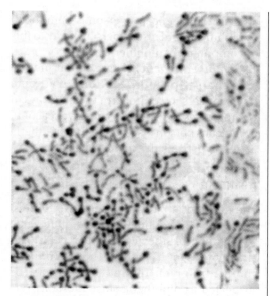

Fig. 23.3: Albert-stained smear of *Corynebacterium diphtheriae* showing metachromatic granules.

days before declaring it negative. Individual strain of *C. diphtheriae* within a biotype can be identified by phage typing, analytic of bacterial polypeptides or DNA restriction patterns, DNA hybridization tests or PCR, ribotyping, etc.

Virulence Test

It may be done *in vivo* (intradermally or subcutaneously) or *in vitro* (Elek test). Besides this, immunoelectrophoresis is also considered reasonably reliable for identification and establishing virulence of *Corynebacterium diphtheriae*.

Subcutaneous test: Overnight growth on Loeffler's slope is mixed in 2 to 5 ml broth and 0.8 ml is injected subcutaneously in 2 guinea pigs. One guinea pig is protected with 500 units of diphtheria antitoxin 8 to 24 hours before. If strain is virulent unprotected animal may die within 4 days. The control animal will remain healthy.

Intracutaneous test: Two guinea pigs are taken. One guinea pig is protected with 500 units of antitoxin the previous day and this animal acts as control. 0.1 ml of emulsion is inoculated at two different sites intracutaneous. To the other animals 50 units of antitoxin is given intraperitoneally 4 hours after skin test in order to prevent death. Toxigenicity is indicated by inflammatory reactions at the site of injection leading to necrosis in 18 to 72 hours while no change in controlled animal occurs.

In vitro: The gel precipitation test is called Elek's test. A rectangular strip of filter paper impregnated with diphtheria antitoxin (1000 unit/ml) is placed on the surface of 20 percent normal horse serum agar in petridish while medium is still in fluid form. When it dries, testing strain is inoculated at right angle to filter paper strip. This plate is incubated at 30°C for 24 to 48 hours. Toxin produced by bacterial growth will diffuse in agar and where it meets optimum concentration will produce line of precipitation. No precipitate will occur in non-toxigenic strain.

Tissue culture test: This may be done by incorporation of *Corynebacterium diphtheriae* into an agar overlay of cell culture monolayers. Toxin produced may diffuse into cells and kills them.

Primary isolates can be rapidly screened for toxigenicity by PCR.

Immunity

In non-immune person (Schick positive), immunity can be produced by active or passive immuni-zation. For active immunization, formal toxoid adjuvant such as alum-precipitated toxoid (APT), purified alum-precipitated toxoid (PAPT) and toxoid antitoxin floccules (TAF) are available.

Adjuvant toxoids give rise to severe reaction in older children and hence not suitable especially at the time of polio epidemic. Toxin-antitoxin floccules contain horse serum which rarely produce serum hypersensitivity. It is used mainly in older children and adults. Generally, children of less than 10 years are immunized with precipitated toxoid.

In endemic areas, active immunization is given at the age of 6 month. A booster dose is given at 18 months and another at school entry (6 years). This gives lasting protection.

Passive immunity: This is an emergency measure when the susceptible are exposed to infection. 500 to 1000 units of antitoxin (anti-diphtheria serum) is given subcutaneously. Being a horse serum, one should take precaution against hypersensitivity.

Combined immunity: All cases that receive ADS prophylactically must get combined immunization. An alum-containing preparation is preferred in combined immunization as the response to plain FT is not satisfactory when given with antitoxin.

Schick test: This is the skin test which is performed to find out susceptibility of a person to diphtheria.

0.2 ml diphtheria toxin is injected intra-dermally on left forearm and same dose of inactivated toxin (70°C for 30 minutes) is injected in right arm. Reading is taken on 1, 4, 7 days' interval. Four types of reactions are observed:

1. *Positive reaction:* An area of erythema and swelling at the site of injection in 24 to 48 hours reaching maximum in 4 to 7 days measuring 1 to 5 cm. The control area injected with heated toxin will show no reaction. Positive test means person is susceptible to diphtheria and antitoxin level is less than 0.01 Lf unit per ml.
2. Negative reaction means no reaction on either arm. It means person is immune to diphtheria *where antitoxin level exceeds 0.02 Lf unit per ml.*
3. Pseudo-reaction is erythema within 6 to 24 hours and disappearing completely in 4 days. This reaction is same on both

arms. This indicates person is immune to diphtheria and also hypersensitivity to this component of diphtheria bacilli.
4. *Combined reaction:* Here initial picture is that of pseudoreaction. Erythema disappears in control arm within 4 days. It progresses in test arm to positive reaction. It means person is susceptible to diphtheria and hypersensitive to the bacillus.

Treatment

The diphtheria bacillus is sensitive to most antibiotics. The antibiotics are of little value in treatment as they cannot deal with toxin already present in patient's body. Antitoxin should be given immediately if case is suspected as diphtheria since mortality rate increased with delay in starting antitoxic treatment. The dosage recommended are 20,000 unit intramuscularly (moderate case) and 50,000 to 100,000 unit for severe cases.

However, penicillin, preferably erythromycin or rifampicin or clindamycin, etc. may be used to prevent infection and to stop cases from becoming carriers. They may be used in dealing with established carriers.

DIPHTHEROIDS

Organism which is distinguished morphologically from *Corynebacterium diphtheriae* is called diphtheroid and is non-pathogenic **(Table 23.1)**. It is found on conjunctiva, mucous membrane of nasopharynx, oral cavity and genitalia.
1. *C. hofmanni* is found in human throat.
2. *C. xerosis* has been isolated from xerosis. Its relation with disease is uncertain. It may be found on skin as normal flora.
3. *Propionibacterium acnes* is found in acne pustule and is anaerobic. It produces lipases, which split off free fatty acids from skin lipids. These fatty acids can produce inflammation and contribute to acne. Tetracycline can inhibit lipolytic action.

Table 23.1: Differences between diphtheria and diphtheroids

Diphtheria	Diphtheroids
A. Morphology	
• Gram-positive and thin	• Gram-positive, short and thick
• Metachromatic granules are more	• They are less or absent
• Pleomorphism present	• Very little pleomorphism
• Chinese letter arrangement	• No such arrangement is seen here
B. Culture	
• Growth on enriched media	• May grow on ordinary media
C. Biochemical reactions	
• Fermentation of glucose only	• May ferment glucose and sucrose
D. Toxicity	
• They are toxic	• Usually non-toxic

Morphology: It is short stumpy 1.5 to 2 μ in length with parallel sides and rounded ends. It does not exhibit pleomorphism and has no metachromatic granules. It occurs in palisades or bundles with uniform shape and staining. Actual differentiation can be made out by biochemical reaction and virulence test.

Mycobacteria

General characters: They are acid-fast, Gram-positive bacilli, slender, rod, aerobic, non-motile, non-capsulated and non-sporing. Growth is generally slow. They do not grow on ordinary media. They require enriched media with egg albumin, e.g., Löwenstein-Jensen's medium.

Classification of Mycobacteria

A. *Tubercle bacilli*
   1. *M. tuberculosis* (human)
   2. *M. bovis* (bovine)
   3. *M. microti* (murine)
   4. *M. avium* (avian)
   5. *M. marinum* (cold blooded)
B. *Lepra bacilli*
   1. Human—*M. leprae*
   2. Rat—*M. leprae murium*
C. *Mycobacteria cause skin lesion*
   1. *M. ulcerans*
   2. *M. balnei*
D. *Atypical mycobacteria*
   Runyon Group I—Photochromogen
   Runyon Group II—Scotochromogen
   Runyon Group III—Non-photochromogen
   Runyon Group IV—Rapid grower
E. *Johne's bacillus*
   M. paratuberculosis
F. *Saprophytic mycobacteria*
   1. *M. butyricum*
   2. *M. phlei*
   3. *M. stercoris*
   4. *M. smegmatis*

MYCOBACTERIUM TUBERCULOSIS

Morphology: *M. tuberculosis* is straight or slightly curved rod 1 to 4 µ long and 0.2 to 0.8 µ wide. It may be arranged singly or in groups. It is non-motile, non-sporing and non-capsulated. *Mycobacterium bovis* is usually straighter, stouter and shorter. It is Gram-positive. It is acid-fast (acid fastness is due to mycolic acid). Beaded or barred staining is seen in *M. tuberculosis*. It is more uniform without any bead in the *M. bovis* **(Table 24.1)**.

Table 24.1: Differentiation between *M. tuberculosis* and *M. bovis*.

Test	M. tuberculosis	M. bovis
• Morphology	Long, thin and curved	Shorter, stout and straighter
• Staining	Barred and beaded	Uniform
• Growth	Eugonic	Dysgonic
• Action of glycerol on growth	Enhanced	Inhibited
• Colony	Dry, rough, raised and wrinkled	Moist, smooth and flat
• Progressive disease in rabbit	–	+
• Niacin production	+	–
• Nitrate reduction	+	–
• Growth in semisolid medium	Grows at surface (aerobic)	Grows 10 to 20 mm below surface (microaerophilic)

Non-acid fast rods and granules from young culture are also reported and when they are injected into susceptible animal they produce tuberculosis. Perhaps these granules are non-acid fast form of tubercle bacilli. These bacilli are called Much's granules.

Cultural Characters

It is aerobic. It grows slowly (generation time 14 to 15 hours). Colonies appear in 2 to 6 weeks. Optimum temperature is 37°C and optimum pH is 6.4 to 7. *M. tuberculosis* grows luxuriantly in culture (eugonic) while *M. bovis* grows sparsely (dysgonic). Addition of glycerol improves the growth of human types. The enriched media is prepared by adding eggs, glycerol, potatoes, meat, bone marrow infusions or aspargine. **Table 24.2** depicts the media for mycobacterial culture.

Liquid media: In liquid media without dispersing agent growth creeps up the side from the bottom, forming surface pellicles extending along the side of tube. Diffused growth is obtained in Dubo's medium (contain Tween 80). Virulent strains tend to form serpentine cords in liquid media.

Liquid media are generally required for sensitivity test, biochemical tests, and preparation of antigen and vaccine.

Solid media: *M. tuberculosis* forms dry, rough, raised and irregular colony. It is creamy white first and becomes yellowish or buff colored later on. It is not emulsified easily. The colony of bovis is flat, smooth and white, breaking up easily when touched.

Egg-based solid media like L.J, Petragnani or American Tradeau Society medium have been used for primary isolation of *Mycobacterium tuberculosis* from clinical samples and have been found more sensitive than agar based media. Otherwise agar based media are more transparent and permit early microscopic detection of colonies. Culture techniques are more sensitive, than staining procedure, but the major limitation are long time taken for their growth.

Solid media used are Dorset egg, Löwenstein-Jensen's medium. Löwenstein-Jensen's medium is most widely used which contains coagulated hen's eggs, salt solution, malachite green, glycerol and aspargine.

Tubercle bacilli may also be grown on chick embryos and in tissue culture. Recently,

Table 24.2: Media for mycobacterial culture.

Media	Composition	Inhibiting agents
Solid media		
1. Löwenstein-Jensen	Coagulated whole eggs with salts, glycerol, potato flour, aspergine, etc.	Malachite green
2. L.J with pyruvic acid	L.J and pyruvic acid	do
3. Petragnani	Coagulated eggs, egg yolks, white milk, potato flour, glycerol, etc.	do
Wallenstain	Egg yolks and glycerol	do
Agar based		
Middlebrook 7H10	Salts, vitamins, co-factors, oleic acid, albumin, catalase, glycerol, dextrose, etc.	do
Middlebrook 7H11	Middlebrook 7H10 and Casium hydrolysate, etc.	do
Liquid		
Dubo's medium	Bovine serum albumin, aspargine, caseine hydrolysase, salts and Tween 80	
Middlebrook 7H9 Broth	Do	

it is reported that selenite medium 5 µg of sodium selenite in agar shortens the time period of growth of colonies of *Mycobacterium tuberculosis* (3 to 5 days) otherwise it takes 2 to 6 weeks for the colonies to appear. Disadvantages of selenite include its toxicity and carcinogenic properties. Rapid growth of *M. tuberculosis* may also be obtained by adding blood or hemoglobin to the medium.

Resistance

It is more resistant to drying and chemical disinfectants. Temperature 60°C for 20 minutes can kill it. Moist heat at 100°C kill it readily. In sunlight the culture may be killed in 2 hours. In sputum it survives 20 to 30 hours even in sunlight.

It is killed by tincture of iodine in 5 minutes and by 80% ethanol in 2 to 10 minutes. Phenol solution (5%) kills it in 24 hours.

Biochemical reactions: The important biochemical tests for its identification are:

1. *Niacin test:* Human tubercle bacilli form niacin when grown on egg medium. Ten percent cyanogen bromide and 40% aniline in 96% ethanol are added to a suspension of culture. Yellow color indicates positive test.
2. *Aryl sulfatase:* Organism is grown, for 2 weeks in media, containing tripotassium phenolphthalein disulphate. Detection of free phenolphthalein is detected by addition of alkali. Red color indicates positive test. It is positive in atypical mycobacteria.
3. *Neutral red:* The virulent strain of tubercle bacilli may bind the neutral red in alkaline buffer more readily and firmly than bovine types.
4. *Catalase test:* A mixture of equal volume of 30 Vol H_2O_2 and 0.2% catechol in distilled water is added to 5 mL of test culture. Effervescence indicates positive catalase test and browning of colonies indicates peroxidase activity.

Most atypical mycobacteria are strongly catalase positive. Tubercle bacilli is peroxidase positive. Catalase and peroxidase activities are lost when tubercle bacilli develop resistance to INH.

5. *Nitrate reduction:* This is positive in *M. tuberculosis* and negative in *M. bovis.*
6. *Amidase test:* Five amides are used, i.e. acetamide, benzamide, nicotinamide, carbamide and pyrazinamide. A 0.00164 M solution of amide is incubated with bacillary suspension at 37°C. 0.1 mL of $MnSO_4$ $4H_2O$, 1 mL of phenol and 0.5 mL of hypochlorite solutions are added. These tubes are placed in boiling water for 20 minutes. A blue color means positive test. The ability to split amides has been used to differentiate atypical mycobacteria.

Antigenic structure: Many antigens have been identified. Group specificity is due to polysaccharide. Type specificity is due to protein antigen. Protein antigen is used for tuberculin test. Tuberculin from *M. tuberculosis, M. bovis* and *M. microtic* appear to be indistinguishable.

Bacteriophage: Fresh isolate can be classified into 4 bacteriophage type A, B, C, AB. The predominant types in South India are A and AB.

Pathogenesis: The basis of virulence of bacillus is unknown. It does not produce toxin. May be the various components of bacillus possess different biological activities influencing pathogenesis, allergy and immunity in disease.

Determinants of Mycobacterium Tuberculosis Pathology

These determinants are as under:
1. Cording factors are actually glycolipid derivatives of mycolic acid. They are present in outer surface of tubercle bacilli. They are responsible for:
   a. Inhibition of migration of polymorphonuclear leukocytes and ultimately results in the formation of granuloma.
   b. Inducing protective immunity as it is immunogenic.
   c. Growth of tubercle bacilli in serpentine cord.

2. Cell surface glycolipids inhibits phagolysome formation. This allows intracellular survival of tubercle bacilli after ingestion by macrophages.
3. Resistance to antituberculosis antibiotics which is acquired by mutation.

The cell wall of bacillus causes, delayed hypersensitivity. Tubercle protein can elicit tubercular reaction and when bound to lipid can induce delayed hypersensitivity. In tissue it leads to formation of monocytes, macrophages, epithelioid cells and giant cells. The bacterial polysaccharide induces immediate hypersensitivity and causes exudation of neutrophils from blood vessels. Lipid causes accumulation of macrophages and neutrophils. Phosphatids induce the formation of tubercle consisting of epithelioid cells and giant cell. The occurrence of eukaryotic like Adenyl cyclase in *M. tuberculosis*, suggest a role for the enzyme in cell signaling and perhaps in the pathogenesis of *M. tuberculosis*.

There are two types of lesion:
1. Exudative.
2. Productive.

Exudative lesion is an acute inflammatory reaction with accumulation of edema fluid, leukocytes and later on monocytes. It may heal by resolution leading to necrosis or develop into productive type.

The productive lesion is predominantly cellular composed of number of tubercles which may enlarge, coalesce, liquefy and undergo caseation.

Route of infection: Tubercle bacilli enter the body commonly by inhalation, ingestion or by inoculation into skin. When inhaled bacilli are lodged in pulmonary alveoli. They are phagocytosed by alveolar macrophages. Inside phagocyte the bacilli keep on multiplying. Phagocytes with ingested bacilli may act as vehicle transporting the infection to different parts of the body. The multiplication of bacilli is stopped only with the development of specific cellular immunity. It occurs in 6 to 8 weeks after infection.

Primary complex or first infection or childhood type of tuberculosis occurs early in life. It consists of subpleural focus of tuberculous pneumonia in lung parenchyma found in lower lobe or in lower part of upper lobe with enlarged draining lymph nodes. Primary complex is an asymptomatic lesion undergoing spontaneous healing resulting in hypersensitivity to tuberculoprotein and acquired immunity. Rarely it may lead to hematogenous spread and development of miliary tubercle meningitis, etc.

The adult type is due to reactivation of primary infection or exogenic reinfection. Lesion may heal by reabsorption, fibrosis and calcification. It may progress to chronic fibrocaseous tuberculosis with tubercle formation, caseation, and shedding of bacilli in sputum.

Laboratory Diagnosis (Table 24.3)

A. *Hematological investigations:*
   1. *Total leukocyte count:* In early acute cases there is leukocytosis. In miliary infection there may be leukopenia.
   2. *Differential leukocyte count:* In early cases there is increase in neutrophils. Later on there is an increase in monocytes and lymphocytes.
   3. *Erythrocytic sedimentation rate* is usually raised which is an index of progress of the disease.
B. *Bacteriological investigations:*
   Microscopy: Smears may be prepared from specimen like sputum, laryngeal swab, pleural fluid, peritoneal fluid, cerebrospinal fluid, pus, urine, gastric lavage, feces and other infected material.

New glass slides should be used for smear. Smear should be made from thick purulent portion of sputum. The smear is dried, fixed and stained by Ziehl-Neelsen technique. The slide is studied under oil immersion objective. Acid-fast bacilli are seen as pink brightened rods, while background is blue **(Fig. 24.1)**. It has been estimated that at least 50,000 to

Table 24.3: Current laboratory diagnostic methods of *Mycobacterium tuberculosis*.

Sl. No.	Method	Advantages	Disadvantages
1.	Microscopy (smear for acid-fast bacilli)	• Low cost • Rapid diagnostic	• Low sensitivity (up to 2/3 of pulmonary tuberculosis cases are negative) • Difficult sample collection
2.	Culture	• Specific	• Time consuming (up to 4–8 weeks) • Not always possible
3.	PCR	• Relatively quick • Very specific	• Relatively expensive • High level of training required • Expensive instrumentation • May detect latent disease
4.	BACTEC	• Specific	• Slow, 2–3 weeks • Expensive
5.	Tuberculosis ELISA test kits	• Quick (procedure time 110 min). • Reproducible with minimal training	• Some equipment required
6.	Rapid tests	• Very quick (procedure time only 15 min). • Minimal training • No special equipment required.	• Lower sensitivity compared to ELISA test kit • No quantitative results

1,00,000 acid-fast bacilli should be present per mL of sputum to get positive report. A negative report should not be given till at least 100 fields are examined taking about 10 minutes time.

Where several smears are to be examined daily, it is more convenient to use fluorescent microscopy. Smears are stained with auramine phenol or auramine rhodamine fluorescent stain. They are examined under ultraviolet light and bacilli appear bright rods against dark background.

Concentration Methods

Following are the methods which concentrate the bacilli without inactivating the bacilli and hence can be used for culture and animal inoculation:

1. *Petroff's method:* Sputum is incubated with equal volume of 4% solution of sodium hydroxide. Shake till it becomes clear. It takes about 20 minutes. Centrifuge it at 3000 rpm for 30 minutes and sediment is neutralized with N/10 HCl. Sediment is used for smearculture and animal inoculation.

2. Homogenization may be achieved with dilute acid (6% H_2SO_4, 3% HCl or 5% oxalic acid).

3. *Flocculation method:* Specimen is treated with digester containing sodium hydroxide and potash alum. It is neutralized with acid. Floccules start appearing. These floccules are sedimented by centrifugation.

4. *Jungmann's method:* Acidic ferrous sulfate and H_2O_2 is used. A bulky deposit is obtained and used for inoculation.

5. Trisodium phosphate is lethal for many contaminating bacteria but tubercle bacilli are unaffected.

6. N-acetyl-l-cysteine with NaOH is considered rapid and effective method for homogenization of mucopurulent specimen. Pancreatin, desogen, zephiran and cetrimide are other homogenizing agent.

7. Addition of 20% clorox to sputum but this method is not suitable for culture.

8. Lauryl sulfate method: Here 1.5% sodium hydroxide and 4.5% lauryl sulfate is used.

Culture: Culture techniques have been estimated to detect 10 to 1000 viable mycobacteria per ml of specimen. The most common media are based on egg and also contain high concentration of malachite green to overcome contamination with other bacteria. The concentrated material is inoculated into 2 bottles of Lowenstein-Jensen (L.J.) media. The tubercle bacilli grow in about 4 to 8 weeks of incubation at 37°C. However, rapid growing mycobacteria may appear in 4 days' time. A negative report is sent if no growth appears by the end of 8th week to 12th week.

Ogawa medium: It is egg-based medium. It is most economical because it replaces aspargine by sodium glutamate. Actually it contains mineral salts (potassium dihydrogen phosphate anhydrous, sodium glutamate), distilled water, malachite green dye and homogenized eggs. The modifed Ogawa medium in addition contains magnesium citrate and glycerol. The pH of modified medium is 6.4. The ingredients are mixed well and dispensed in 6 to 8 ml volume in MacCortneys bottles. Now medium in MacCortneys bottle is insipissated at 80°C to 85°C for 45 minutes. The inspissation is repeated for 2nd and 3rd time. This medium may be stored in refrigerator for several weeks.

In laboratories where centrifuges are not available, sputum specimens are deconta-minated with 4% of sodium hydroxide and inoculated directly on modified Ogawa medium.

Middlebrook 7H 10 and 7H 11 are agar based media. They achieve slightly higher isolation yield than egg-based media but are quite expensive.

Blood agar is an alternative culture medium for the isolation of mycobacterium. *Mycobacterium tuberculosis* grows within one or two weeks on blood agar plates. Average number of colonies isolated from clinical specimens on blood agar is significantly higher than the number of colonies on egg-based medium. It can also be used as alternative medium for drug sensitivity testing of *Mycobacterium tuberculosis* against anti-tubercular drugs like isoniazid, rifampicin, streptomycin and ethambutol. Results are obtained much earlier with blood agar. However, they require 5 to 10% carbon dioxide. Desiccation may be prevented by sealing the plates with tapes or by using tubes instead of plates.

Colonies that develop are smeared and stained by Ziehl-Neelsen method and examined. For routine purpose, slow growing, non-pigmented, acid fast and niacin positive is taken as *M. tuberculosis*. Confirmation is done by animal inoculation and biochemical tests.

Allergy tests: Hypersensitivity to tuberculo-protein by tuberculin test is of limited value as it does not differentiate between clinical disease and sub-clinical disease. It is of some value in indicating active infection in children below 5 years ago. A negative tuberculin test is often helpful to exclude the diagnosis of tuberculosis.

Serology: No serological test is helpful in the diagnosis of tuberculosis. IHA may be positive in cases of established tuberculosis. However, high titers of IgG antibody to PPD, detectable by ELISA test, are considered to exist in many patients with active pulmonary tuberculosis. The soluble antigen fluorescent antibody (SAFA), ELISA and IHA tests are proving of considerable diagnostic significance.

DNA probe for detection of tubercle bacilli is quite rapid and specific.

Rapid techniques for establishing the diagnosis of *Mycobacterium tuberculosis* are polymerase chain reaction and detection of antigen A 60.

Immunity: Infection with tubercle bacillus induces delayed hypersensitivity and resistance to infection. Cell mediated immunity is the only immunity operative in tuberculosis. Humoral immunity has no influence on the course of disease. In non-immune host bacillus is able to multiply inside phagocyte and destroy the cell. In immune host activated T lymphocytes release lymphokines which make the macrophages bactericidal.

The main cell is the activated CD4 and helper T cell. They may develop along the Th-1 or Th-2 cells. Thus, they release cytokines like interferon gamma, interleukins-1, interleukins-2, toxic necrosis factor alpha-Th-1 dependent cytokines. Above mentioned factors activate macrophages causing protective immunity and containment of the infectivity. Th-2 cytokines induce delayed type hypersensitivity, tissue destruction and progressive disease.

Subcutaneous injection of virulent tubercle bacilli in normal guinea pig produces no immediate response. At the site of injection a nodule appears after 10 to 14 days. The nodule bursts into non-healing ulcer which persists till the animal dies of progressive tuberculosis. Draining lymph nodes are enlarged and caseous. If subcutaneous injection of tubercle bacilli is given to guinea pig infected with *Mycobacterium tuberculosis* 4 to 6 weeks earlier, indurated lesions appear at the site of injection. It undergoes necrosis and shallow ulcer appears which heals rapidly without involving lymph nodes. This is called Koch's phenomenon and is a combination of hypersensitivity and immunity. Koch's phenomenon has 3 components:
1. Local skin reaction.
2. Focal response causing congestion and hemorrhage around tuberculous foci.
3. Systemic response of fever which may be fatal.

Tuberculin

1. Old tuberculin (OT) consists of filtrate of glycerol broth culture of bacilli concentrated to 1/10th of volume by evaporation on water bath.

2. Purified protein derivative (PPD) is prepared by precipitation of tubercle bacilli culture grown in synthetic medium with trichlor acetic acid. PPD is superior to OT because it is stable, and constant in activity. Tuberculin prepared from bovine type is as active as tuberculin prepared from human type.

In Mantoux test, widely used in graded doses of tuberculin which is injected intradermally on forearm. After 48 to 72 hours positive reaction is indicated by erythema, edema and induration of the size measuring 6 to 10 mm in diameter. The graded dose ranges from 1 tuberculin unit (0.01 mg OT or 0.00002 mg PPD) to 100 or 250 TU. Tuberculin injected into hypersensitive host may give rise to severe local reactions and flare up of inflammation and necrosis at main site of injection. So, tuberculin is injected in the doses, i.e. 5 TU dose in surveys, 1 TU in person suspected of hypersensitivity and up to 250 TU if reaction is negative. The tuberculin test becomes positive within 4 to 6 weeks after infection or injection of a virulent bacilli.

Interpretation of Mantoux Test

Note the area of inoculation for erythema, edema and palpate the area for any hard nodular feeling. In case there is nodular feeling measure its diameter in both the directions using centimeter scale.

1. No erythema or edema or induration	Negative
2. Slight redness, trace of edema of 5 mm or less	Doubtful 1+ reaction
3. Redness, definite edema, dense hard elevated borders with bulbous or dotted vesicles more than 5 mm diameter but less than 10 mm.	2+ reaction
4. Marked redness, edema, hard elevated borders of 10 mm diameter	3 + reaction
5. Marked redness, edema, necrosis and hard elevated borders of more than 10 mm diameter	4 + reaction

False Negative Tuberculin Test

It is seen in miliary tuberculosis, malnutrition, malignancy, viral infection (measles), sarcoidosis and immunosuppressive therapy or defective CMI.

False Positive

It is seen in *M. avium* or atypical mycobacterium.

Uses of Tuberculin Test

1. Diagnosis of active infection in infants.
2. Measure prevalence of infection in community.
3. Susceptibility of BCG vaccination.
4. Indication of successful vaccination.

Rapid laboratory methods to diagnose tuberculosis: Faster culture methods using radiometric systems such as BACTEC nonradiometric like MGIT are being used increasingly mainly because they reduce the time of culture and drug sensitivity testing to about 2 to 3 weeks. Nucleic acid amplification techniques are used mainly for the cases where there is a chance of infection other than *Mycobacterium tuberculosis*. Undoubtedly many of these techniques are quite expensive.

BCG (Bacille Calmette-Guérin)

This is a bovine strain of tubercle bacillus rendered completely avirulent by culturing repeatedly (*M. bovis* maintained for 13 years by 239 subculture on glycerine potato medium). The strain is used in inducing active immunity to tuberculosis. The vaccine contains live avirulent bacilli and is administered to tuberculin negative individual.

The vaccine is given intradermally over deltoid region. It confers 60% protection in India and 80% protection in USA and UK. Immunity lasts for 10 to 15 years. After BCG vaccination a positive tuberculin test may last for 3 to 7 years.

■ BCG VACCINE

One possible explanation for poor efficiency of BCG vaccine is a shortage of antigens that elicit a protective response against *Mycobacterium tuberculosis*. As we know, the attenuated BCG vaccine was originally derived by serial passage of virulent strain of *Mycobacterium bovis*. In the process there was loss of many coding sequences including a group of nine genes known as the region of difference 1 (RD 1). There is a report that immunization with recombinant BCG strain with RD 1 replaced improves protection against *Mycobacterium tuberculosis* in animal models. It appears that the presence of two extra antigens (ESAT 6 and CPF 10) involve more rebust CD4 T cell response coupled with possible role for these molecules allowing vaccine strain to persist in host might be contributing factors towards improved efficacy and hence enhanced protection.

Complications of BCG

Local

1. Abscess
2. Ulcer
3. Keloid
4. Tuberculoid
5. Confluent reaction to Heaf's multiple punctures
6. Lupis vulgaris
7. Lupoid lesion

Regional

1. Enlargement of draining lymph node.
2. Abscess formation in lymph node.

General

1. Fever
2. Mediastinal adenitis
3. Erythema nodosum
4. Otitis media

BCG also confers immunity against leprosy. It is also used in the treatment of leprosy and malignancy.

Mycobacterium habana has been identified as a possible source of vaccine against tuberculosis. It may become alternative to BCG whose efficiency has been questioned of late. It elicits cell-mediated response *in vitro* and *in vivo*.

Other different BCG strains are:
1. Glaxo freeze dried BCG vaccine 1077
2. Danish BCG vs vole bacillis
3. Isoniazid sensitive strains of BCG
4. 1173-P$_2$
5. Tokyo 172
6. Copenhagon 1331.

Clinical trials of *Mycobacterium vaccae* vaccine in tuberculosis are in progress.

Treatment: Streptomycin, PAS and INH are first line drugs. The reserve drugs are ethambutol, rifampicin, pyrazinamide, procainamide, cycloserine, capreomycin and thiocetazine.

ATYPICAL MYCOBACTERIA (TABLE 24.4)

They are also called opportunistic, tuberculoid or mycobacteria other than typical tubercle bacilli (MOTT) or environmental organisms.

They resemble *M. tuberculosis* but exhibit number of atypical characters:
1. They grow much faster than *M. tuberculosis.* Colonies may appear within 7 to 10 days.
2. They may grow on simple media like nutrient agar.
3. They are capable of growing at low temperature (20°C to 25°C) and high temperature 45°C.
4. Most of these bacteria are resistant to antitubercular drugs.
5. Organism is either longer than *M. tuberculosis* or smaller.
6. They are pigmented.
7. They are catalase positive.
8. Aryl sulfatase test is always positive.
9. Cord formation is absent.

Atypical mycobacteria are classified into following 4 groups according to *RUNYON:*

Group I: It is known as photochromogens. It produces no pigment in the dark but when young culture is exposed to light for 1 hour in presence of air and reincubated at 24 to 48 hours yellow orange pigment appears. It is slow growing, e.g., *Mycobacterium kansasii* which produces chronic pulmonary infection in man.

Table 24.4: Difference between typical and atypical *Mycobacterium.*

Group	Growth time	Colonies	Morphology	Pigment	Catalase	Niacin	Neutral red	Cord test
Human	6 to 9 weeks	• Dry	• Slender	None	Moderate	+	+	Tight
Bovine	3 to 6 weeks	• Dry • Smooth • Dysgonic	• Short and thick	None	Moderate	–	+	Tight
Group I	3 to 6 weeks	• Dry • Eugonic	• Larger • Beaded	Yellow or light yellow	Violent	–	+	Slight
Group II	2 to 3 weeks	• Moist • Smooth • Eugonic	• Large • Coarse • Beaded	Yellow to orange in dark	Violent	–	–	None
Group III	3 to 4 weeks	• Dysgonic • Doomed	• Small • Bipolar beads	None rarely light yellow	Moderate	–	–	None
Group IV	3 to 5 days	• Usually moist and spreading	• Large • Incompletely acid fast	White to all colors	Variable	–	–	None

Group II: It is known as scotochromogens. It forms pigmented (orange) colonies even in the dark. It sometimes contaminates culture of tubercle bacilli. It is usually non-pathogenic. However, *M. scrofulaceum* causes cervical adenitis (scrofula) in children.

Group III: It is non-photochromogen. It does not form pigment even on exposure to light. The colonies are buff colored, e.g., *M. intracellulare* (chronic pulmonary infection, renal infection and lymphadenopathy), *M. avium* (cervical adenitis in children and lung infection in adults) and *M. xenopi* (chronic lung infection in man). It can grow even at 45°C. Actually *Mycobacterium avium* and *Mycobacterium intracellulare* are closely similar that they have been considered as one group called *Mycobacterium avium* complex (MAC). In diseases like AIDS, they may cause lymphadenopathy, pulmonary disease, etc.

Group IV: It is also called rapid growers. Colonies appear within 7 days of incubation at 37°C or 25°C. All the chromogenic rapid grower are saprophyte. *M. fortuitum* (pulmonary lesion for which no effective chemotherapy is available) and *M. chelonei* may cause abscesses in man.

▌SKIN PATHOGENS

Two species, *M. ulcerans* and *M. marinum* are skin pathogens causing chronic ulcer and granulomatous lesion of skin (**Table 24.5**). Cutaneous localization is because they multiply at skin temperature.

M. ulcerans: It forms large clumps of bacilli which are acid fast and alcohol fast. It grows on LJ media slowly in 4 to 8 weeks. Growth occurs between 30°C and 33°C.

It causes ulcer usually on legs and arms following infection through minor injuries. After few weeks area become indurated and breaks down forming indolent ulcer which slowly extends under the skin. It is non-pathogenic to guinea pig and rabbit. In foot pad of mice if injected, forms edema of leg.

Table 24.5: Difference between *M. ulcerans and M. marinum.*

Characters	M. ulcerans	M. marinum
• Distribution	Tropics	Temperate zone
• Clinical course	Chronic progressive ulcer	Self-limited ulcer
• Bacilli in ulcer	Abundant	Scanty
• Rate of growth	Slow, 4 to 8 weeks	Faster, 1 to 2 weeks
• Growth at 25°C	–	+
• Growth at 37°C	–	+
• Culture film	Bacillus in cord	No cord formation
• Pigment in light	–	+
• Mouse pad lesion	Edema, and rarely ulcer	Marked inflammation and purulent ulcer

M. marinum: It is also called *M. balnei*. It causes tuberculosis in fish and amphibia. It occurs as saprophytes in fresh or salt water. Human infection may occur in epidemic form. The ulcers produced are self limited and undergo spontaneous healing. Growth occurs in 1 week at 30°C. Colonies are non-pigmented in dark and golden yellow on exposure to light.

Footpad inoculation in mice causes severe and purulent ulcer formation.

▌MYCOBACTERIUM LEPRAE (FIG. 24.1)

India today, has over 40 lakh leprosy cases, or half the world's total. The maximum number are in UP. In some areas of the country, 1–3% of the population has the disease.

About 20,000 people are reported suffering from leprosy in Jammu and Kashmir state.

Morphology: It is long 4 to 5 µ, slender, slightly curved or straight, occurring in bundles of parallel packets. It is weakly acid fast (5% H_2SO_4 is used for decolorization). In smear living bacilli are uniformly stained while dead bacilli are fragmented and irregular.

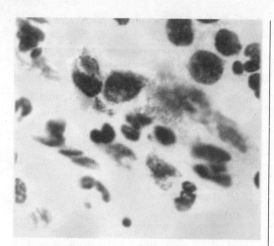

Fig. 24.1: *Mycobacterium leprae* (modified Ziehl staining).

Bacteriological index is defined as number of viable bacilli in a lesion. Their viability is assessed from stained smear. Internationally agreed bacteriological index is 6+. Scale commonly used is × 100 oil immersion. It may be expressed as under:

6+ 1000 or more bacteria in every microscopic field.

5+ 100 or more bacteria in every microscopic field.

4+ 10 or more bacteria in every microscopic field.

3+ 1 or more bacteria in every microscopic field.

2+ 1 or more in every 10 microscopic field.

1+ 1 or more in every 100 microscopic field.

Morphological index is more significant and meaningful for assessing the progress of patient on chemotherapy. It is defined as the percentage of uniformly stained bacilli in the tissue.

Cultural characters: It has not been cultured in bacteriological media or tissue culture. However, there are reports of successful cultivation:

1. In Indian Cancer Research Centre Bombay (1962), acid-fast bacilli was isolated from lepromatous patient. They employed human fetal spinal ganglion cell culture.

The ICRC bacilli has been adapted to grow on L. J. media.

2. Shepard (1960) found that leprae bacilli can multiply in footpad of mice.

3. Armadillo has also been found susceptibility to experimental infection. *Mycobacterium leprae* from armadillo or human tissue contains a unique O-diphenoloxidase, perhaps an enzyme characteristic of leprosy bacilli.

Generation time of leprae bacilli is 20 days.

4. European hedgehog animal model is evaluated and can be kept to be bred in captivity. It is found quite useful for multiplication of leprae bacilli.

Pathogenesis: Leprae bacilli are obligate parasite of man. Portal of entry is most probably skin and nasal mucosa. It needs close and prolonged contact with infective patient for contact. Incubation period is 5 to 8 years.

One Gram of lepromatous tissue may contain about 7000 million leprosy bacilli.

The habitat of leprosy bacilli in nerves is the Schwann cell or occasionally the axon which it ensheathes. Under adverse conditions, it may find a retreat in a nerve for which it has great affinity and in which it is not readily detected by immunological means. Sites of multiplication of leprosy bacilli include Schwann cells, smooth and striated muscles. Leprosy bacilli are found in arector pili in skin hair follicles, sweat gland, muscular media of arterioles, endothelial lining of small blood vessels, dartos muscle of scrotum and smooth muscles of iris. Nasal secretions, nasal mucosa, erosions, ulcers and blisters of BL and LL also contain leprosy bacilli. They are found in the sputum, semen, sweat, sebum, tears and breast milk of person with untreated lepromatous leprosy.

The disease occurs in two forms **(Table 24.6):**
1. Tuberculoid.
2. Lepromatous.

Tuberculoid leprosy is seen in patients with high degree of resistance. The lesions are

Table 24.6: Difference between lepromatous leprosy and tuberculoid leprosy.

Characters	Lepromatous leprosy	Tuberculoid leprosy
• Cell-mediated immunity	Deficient	Adequate
• Lepromin test	Negative	Positive
• Lepra bacilli in lesion	Numerous	Scanty
• Inflammatory cells	Extensive infilteration with mononuclear leukocytes and plasma cells	Infilteration with few inflammatory cell
• Lesions	Serious disease with lesion about 1 to 2 cm appearing first on face, ear lobes and situated in skin and subcutaneous tissue	Chronic but benign disease with asymmetrical small patch lesion having raised edges. Patches can also be larger and elevated
• Sites involved	May occur on face, extremities, neck (axillae, groin and perineum spread)	Involves face, gluteal region and limbs
• Mucous membrane, lymph nodes, eyes and internal organs involvement	Common	Not rare
• Nerve involvement	Symmetrical	Thickened peripheral nerve (ulnar, peroneal and greater auricular nerves)
• Leonine face	Present	Absent
• Mycobacterial antibodies	Present	May be present
• Prognosis	Bad	Good

few, well demarcated consisting of macular anesthetic patches. Neural involvement occurs early and may lead to deformity. Cell mediated immunity is adequate and lepromin test is positive. Prognosis is good.

Lepromatous leprosy, where host resistance is very low, the lepromin test is negative and prognosis is poor. Here we find infiltrating skin lesion. Peripheral nerve trunk becomes involved with the progress of diseases. There may be erythematous patch and diffuse infiltrate of nodular lesions.

The borderline type refers to lesions possessing characteristics of both tuberculoid and lepromatous lesion. It may shift to lepromatous or tuberculoid depending upon chemotherapy or change in host resistance.

The indeterminate type is early unstable tissue reaction which is not characteristic of lepromatous or tuberculoid type. In many persons the lesion heals spontaneously. In others, lesion may progress to tuberculoid or lepromatous type.

Lepromin test: The hypersensitivity in a leper may be demonstrated by intradermal inoculation of a material prepared from leprosy nodules. Two types of reactions are known:

1. Fernandes reaction is an early reaction occurring within 24 to 48 hours may last for 3 to 5 days. There is erythema and induration about 10 to 30 mm in diameter.
2. Mitsuda reaction occurring 3 to 4 weeks after the test. It is expression of immunity and is non-specific. It also occurs in tuberculosis and BCG vaccinated person. It is negative in lepromatous leprosy and is positive in tuberculoid leprosy.

0.1 mL of antigen is injected intradermally and then early reaction and delayed reactions are studied.

Lepromin test is done for following purposes:
1. To classify the lesion of leprosy. It is positive in tuberculoid leprosy and negative in lepromatous leprosy.

2. To assess the prognosis and response to treatment. A positive reaction indicates good prognosis. Conversion to lepromin positivity during treatment indicates improvement.
3. To assess the resistance of individual to leprosy. It is desirable to recruit only lepromin positive persons for work.
4. To verify the identity of candidate leprae bacilli. Cultured acid-fast bacilli claimed to be leprae bacilli should give the results similar and parallel to standard lepromin.

Laboratory Diagnosis

❖ Smear from lepromatous nodules, skin scraping or nasal mucosa are stained with Ziehl-Neelsen method using 4 to 5% H_2SO_4, for decolorization. Smear shows acid-fast bacilli arranged in packed bundles in lepra cells.

❖ *Lepromin skin test:* 0.1 mL of lepromin antigen is injected intradermally. The early reaction is seen as induration which increases in size up to 10 mm in diameter till 3 to 5 days. Later it becomes nodules of 2 to 4 mm in diameter in 3 to 4 weeks' time. The center of nodule is necrosed resulting ulcer which heals up in several weeks. This test is useful only in assessing the prognosis of disease. It has no diagnostic value.

❖ The immunodiagnostic tests are quite useful for: (a) epidemiological study, (b) identification of individuals at high risk, (c) early detection of disease among patients with symptoms, (d) prognosis of patients, and (e) evaluation of the effect of disease. A number of immuno-diagnostic tests are further developed. An ELISA test of comparable sensitivity to the radioimmuno-assay test to *M. leprae* has been established. A method has also been developed for early detection of systematic infection in armadillos, and monoclonal antibody are being evaluated for their specificity for *M. leprae*.

Several other new techniques based on different principles are available, e.g., Dot, ELISA, fluorescent leprosy antibody absorption (FLA-ABS) test, passive hemagglutination test, specific carbohydrate epitope found in phenolic glycolipid-1 (PGL-1) of *Mycobacterium leprae*.

At present FLA-ABS is the most sensitive test for detection of presence of *Mycobacterium leprae* in the community and also useful for monitoring the transmission of disease.

Treatment and prophylactic measures: Dapsone is the mainstay of antibacterial treatment of leprosy and is administered for at least 3 to 4 years. However, acedapsone which is administered at 75 days' interval is good in treatment and prophylactically as well. Rifampicin is reported bactericidal to *Mycobacterium leprae*. Recently Clofazimine is also found bactericidal to this organism. A lot of research work is undertaken to prepare vaccine against leprosy. Many quarters claim successful vaccine preparation which is under trial.

General characters: They are rod shaped, sporogenous classified into two groups:
a. Aerobic bacillus.
b. Anaerobic clostridia (Discussed in Chapter 29).

Aerobic bacilli are Gram-positive, non-motile, spore bearing bacilli occurring in chains. They are thick with truncated or convex ends. They include psychrophilic, mesophilic and thermophilic species. The salt tolerance varies from less than 2 to 25% of NaCl.

Bacillus anthrax is the only pathogenic species causing anthrax whereas *B. subtilus* is opportunist and *B. cereus* may produce food poisoning.

BACILLUS ANTHRAX

It remains in parasitic form in cattle and sheep. Infection in man is the result of accidental contact with infected animal.

Morphology: It is non-motile, non-acid fast, Gram-positive measuring 1 × 3 to 4 μ. They may be arranged singly or in short chains. The entire chain may be surrounded by capsule. Capsule is polypeptide in nature (D-glutamic acid). Capsule production depends upon a 60 megadalton plasmid, p × O_2.

In culture the bacilli are arranged end to end in chains. The chain of bacilli presents bamboo stick appearance. Spores are formed in soil only in presence of oxygen and not in animal body. Sporulation may be brought about by:
1. Distilled water.
2. 2% NaCl.
3. Growth on oxalated agar shows spores which are central, oval and of the same

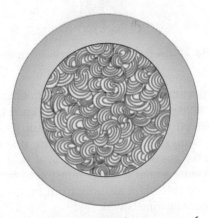

Fig. 25.1: Medusa head appearance of colony on nutrient agar.

width as the bacillary body.

Cultural characters: It is aerobic growing at optimum temperature of 37°C (range being 12°C to 45°C). The optimum temperature for spore formation is 25°C to 30°C. Growth may occur on ordinary media.

a. *Nutrient broth:* There may be floccular turbidity or no turbidity.
b. *Agar plate:* Colony is irregular, around 2 to 3 mm in diameter, raised, dull opaque, grayish white with a frosted glass appearance and cut glass appearance (in transmitted light). With magnifying glass they look like tangled mass of long hair like curls (barrister wig or medusa head appearance) **(Fig. 25.1)**.
Virulent capsulated strain forms rough colonies whereas avirulent forms smooth colonies.
c. *Blood agar:* The colony is non-hemolytic.
d. *Gelatin stab:* A characteristic "inverted tree"

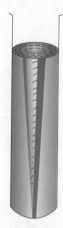

Fig. 25.2: Gelatin stab showing inverted tree appearance.

appearance is seen with slow liquefication starting from the top as shown in **Figure 25.2**.

e. *Selective medium (PLET):* It consists of polymyxin, lysozyme, ethylene diamine tetra acetic acid (EDTA) and thallous acetate added to heart infusion agar. It is used to isolate anthrax from mixture of spore bearing bacilli.

Biochemical Reactions

Glucose, maltose and sucrose are fermented with acid production only. Nitrates are reduced to nitrite, catalase is positive and gelatin is liquefied.

Resistance: Vegetative form is killed within 30 minutes at 56°C. Anthrax spore remains viable for years in dry state. Dry heat at 40°C requires 3 hours and steam 5 to 20 minutes for sterilization. They survive in 5% phenol for weeks. They are killed in 4% potassium permanganate and destroyed in 2% formaldehyde. They are susceptible to penicillin, sulfonamide, erythromycin, streptomycin, tetracycline and chloramphenicol.

Antigenic structure: Three antigens have been recognized.

a. Capsular antigen is found in virulent strain. It consists of polypeptide of high molecular weight composed of D-glutamic acid. It is a hapten. Antibodies against this antigen are not protective.

b. Somatic polysaccharides are found as a complex in cell wall. It cross reacts with capsular polysaccharide of type 14 pneumococcus. Antibody to this antigen is not protective.

c. Somatic protein (protective antigen) is present in edema fluid of anthrax lesion. It is heat labile. Its antibody is protective.

Toxin: *Bacillus anthrax* produces substance having exotoxin like properties. They are:
1. Protective antigen or protein.
2. Edema factor.
3. Lethal factor.

The specific toxin is lethal, edema producing and is produced by virulent strain. This toxin seems to have an affinity for cell of reticulo-endothelial system.

Pathogenicity: In susceptible animals, the organisms proliferate at the site of entry. The capsules remain intact, and the organisms are surrounded by a large amount of proteinaceous fluid containing few leukocytes from which they rapidly disseminate and reach bloodstream.

In resistant animals, the organisms proliferate for a few hours by which time there appears massive accumulation of leukocytes. The capsule gradually disintegrates and disappears. Thus, organisms remain localized.

In nature anthrax is primarily a disease of cattle and sheep, less often of horses and swine. Experimentally fatal infection can be produced in mouse, guinea pig, rabbits, etc. Infection can be produced by cutaneous, subcutaneous, intracutaneous, intramuscular, ingestion and inhalation. Guinea pig dies within 2 to 3 days after subcutaneous injection. Autopsy of dead animal shows hemorrhage, local edema, congested viscera and blood coagulates less firmly. Microscopically bacilli are found in large numbers in the local lesion in blood and viscera. The bacilli are confined to interior of capillaries and tissues and may rarely penetrate.

Route of infection in man: The persons most commonly involved are butchers, shepherds, handlers of hides, hair and laboratory workers. There are three routes of infection:

a. Through skin it results in malignant pustule. The spores enter the skin through cuts, abrasion or hair follicle. This lesion starts as papule in 1 to 3 days after infection. It becomes vesicular containing fluid. The whole area is congested and edematous and several satellite lesions, filled with serous fluid are arranged around central necrotic area covered by a black eschar. Cutaneous anthrax generally resolves spontaneously but may lead to septicemia.

b. Pulmonary anthrax is called woolsorter's disease. It is due to inhalation of dust (containing spores) from infected wool. Hemorrhagic meningitis may occur as a complication.

c. Intestinal anthrax occurs very rarely from ingestion of cooked or partly cooked meat. A violent enteritis with bloody diarrhea occurs with high fatality.

Laboratory Diagnosis

A. Hematological Investigations

Leukocytosis occurs when tissues are invaded otherwise total leukocyte count is within normal limit.

B. Bacteriological Investigations

Microscopic examination: Smear prepared from exudate, sputum, etc. on Gram's staining shows Gram-positive non-sporing bacilli occurring in chain.

Culture: The material is inoculated on nutrient agar plate. Smear shows Gram-positive spore bearing bacilli.

Animal inoculation: A small amount of exudate or isolated culture from infected man is injected subcutaneously in guinea pig. Guinea pig dies within 36 to 48 hours. Smear from heart blood and spleen shows typical Gram-positive bacilli.

Serological test: It is a precipitation test. It is used in making rapid diagnosis. The infected tissues are grounded in saline, boiled for 5 minutes and filtered. This tissue extract is layered over anthrax antiserum. Zone of precipitate at the junction of tissue extract and antiserum within 5 minutes at room temperature means test is positive. It is called ASCOLI TEST.

McFadyean reaction: When blood films containing anthrax bacilli are stained with polychrome methylene blue for a few seconds and examined under the microscope, amorphous purplish material is seen around bacilli. This represents capsular material and is characteristic of anthrax bacilli.

Polymerase chain reaction: Using this technique *Bacillus anthracis* may be confirmed.

Treatment: Ciprofloxacillin, penicillin, streptomycin and tetracyclines are effective. Scalvo's serum may be used in serious toxic cases. Persons with high occupational risk should be immunized with a cell-free vaccine (Sterne strain cell culture) which is available from Centers for Disease Control, Atlanta 30333.

Current strategies for vaccine development include purification of protective antigen, expression of protective antigen in recombinant microbial vaccines and construction of improved live attenuated strains of *Bacillus anthracis.*

Non-living vaccine consisting of alum precipitated or aluminium hydroxide absorbed extracellular components of unencapsulated *B. anthracis* are used in USA for army personnel, agricultural workers, veterinary personnels, etc. The major active component of these vaccines is protective antigen. Live attenuated vaccines having *B. anthracis* (spores) are used. Sterne spore vaccines (loss of plasmid that encodes capsular polypeptide) may be used.

A mutant form of protective antigen that lacks the protease sensitive sequence and that cannot be processed to interact with *E. coli* for LF to mediate toxicity has been produced by

Table 25.1: Differences between *B. anthrax* and *B. anthracoid*.

B. anthrax	*B. anthracoid*
• Non-motile	• Generally motile (by swarming, e.g. B. cereus)
• Capsulated	• Non-capsulated
• Grows in long chain	• Grows in short chain
• Medusa head colony	• Not present
• Hemolysis of sheep RBC absent	• Usually well-marked
• Inverted fir-tree growth in gelatin	• Fir-tree growth absent
• No turbidity in broth	• Turbidity usually present
• No growth in penicillin agar (10 unit/mL)	• Grows usually
• No growth at 45°C	• Grows usually
• Growth inhibited by chloral hydrate	• Not inhibited
• Susceptible to gamma phage	• Not susceptible
• Salicin fermentation negative	• Positive
• Pathogenic to man and laboratory animals	• Not pathogenic
• Methylene blue reduced weakly	• Methylene blue generally reduced strongly
• Liquefaction of gelation slow	• Liquefaction of gelatin rapid
• Lecithinase reaction weakly positive	• Strongly positive with *B. cereus*
• Culture filtrates non-toxic to tissue culture cells	• Culture filtrates (*B. cereus*) toxic to tissue culture cells
• Produces toxin, neutralized by *B. anthrax* antitoxin	• Any toxic substance produced not neutralized by *B. anthrax* antitoxin

genetic engineering as one candidate vaccine against anthrax.

BACILLUS SUBTILIS

It is Gram-positive about 1.5 μ × 4.5 μ, straight occurring singly or chain, motile and non-capsulated.

It grows on blood agar producing wider zone of beta hemolysis. It may grow in broth culture and on nutrient agar, etc.

It does not produce any toxin. Some strains may produce soluble hemolysin. They are opportunist pathogens. They cause egg infection and septicemia. They may contaminate blood transfusion bottle and thus hemolyse the blood.

BACILLUS CEREUS

They are responsible for food poisoning. They can grow in food and produce an enterotoxin that causes diarrhea by a mechanism similar to that of *Escherichia coli* enterotoxin.

Aerobic spore bearer having resemblance with *B. anthracis* are called anthracoid bacillus. They differ from each other as shown in **Table 25.1**.

Clostridium

General characters: The genus *Clostridium* consists of Gram-positive, anaerobic, spore forming, spindle-shaped and highly pleomorphic bacilli. Spores are wider than bacillary bodies. The genus contains bacteria causing 3 major diseases of man; tetanus, gas gangrene and food poisoning. Some pathogens, e.g., *Clostridium welchii* now a days called *Clostridium perfringens* and *Clostridium tetani* are found normally in human and animal intestine.

Clostridia are motile with peritrichate flagella, except *Clostridium perfringens* and *Clostridium type VI. Clostridium perfringens* and *Clostridium butyricum* are capsulated while others are not so. Pathogenic clostridia forms powerful exotoxins. *Clostridium botulinum* is non-invasive while *Clostridium tetani* has slight invasive properties. Tetanus results from the action of powerful exotoxin of *Clostridium tetani*. The gas gangrene clostridia are toxigenic and invasive causing even septicemia.

CLOSTRIDIUM TETANI

It is widely distributed in soil and in intestine of man and animals.

Morphology: It is slender, long, slightly curved, Gram-positive 4.8 µ × 0.5 µ and occurring singly or in chain. It shows considerable variation in length. Spores are spherical, terminal and bulging, giving the bacilli drumstick appearance **(Fig. 26.1)**. It is non-capsulated and motile.

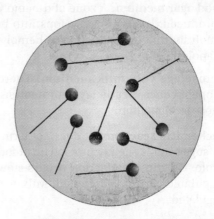

Fig. 26.1: *Clostridium tetani.*

Cultural characters: It is an obligatory anaerobe that grows only in absence of oxygen. The characteristic of anaerobic bacilli is their inability to utilize oxygen as the final hydrogen acceptor. It lacks cytochrome and cytochrome oxidase and is unable to break down hydrogen peroxide because it lacks catalase and peroxidase. Therefore, hydrogen peroxide tends to accumulate to toxic concentration in the presence of oxygen. It also lacks superoxide dismutase and consequently permit the accumulation of toxic-free radical superoxide. Hence, it can carry out its metabolism only at negative oxidation reduction potential which means an environment that is strongly reducing. The optimum temperature is 37°C and pH 7.4. It grows fairly well in ordinary media. Cultures have burnt organic smell.

Cooked meat medium: It grows well in this medium with turbidity and gas formation. The meat is not digested but is turned black after prolonged incubation.

Nutrient agar medium: It produces swarming growth forming fine film over the medium. By increasing the concentration of agar in the medium after 2 to 4 days' incubation, colonies are irregularly round, 2 to 5 mm in diameter, translucent, grayish yellow with granular surface and ill-defined edges.

Blood agar medium: A zone of α hemolysis is produced. It later on develops into beta hemolysis, due to production of hemolysin (tetanolysin).

Lactose egg yolk milk medium: There is no opalescence, pearly layer, proteolysis or lactose fermentation.

Biochemical reactions: It does not ferment any sugar and is slightly proteolytic. It forms indole. Gelatin liquefaction occurs slowly. Coagulated serum is softened. Milk is not coagulated.

Resistance: Spores of *Clostridium tetani* withstand boiling for 15 to 90 minutes. Autoclaving at 121°C for 20 minutes kills spores. Spores otherwise can survive in soil for years. Iodine (1% aqueous solution) and H_2O_2 (10 volumes) kill spores within a few minutes.

Antigen structure: The flagellar antigen differentiate *Clostridium tetani* into 10 types but toxin (neurotoxin) produced is pharmacologically and antigenically identical.

Toxin: *Clostridium tetani* produces three types of toxin:
a. Hemolysin (tetanolysin)
b. Neurotoxin (tetanospasmin)
c. Non-spasmogenic peripherally active neurotoxin.
  a. *Tetanolysin:* It is heat labile and oxygen labile and is active against RBC of many animals (rabbit, horse, etc.). Its pathogenic role is not known. May be it acts as a leukotoxin.
  b. *Tetanospasmin:* It is oxygen stable and gets inactivated at 66°C in 5 minutes (heat labile). Toxin has been crystallized. Horse is most susceptible. Birds and reptiles are highly resistant. It gets toxoided in presence of low concentration of formaldehyde. It is a good antigen and specifically neutralized by antitoxin. It is protein with 67,000 molecular weight. It acts like strychnine by inhibiting the synthesis and liberation of acetylcholine, thus, interfering with neuromuscular transmission. It can be fixed to cerebral gangliosides. It can cause inhibition of postsynaptic spinal neuron by blocking the release of inhibitory mediator. This results in generalized muscular spasms, hyper-reflexia and seizures.
  c. A third toxin is a non-spasmogenic peripherally active neurotoxin.

Pathogenesis: Spores implanted in wound multiply only if conditions are favorable. Toxin so produced is absorbed by motor nerve ending. Toxin travels along the axis cylinders of peripheral nerve and reach central nervous system. It is fixed specifically by ganglioside of gray matter of nervous tissue. Its exact mode of action is not known but it may act at synaptic junctions between anterior horn cells and related internuncial neurons leading to abolition of spinal inhibition. As a result, muscle rigidity and spasm occurs.

If given orally it is destroyed by digestive enzyme and so is not effective. Subcutaneous, intramuscularly and intravenous route is equally effective. Intraneural route is more lethal.

If toxin is injected intramuscularly in one of the hind limbs of guinea pig or mice, spasm of inoculated limb appears. This is due to toxin acting on the segment of spinal cord. Subsequently spread of toxin up to the spinal cord causes ascending tetanus and likewise opposite hind limb is involved. If toxin is injected intravenously spasticity develops in the muscles of head and neck first and then spreads downwards (descending tetanus).

Tetanus: Tetanus results from contamination of wound by *Clostridium tetani*. The spores are found in soil. Germination and multiplication occur if certain factors like necrotic tissue, ionisable calcium salts and lactic acid are present. Infection of wound with pyogenic organisms increases the risk of tetanus. Toxin is probably absorbed from the area of infection and through motor nerve endings reach anterior horn cell. Other views are that toxin is absorbed through bloodstream and perineural lymphatics.

The incubation period is 2 days to several weeks and it depends upon site, nature of wound, doses, toxigenicity of organism and immune status of patient. In rural India tetanus is estimated to be the most common cause of death.

There are many clinical types of tetanus:

Tetanus neonatorum: It occurs from contamination of cut surface of umbilical cord in infants. It has high rate of fatality.

Postabortal and puerperal tetanus: It results from infection of genital tract with unsterile instrument and dressing. Puerperal tetanus is rare but most dangerous.

Splanchnic tetanus: There is involvement of muscle of deglutition and respiration with dysphagia.

Cephalic tetanus: It occurs from the wounds of head. There is unilateral and bilateral contraction of muscles of face.

Laboratory Diagnosis

The diagnosis is always clinical and bacteriological findings confirm the diagnosis.
1. *Microscopic examination:* Smears from wound material after Gram's staining show Gram-positive bacilli with typical drumstick appearance.
2. *Culture:* Diagnosis by culture is more dependable. Excised bits of tissue from necrotic depth of wound is inoculated into cooked meat broth, blood agar and lactose egg yolk medium. The addition of polymyxin B to which clostridia resist, make the medium more selective.

If the material is grossly contaminated with other organisms, heating at 80°C for 10 minutes may be useful for destroying non-sporing organisms.

Animal inoculation: Mouse is a suitable laboratory animal for demonstration of toxigenicity. 2 to 4 days' old cooked meat culture (0.2 mL) is inoculated into the root of tail of a mouse. A second mouse which has received tetanus antitoxin (1000 units) an hour earlier serves as control. Symptoms appear in test animal in 12 to 24 hours with stiffness of tail. Rigidity develops to the inoculated side of the leg, opposite leg, trunk, forelimb in this order. The animal dies within 2 days. However, appearance of ascending tetanus in animal is diagnostic.

Prophylaxis: It is a preventable disease. Immunity to tetanus may result from infection or by immunization **(Table 26.1)**.

Active immunization: Usually two injections 1 mL each of tetanus toxoid is given intramuscularly at the interval of 6 weeks. Third injection is given after 6 to 12 months. A full course of immunization confers immunity for 10 years. Toxin is given either alone or along with diphtheria toxoid and pertussis vaccine (triple vaccine) in which pertussis vaccine acts as adjuvant.

Passive immunization: It is an emergency procedure to be used only once. It is done by giving antitetanus serum (ATS). The recommended dose is 1800 IU subcutaneously or intramuscularly as early as possible after wounding. Unfortunately, it carries the risk of hypersensitivity and immune elimination (half life is 2 days).

Passive immunity without risk of hypersensitivity be obtained by use of human antitetanus immunoglobulin (ATG). This is effective in smaller dose (280 units) and has longer half life (3 to 5 weeks).

Combined immunization: It consists of administering to non-immune person ATS at one site along with a dose of toxoid at

Table 26.1: Tetanus prophylaxis in wound.

Nature of wound	Immune status		
	Immune	Partial immune	Non-immune
Clean (wound toilet performed within 6 hours)	Toxoid × 1	Toxoid × 1	Toxoid × 3
Contaminated (soil, necrotic material present)	Toxoid × 1	Toxoid × 1 ATS Antibiotics	Toxoid × 3 ATS Antibiotics
Infected	Toxoid × 1 Antibiotics	Toxoid × 1 ATS Antibiotics	Toxoid × 3 ATS Antibiotics

Note: Immune patients having full course of 3 injections of toxoid. Partial immune patient has had 2 injections of toxoid. Non-immune patient has had no injection of toxoid or his immune status is not known.

other site followed by other doses of toxoid at appropriate intervals. Ideally in emergency, combined immunization should be performed instead of passive immunization alone.

CLOSTRIDIUM PERFRINGENS (CLOSTRIDIUM WELCHII)

It is a normal inhabitant of the large intestine of man and animals. It is found in feces and contaminates the skin of perineum, buttocks and thigh. It also produces food poisoning and necrotic enteritis in man.

Morphology: It is a plump, Gram-positive bacillus with straight, parallel sides, rounded or truncated ends about 4 to 6 μ × 1 μ. It may occur singly or in chains. It is pleomorphic. Filaments and involution forms are common. It is capsulated and non-motile. Spores are central or subterminal.

Cultural characters: It is an anaerobe, growing rapidly at 37°C.
a. *Cooked meat medium:* Fairly good growth occurs at 37°C. The medium becomes turbid within 24 hours with production of gas. The meat is turned pink without digestion **(Fig. 26.2)**. The culture has sour odor.
b. *Nutrient agar:* Two types of colonies appear after 24 hours of incubation; (i) 2 to 4 mm round, smooth, butyrous emulsifiable colonies, (ii) Umbonate colonies with

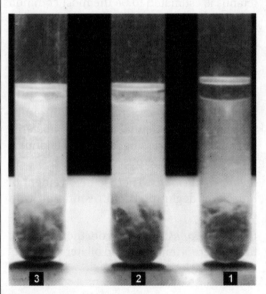

Fig. 26.2: Cooked meat medium: (1) Control; (2) *Clostridium sporogenes;* (3) *Clostridium perfringens.*

brownish opaque center and lighter radially striated periphery having crenated edges.

Biochemical reactions: Glucose, maltose, lactose and sucrose are fermented with production of acid and gas. In litmus milk it produces acid with gas **(Fig. 26.3)**. Milk is disrupted due to vigorous production of gas. This is called stormy clot. Indole is negative and H$_2$S is formed abundantly.

Resistance: Autoclaving at 121°C for 18 minutes destroys the spores. Spores are

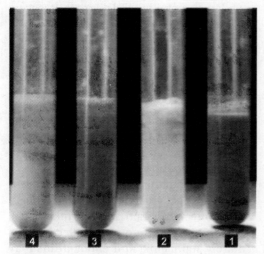

Fig. 26.3: Litmus milk: (1)Control; (2) *Clostridium perfringens;* (3) *Pseudomonas aeruginosa;* (4) *Escherichia coli.*

resistant to antiseptics and disinfectants in common use.

Antigenic structures: *Clostridium perfringens* are differentiated into 6 types (A,B, C, D, E, F) on the basis of toxin produced by the strains. Toxins are antigenic and antitoxic sera are used for routine typing of strain.

Toxin: *Clostridium perfringens* produces at least 12 distinct toxins, besides many other enzymes and biological active soluble substances. According to kind and quantity of toxins produced, different strains of *Clostridium perfringens* are divided into 6 types, i.e., A to F. The 4 major toxins, alpha, beta, epsilon and iota are responsible for pathogenicity.

Alpha toxin is more important and is produced by all strains of *Clostridium perfringens.* Type A strains produce it more abundantly. It is responsible for toxemia of gas gangrene. It is lethal, dermonecrotic and hemolytic. It also shows lecithinase activity and gives positive Nagler's reaction.

NAGLER'S REACTION

Clostridium perfringens are cultured on plates containing 20% of human serum or egg yolk.

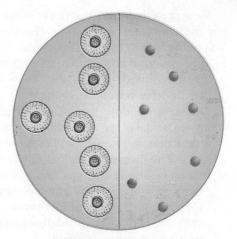

Fig. 26.4: Nagler's reaction.

The organism produces opalescence in media containing human serum and egg yolk. The opalescence is due to lecithinase activity of alpha toxin. Alpha toxin splits lipoproteins and liberates lipids. The lipid deposits around the colony to give opalescence **(Fig. 26.4)**. The reaction is specific and is inhibited by alpha toxin antitoxin sera. It is a useful test for the rapid detection of *Clostridium perfringens* in clinical specimen.

Beta, epsilon and iota toxins have lethal and necrotizing properties.

Besides toxins, *Clostridium perfringens* also produces soluble substances with enzymatic properties, e.g., neuraminidase, hemagglutinin, fibrinolysin, hemolysin, histamine, etc.

Pathogenicity: Only type A and F are pathogenic for man. Type A is responsible for gas gangrene and food poisoning.

A. *Gas gangrene: Clostridium perfringens* type A is the predominant agent causing gas gangrene. Other organisms associated with gas gangrene are *Clostridium septicum, Clostridium edematiciens* and anaerobic streptococci.

Organisms enter the wound usually along with foreign particles, e.g., soil, dust, etc. Clostridia may be present on normal skin. Infection may be endogenous.

Mere presence of clostridium in wound does not constitute gas gangrene. There are 3 types of anaerobic wound infection:

1. Simple wound contamination with no invasion of underlying tissue. There is usually delay in wound healing.
2. *Anaerobic cellulitis:* In which clostridia invade fascial plane with minimal toxin production and no invasion of muscle tissue. The disease is gradual in onset. It may be limited to gas abscess or extensive involvement of a limb occurs. Infecting clostridia is of low invasive power and poor toxigenicity. Toxemia is absent and prognosis is good.
3. *Anaerobic myositis:* It is most serious and is associated with abundant formation of exotoxin. The clostridia multiply and elaborate toxin which causes further damage. The lecithinase (toxin) damages cell membranes, muscle fibers and increases capillary permeability. Resulting edema may cause increased tension and anoxia in affected muscle. Hemolytic anemia and hemoglobinuria are due to lysis of RBC by a toxin.

    The collagenase destroys collagen barriers in tissue. Hyaluronidases break down intercellular substances. Abundant production of gas reduces blood supply by pressure effect extending the area of anoxic damage. Thus, there is spread of infection and lesion is progressive one.

    The incubation period is 7 hours to 6 weeks. The disease develops with increasing pain, tenderness, edema of affected part with systemic signs of toxemia. Profound toxemia and prostration develops and death occurs due to circulatory failure.

B. *Food poisoning:* Some strains of type A produce food poisoning. They are characterized by marked heat resistance of spores and production of alpha and beta toxin. They are non-hemolytic strains. Incubation period is 10 to 12 hours. It starts with pain in abdomen, vomiting and diarrhea. Recovery takes place in 24 to 48 hours.

C. *Enteritis necrotican:* A severe and fatal enteritis due to F type strain may occur. The pathogenesis of this disease is suggested to be a low protein diet that predisposes to decreased levels of digestive proteases with subsequent mobility to degrade the clostridia beta toxin. The proteases are further blocked by ingestion of trypsin inhibitors found in sweet potatoes.

Apart from this *Clostridium perfringens* may cause gangrenous appendicitis, biliary tract infection, brain abscess, meningitis, panophthalmitis, urogenital infection, etc. Rarely septicemia and endocarditis may occur.

Laboratory Diagnosis

A. Hematological investigation:
   a. Total leukocyte count usually shows no change. Increased count occurs in secondary infection.
   b. Differential leukocyte count shows no change.
   c. Anemia, increased serum, bilirubin and hemoglobinuria may occur due to excessive RBC destruction.

B. Bacteriological investigation:
   Specimens: They are collected from:
   1. Muscles at the edge of affected area.
   2. Exudate from area where infection appears more active.
   3. Necrotic tissue and muscle fragment.

Microscopic Examination

Gram-stained smear shows Gram-positive, long and thick bacilli. Gram-positive bacilli without spore are suggestive of *Clostridium perfringens.*

Culture: Material is inoculated on fresh blood agar and cooked meat media. Surface culture is incubated aerobically and anaerobically. Anaerobic culture is studied after 48 to 72 hours of incubation. Further identification is done by:

1. Nagler's reaction.
2. Biochemical reaction.
3. Animal pathogenicity.

Blood collected during bacteremia is cultured in cooked meat medium and glucose broth. It is identified in usual way.

Animal Pathogenicity

On the hind limb of guinea pig 0.1 mL of 24 hour cooked meat broth is injected intramuscularly. Death of animal occurs in 24 to 48 hour. Autopsy shows swelling of injected limb with crepitation due to gas formation. The muscle becomes pink. Organism can be recovered from heart and spleen.

Bacteriological Diagnosis of *Clostridium perfringens* Food Poisoning

From the feces of patient and suspected food, isolation of non-hemolytic, non-motile anaerobic and Gram-positive bacilli is suggestive of *Clostridium perfringens* infection.

Treatment: Antibiotics and surgery in gas gangrene.

CLOSTRIDIUM BOTULINUM

Clostridium botulinum spores are widely distributed in soil, animal manure, sea mud, vegetables, etc. It causes botulism, a severe form of food poisoning.

Morphology: It is Gram-positive about 5 μ × 1 μ, non-capsulated motile by peritrichate flagella producing subterminal, oval and bulging spores. It shows pleomorphism and occurs either singly or in pairs or chains.

Culture characters: It is strict anaerobic. There are 6 different types (A to F). They differ from one another in their culture characters. These types are identified on the base of immunological difference in toxin production. It grows at 20 to 35°C in neutral or slightly alkaline medium.

a. *Cooked meat medium:* After 2 to 4 days' incubation there is abundant growth. There is blackening of meat particles and gas is also produced.

b. *Nutrient agar medium:* Single colony is difficult to get because of tendency to spread. Colonies develops after 48 hours. Colony is irregular, 3 to 8 mm, glistening and with granular surface. Consistency of colony is butyrous and is emulsified easily.

c. *Blood agar:* Colonies on blood agar medium are hemolytic.

d. *Lactose, egg yolk, milk agar medium:* All types of this organism produces opalescence and pearly layer. All are lactose negative.

Resistance: Spore is highly resistant, surviving several hours at 100°C. It withstands 120°C for 20 minutes. However, heat resistance is diminished at acid pH or high salt concentration.

Biochemical reactions: All types ferment glucose, maltose with acid and gas. There are two biochemical types of *Clostridium botulinum:*

a. Proteolytic (types A, B and F).
b. Saccharolytic and non-proteolytic (type C, D and E). H_2S is produced by all types.

Antigenic structure: Six types are distinguished by their toxin production. The toxins are antigenically distinct.

Toxin: It produces powerful exotoxin responsible for pathogenicity. Toxin has been isolated as crystalline protein which is most toxic substance known, i.e., 0.000,000,003 mg is the lethal dose of mice. It is a neurotoxin which acts slowly by inhibiting release of acetylcholine at synapses and neuromuscular junctions. Flaccid paralysis results.

Toxin is stable. It resists digestion in the intestine and is absorbed through intestinal mucosa in an active form. It can be toxoided. The most important and potent exotoxin is that of type A. The other types of toxin are less toxic.

Botulinum toxin is now found useful in strabismus, blepharospasm, hemifacial spasm, tremors (dystonic one), spasmodic torticolis, vocal muscle spasm, stuttering, spasticity and writer's cramp.

Pathogenesis: *Clostridium botulinum* is non-invasive and its pathogenicity is due to toxin, produced in contaminated food. Botulism is because of ingestion of preformed toxin in food. Human botulism is caused by type A, B and E. Source of this toxin is preserved food, meat, canned vegetable and fishes, etc.

Incubation period is 12 to 36 hours. Vomiting, thirst, constipation, difficulty in swallowing, speaking and breathing are the manifestations which may be followed by coma, delerium and death in 1 to 7 days.

Laboratory Diagnosis

Bacteriological Investigations

Specimen: Diagnosis is based on demonstration of bacillus or toxin in food or feces. In early stages toxin may be detected from patient's blood.

Culture: Isolation of organism (toxigenic strain) from vomit, food or feces in absence of toxin is of no significance.

Demonstration of *Clostridium botulinum* toxin: Specimen like food, vomit, etc. are grounded up and soaked overnight in equal volume of isotonic saline solution. It is centrifuged, and supernatant is divided into 3 parts. One portion is heated at 100°C for 10 minutes. Penicillin is added (concentration being 100 units/mL).

One of the guinea pig is protected with polyvalent botulinum antitoxin and 2 mL of unheated material is injected intraperitonially only. Unheated material (2 mL) is injected into second guinea pig. The third animal is injected with 3 mL of heated material.

Second guinea pig develops toxin symptoms like dyspnea, flaccid paralysis and dies within 24 hours. First and third animals show no toxic symptoms.

Typing is done by passive protection with type specific antitoxin. A retrospective diagnosis may be made by detecting of antitoxin in patients serum.

Treatment: Active immunization with toxoid is effective. However, antitoxin is of no use in treatment as toxin already get fixed up to nervous tissue by the time disease becomes apparent. Trivalent antitoxin must be promptly administered intravenously. However, early administration of potent antitoxin (intravenously) with guanidine hydrochloride as an adjunct is recommended. Such measures with artificial respiration have reduced fatality rate from 65 to 25%.

■ CLOSTRIDIUM DIFFICILE

Clostridium difficile is a commensal bacterium of the human intestine found in 2–5% of the population. It was first isolated from the feces of neonates and was named so due to the difficulties in isolating the organism.

Morphology

It is an anaerobic, sporeforming, long slender, Gram-positive bacillus containing oval and terminal spores. It has a tendency to lose its Gram reaction.

Toxins

Two types of toxins are produced by *Clostridium difficile*, an enterotoxin (toxin A) and a cytotoxin (toxin B). Toxin A usually results in diarrhea and toxin B produces cytopathogenic effects in several tissue culture cell lines.

Pathogenesis

Prolonged use of antibiotics, especially those with a broad spectrum of activity can result in disruption of normal intestinal flora, leading to an overgrowth of *Clostridium difficile*, which flourishes under these conditions. It thereby results in acute colitis with (Pseudomembranous colitis) or without membrane formation. It is usually a fatal disease if not treated promptly.

Laboratory Diagnosis

Toxigenic culture, in which organisms are cultured on selective medium and tested for toxin production, remains the gold standard and is the most sensitive and specific test, although it is slow and requires a considerable effort.

Toxin production can be demonstrated in the faeces by its characteristic effect on human diploid cells and Hep-2. ELSIA is also helpful in detecting the toxin production.

Treatment

Metronidazole is the drug of choice. Other antibiotics that may be effective against *Clostridium difficile* include vancomycin and linezolid. Drugs traditionally used to stop diarrhea should not be used as they frequently worsen the course of *Clostridium difficile* related pseudomembranous colitis.

Chapter 27

Enterobacteriaceae

General characters: Numerous interrelated bacterial flora of intestine are Gram-negative rods, motile only with peritrichate flagella or non-motile, non-sporing, non-acid fast, ferment glucose with or without formation of gas, reduce nitrates into nitrites, form catalase, oxidase negative and aerobic or anaerobic.

Classification

I. *Based on action on lactose:*
It is an old method. It has practical value in diagnostic bacteriology.
a. Lactose fermenter
e.g. *Escherichia coli*
Klebsiella
b. Late lactose fermenter
e.g. *Shigella sonnei*
Paracolons
c. Non-lactose fermentation
e.g. *Salmonella*
Shigella
II. *Modern taxonomical concept:*
Enterobacteriaceae may be classified into tribes, genera and species by their cultural and biochemical characters. The species are further classified as: biotypes, serotypes, bacteriophage types and colicin types. At present there are five tribes as under:

Enterobacteriaceae

Tribe I   Escherichieae
Genus: *Escherichia*
Edwardsiella
Citrobacter
Salmonella
Shigella
Tribe II   *Klebsielleae*
Genus: *Klebsiella*
Enterobacter
Hafnia
Serratia
Tribe III   Proteeae
Genus: *Proteus*
Tribe IV   Erwinieae
Genus: *Erwinia*
Tribe V   Yersinae
Genus: *Yersinia pestis*
Yersinia enterolitico
Yersinia pseudotuberculosis

ESCHERICHIA COLI

It lives only in human or animal intestine. Detection of *Escherichia coli* in drinking water is taken as evidence of recent pollution with human or animal excreta. *Escherichia coli* in contaminated water may be detected using PCR (rapid and sensitive), DNA probes, plating and biochemical tests.

Morphology: It is Gram-negative, non-capsulated, short, plump bacilli 2 to 4 µ × 0.4 to 0.7 µ in diameter and are motile. Spores are not formed.

Cultural characters: It is aerobic and facultative anaerobe growing on simple media. Optimum temperature is 37°C.
1. *Liquid broth:* It shows uniform turbidity after 8 to 24 hours' incubation.

2. *Nutrient agar:* Colonies appear after 12 to 18 hours of incubation. They are circular 1 to 3 mm in diameter, smooth, colorless, having entire edge with butyrous consistency. Colonies are emulsified easily.
3. *MacConkey medium:* The colonies are pink due to lactose fermentation.
4. *Blood agar:* Some strains may show zone of beta hemolysis.

Biochemical reactions: It ferments lactose, glucose, sucrose, maltose and mannitol forming acid and gas. Indole and methyl red (MR) is positive. VP and citrate is negative. Urease is not hydrolyzed. H_2S is not produced.

Resistance: It can survive for months in soil and water. It is killed at 60°C in 20 minutes and chlorine (0.5 to 1 part per million). It is sensitive to streptomycin, tetracycline, chloramphenicol, furadantin and nalidixic acid.

Antigenic structure: There are 4 types of antigens:
1. *Somatic antigen* (O antigen): They are heat stable. They are divided into 175 groups designated as 1, 2, 3 and so on.
2. *Surface antigen* (K antigen). They are heat labile. They interfere with O agglutination unless destroyed by heating at 100 to 121°C. They are of 3 types:
   a. L antigen is destroyed by heating at 100°C for 1 hour and its capacity to combine with antibody is lost.
   b. A antigen is capsular antigen and is heat stable and is associated with well-marked capsule.
   c. B antigen is destroyed by heating at 100°C for one hour. Still they retain the capacity to combine with antibody.
      Only one of L, A and B surface antigen is present in a strain. 100 K antigens are recognized so far. Now K antigen is divided into two types i.e., Type I and Type II.
3. *Flagellar antigen* (H antigen): They are thermolabile and monophasic. About 75 types have been described.

4. *Fimbrial antigen* (F antigen): They are thermolabile and have no significance in antigenic classification of *E. coli*.

The antigenic pattern of a strain is recorded as number of particular antigen it carries, e.g., $O_{111} K_{58} H_2$. The normal colon strain belongs to early O group (1, 2, 8, 4, etc.), while enteropathogenic belongs to later O group (26, 55, 86, 111, etc.).

Toxin production: It produces endotoxin. Besides that, it also produces two types of exotoxins:
a. Enterotoxin which is heat labile, filtrable and causes fluid accumulation in rabbit ileal loop. The mode of action is by activation of adenyl cyclase thereby raising level of cAMP in cell thus causing excretion of fluid and electrolytes in the lumen of intestine.
   Two types of *E. coli* enterotoxins have been recognized, i.e., heat labile toxin (LT) and heat stable toxin (ST). A strain of *E. coli* may produce one or both types of enterotoxins. The production of enterotoxins is under genetic control of transmissible plasmids. Heat labile toxin (LT) is of large molecular weight (80,000) protein which gets inactivated by heating at 60°C for 10 minutes. On the other hand, heat stable toxin (ST) is of low molecular weight (8,000 to 8,500). ST is non-antigenic toxin which seems to stimulate fluid secretion in the gut through mediation of cyclic guanosine monophosphate (cGMP).
b. Hemolysin which may be:
   i. Heat labile, filtrable and lethal for animals.
   ii. Associated with bacterial cell and is not filtrable.

Pathogenesis

Endotoxin may cause fever, leukopenia, hypotension, disseminated intravascular coagulation (DIC), etc.

Other lesions produced are:
1. *Gastroenteritis:* Certain serotypes produce fatal type of gastroenteritis in infants, e.g., 4, 26, 46, 55, 86, 111, 112, 119, 127 and 129.

Sporadic summer diarrhea occurs in children during second or third summer of life in non-epidemic form. Lactic acid produced from lactose fermentation may cause irritation of the colon. Result is violent nausea, vomiting and diarrhea.

There are six groups of *E. coli* which can cause diarrheal diseases:

a. *Enteropathogenic E. coli also called EPEC:* They are carrying β type of surface (K) antigen. They have caused several serious institutional outbreaks of diarrhea in babies less than 18 months old. Over 25 serotypes are identified, e.g., $O_{26}:B_6; O_{55}:B_5; O_{86}:B_7$, etc. The pathogenic mechanism of EPEC is their tight adherence to enterocytes resulting in the loss of microvilli and cupping of enterocyte membrane to bacteria.

b. *Enterotoxigenic E. coli also called ETEC:* They produce heat labile and heat stable enterotoxin and thus producing diarrhea. They cause diarrhea in children and also travellers' diarrhea. No biochemical markers are available to identify ETEC strains. Their identification depends on the demonstration of the toxins. They possess surface properties called colonization factors which promote their virulence. Colonization factors may be pili or special type of protein K antigen. Most strains of ETEC belong to O serotypes 6, 8, 15, 25, etc. They are known to cause:

1. Mild or moderately severe childhood diarrhea in developing countries.
2. Cholera-like syndrome in adults living in areas where cholera is endemic.
3. Travellers' diarrhea in persons from developed country who visit developing countries.
4. Outbreaks of diarrhea in newborn nurseries in developed countries.
5. Outbreak of diarrhea due to fecal contamination of food and water in developed countries.

c. *Enteroinvasive E. coli also called EIEC:* They invade intestinal epithelium like other dysentery causing bacilli. They are biochemically atypical as they may be late lactose fermenter or non-lactose fermenter. They cause keratoconjunctivitis when instilled in the eyes of guinea pig (Sereny test). The invasion of HeLa cells in tissue culture also provides another test for its demonstration. They belong to serogroup like O_{28}ac, O_{112}ac, O_{124}, etc.

d. *Enterohemorrhagic E. coli also called EHEC:* They were identified in 1983 following foodborne outbreaks of hemorrhagic colitis caused by *E. coli* O_{157} : H_7. Here there is usually no fever but hemorrhage is marked. EHEC produces a cytotoxin. It is also called "Vero toxin" because of its affects on vero cells in culture.

e. Enteroaggregative *E. coli* (EAEC)

f. Diffusely adherent *E. coli* (DAEC)

2. *Urinary tract infection,* e.g., cystitis, pyelitis and pyelonephritis. Infection may be precipitated by urinary obstruction due to prostatic enlargement, calculi and pregnancy.

Escherichia coli serotype commonly responsible for urinary tract infection are 0, 1, 2, 4, 6 and 7. Strains carrying K antigen are responsible for pyelonephritis while strains from cystitis lack "K" antigen.

Urinary tract infection causing Escherichia coli possess certain characters like binding of *Escherichia coli* to epithelial cell receptors by means of adhesion. Almost all *E. coli* strains that cause pylonephritis in patients with anatomically normal urinary tracts possess a particular pilus (P pilus or gal pilus that mediates attachment to the digalactoside portion of glycosphingolipids present on uroepithelium. The strains that produce pyelonephritis are also hemolysin produce, have aerobactin (a siderophore for scavenging iron) and are resistant to the bactericidal action of human serum.

As such, uroepithelial adhesion assay has become one of the important parameters. Six antigenic types F_7 to F_{12} of fimbrial have been identified from uropathogenic.

3. *Pyogenic infection,* e.g., wound infection, abscess, peritonitis, cholecystitis and meningitis.
4. *Septicemia:* It is one of the most common cause of septicemia. The manifestations are fever, hypotension, disseminated intravascular coagulation (endotoxin shock), etc. Mortality is significantly high.

Laboratory Diagnosis

1. *Hematological investigations:*
   a. Total leukocyte count is usually within normal limits. In tissue invasion moderateleukocytosis may be there.
   b. *Differential leukocyte count:* There may be increase in polymorphonuclear cells in tissue invasion.
2. *Bacteriological investigations:*
   Specimen: In urinary tract infection midstream urine is collected under aseptic conditions. Immediately the urine is examined and in case of delay it should be stored at 4°C.
   In acute diarrhea a sample of feces or a rectal swab is collected. Pus may be collected on sterile cotton swab or sterile container.

Smear Examination

Centrifuged urine deposit is examined for pus cell, RBC and bacteria. Gram-stained smear from centrifuged deposit shows moderate to large number of pus cell and Gram-negative bacilli.

Examination of wet and stained smear of fecal matter is of little use. Treatment of fecal matter with fluorescent labeled O group antisera is useful for an early provisional diagnosis of infantile diarrhea. Here, DNA probes for different enteropathogenic forms are quite reliable and useful. ELISA, precipitin test, radioimmunoassay are other useful tests to establish the identity of enteropathogenic strains.

Culture

Material is inoculated on blood agar plate and MacConkey plate. Lactose fermenting, Gram-negative, motile, indole positive, MR positive, VP negative and citrate negative is suggestive of *Escherichia coli.*

The count of organism should be more than 1 lakh per mL (10^5 per mL) in urinary tract infection. It is called significant bacteriuria.

Treatment: It is sensitive to sulfonamides, trimethoprim, tetracyclines, chloramphenicol and aminoglycosides. Resistance to one or more drug is quite common. Nitrofurantin and nalidixic acid may be useful for treating urinary tract infection. In septicemia or serious infection, treatment is required to be started immediately without waiting for even drug sensitivity tests and drug of choice (unlikely to be resistant) is gentamicin.

Towards preparation of vaccine against *E. coli* colonization factor antigen (CFA) is being considered. This prototype vaccine includes CFA I, II and IV and is under evaluation in Sweden.

▌EDWARDSIELLA

It is non-capsulated, motile bacillus with weak fermentation of sugar (glucose, maltose). It forms indole, H_2S and utilizes citrate.

Edwardsiella tarda is intestinal flora of snake. It has also been isolated from human diarrheaic feces. However, its pathogenic role is not known.

▌CITROBACTER

It occurs as intestinal commensals in man. It is motile, utilizes citrate, grows in KCN, produces H_2S and may ferment lactose. It has two species:
1. *C. freundii.*
2. *C. intermedius* (H_2S negative).

It has been isolated from enteric fever cases. It may cause urinary tract infection, infection of gallbladder and meninges, etc.

KLEBSIELLA

It is found in the mucosa of upper respiratory tract, intestine and genitourinary tract. It is non-motile, capsulated, growing in ordinary media forming large mucoid colonies of varying degree of stickiness. It has been classified into 3 species on the basis of biochemical reactions.

1. *K. pneumoniae:* It ferments sugar (glucose, lactose, mannitol) with production of acid and gas. Indole and MR are negative, VP and citrate are positive. It hydrolysis urea. It may cause pneumonia, urinary tract infection and pyogenic infections. Serotype 1, 2 or 3 is usually responsible for pneumonia.
2. *K. ozaenae:* It causes foul smelling nasal discharge (ozaena). Biochemical reactions are variable. It belongs to capsular type 3, 4, 5, 6.
3. *K. rhinoscleromatis:* It causes rhinoscleroma. Organisms are seen intracellulary in lesion. It belongs to capsular type 3.

Difference between Klebsiella and Escherichia Coli

E. coli	Klebsiella
• Non-capsulated	• Capsulated
• Motile	• Non-motile
• Indole and MR positive	• Indole and MR negative
• Citrate and VP negative	• Citrate and VP positive
• Urease negative	• Urease positive
• Colonies not mucoid and string test negative	• Colonies mucoid with string test positive
• Slender and long	• Short and thick
• Gas from glucose fills 1/3rd of Durham's tube	• Gas from glucose fills more than 2/3rd of Durham's tube

ENTEROBACTER

It is motile, non-capsulated, lactose fermenting, indole and MR negative, VP and citrate positive. It liquefies gelatin. There are 2 species.

1. *E. cloacae.*
2. *E. aerogenes* found in human and animal feces, soil, etc.

HAFNIA

It is also intestinal commensal. It is non-capsulated, motile, non-lactose fermenter, indole and MR negative. VP and citrate positive. Only one species is known *H. alvei.*

SERRATIA

It forms pink red or magenta non-diffusible pigment, i.e., prodigiosin. Only one species is recognized, *S. marcescens*. It has been isolated from cases of meningitis, endocarditis, septicemia and respiratory infection. It may be an opportunist pathogen infecting debilited patients of hospital.

PROTEUS

Morphology: It is Gram-negative rods showing great variation in size, 0.5 × 1 to 3 μ. It may be in long filaments or in granular form. It is actively motile and show swarming motility, best seen at 20°C (**Fig. 27.1**). It is non-sporing and non-capsulated.

Cultural character: It is aerobic and facultative anaerobic. Culture emits characteristic putrefactive (fishy or seminal) odor. *Proteus vulgaris* and *Proteus mirabilis* show swarming type of growth at 37°C while swarming is absent in other species.

Broth: It shows uniform and moderate turbidity after 18 to 24 hours of incubation. There is powdery deposit and ammonical odor.

Nutrient agar: *Proteus vulgaris* and *Proteus mirabilis* swarm on solid media at 37°C after 12 to 18 hour incubation.

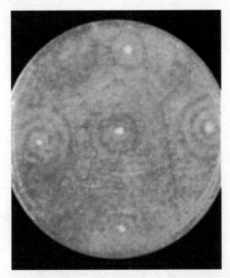

Fig. 27.1: Swarming *Proteus* on blood agar media.

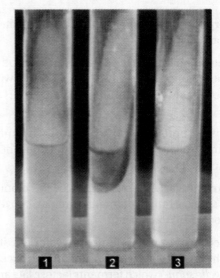

Fig. 27.2: Phenylalanine agar: (1) Control; (2) *Proteus vulgaris;* (3) *Escherichia coli.*

Swarming may be due to progressive surface growth spreading from the edge of parent colony.

Swarming can be suppressed by:
1. Six percent agar in media.
2. Chloral hydrate.
3. Sodium azide (1 : 500).
4. Alcohol (5 to 6%).
5. Sulfonamide.
6. Boric acid (1 : 1000), etc.

Swarming does not occur on MacConkey agar medium.

Biochemical reactions: It forms acid and gas from glucose (except *Proteus rettgeri*). It characteristically deaminates phenylalanine to phenylpyruvic acid (PPA) **(Fig. 27.2).** Hydrolysis of urea is another characteristic property of proteus.

It is MR positive and VP negative. It is non-lactose fermenter. H_2S is produced in *Proteus vulgaris* and *Proteus mirabilis.* Indole is not produced by *Proteus mirabilis. Proteus morganii* and *Proteus rettgeri* are H_2S negative. Citrate is positive in *Proteus rettgeri* and negative in *Proteus morganii.*

Antigenic structure: A number of O and H antigens are produced in proteus. *Proteus vulgaris* is divided into 12 types X_2, X_{19}, XK, XL and A to H. All of these have distinct O antigen (alkali labile polysaccharide). Strain X_{19}, X_2 and XK agglutinate with the sera of typhus patient because of common antigenic factor in O antigen of proteus and antigen of rickettsiae.

Pathogenicity: It is an opportunist pathogen. It may cause urinary tract infection. It may produce pyogenic lesions like abscess, infection of wound, ear or respiratory tract. *Proteus morganii* is reported to cause infantile diarrhea.

Laboratory Diagnosis

Hematological investigations: Leukocytosis with increase in polymorphonuclear cells may occur when tissues are invaded.

Bacteriological investigations: On culture of material (urine, pus, sputum, etc.) we find swarming type of growth. It can be further identified by biochemical tests.

SHIGELLA

It is found exclusively in the intestinal tract of man.

Morphology: It is non-motile, non-capsulated, about 0.5 × 1 to 3 μ in size.

Cultural character: It is aerobic and facultative anaerobic, grows readily in simple media with an optimum temperature of 37°C and pH of 7.4.

Broth: There is uniform growth with mild turbidity after 12 to 24 hours' incubation. There is no pellicle formation.

Nutrient agar: After overnight growth, colonies are small, 2 mm in diameter, circular, convex, smooth and translucent.

MacConkey agar: Colonies are colorless due to the absence of lactose fermentation except *Shigella sonnei* which ferments lactose late and forms pink colonies.

Desoxycholate citrate agar (DCA): It is a useful selective medium for *Shigella*.

Resistance: It is killed at 56°C in 1 hour and 1% phenol in 30 minutes. Boiling, pasteurization and chlorination kill the organism. In water and ice it survives and remains viable for 1 to 6 months.

Biochemical Reactions (Fig. 27.3)

It is MR positive and reduces nitrates to nitrites. It does not form H$_2$S, cannot utilize citrate and is inhibited in KCN. Catalase is positive except *Shigella dysenteriae* type I. Glucose is fermented with production of acid and no gas (except Newcastle and Manchester biotypes of *Shigella flexneri* type 6). Fermentation of mannitol forms the basis of classification as shown above.

Antigenic structure: It has one or more major antigens and large number of minor somatic antigens. There is antigenic sharing between some members of genus and between *Shigella* and *E. coli*. The somatic O antigen of *Shigella* is lipopolysaccharide. Their serologic specificity depends on the polysaccharides. Common fimbrial antigen may occur. For identification of *Shigella* both antigenic and biochemical properties should be considered.

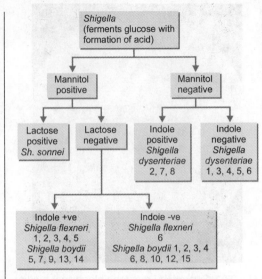

Fig. 27.3: Biochemical reactions.

TOXIN

Following toxins are produced:
a. *Endotoxin:* On autolysis endotoxin is released which is lipopolysaccharide and contributes to the irritation of bowel wall.
b. *Enterotoxin of Shigella dysenteriae* inhibits sugar and amino acid absorption in small intestine of man.

Classification: On the basis of biochemical and serological properties shigella are classified into 4 groups as discussed below:

Shigella dysenteriae: It consists of 10 serotypes. It is unique in forming powerful exotoxin (neurotoxin). It can be toxoided. This shiga exotoxin is found to be immunologically resembling verocytotoxin (VT-1). This VT-1 is also known as Shiga like toxin (SLT1 and SLT2). *Shigella dysenteriae* type I causes most severe bacillary dysentery and also called *Shigella shigae*.

Shigella flexneri: It consists of 6 antigenic types (1 to 6) and several subtypes. Serotype 6 is always indole negative and occurs in three biotypes (Boyd 88, Manchester and Newcastle).

Shigella boydii: Eighteen serotypes are known. This species resemble *Shigella flexneri* biochemically and differs from it serologically.

Shigella sonnei: It is late lactose and sucrose fermenter. Indole is not produced. On the basis of their capacity to form colicine, it is divided into 17 types. Each type being characterized by the production of specific colicine. It causes mild dysentery.

Pathogenesis: Shigellae cause bacillary dysentery. Ingested bacilli may infect villi of large intestine and multiply inside them. It spreads and ultimately involves lamina propria. Inflammatory reaction results in epithelial necrotic patch which later on become transverse superficial ulcers.

Shigella bacilli are highly infectious. The infecting dose is 103 organisms. There is invasion of mucosal epithelium; microabscesses appear in the wall of the large intestine and terminal ileum leading to necrosis of mucous membrane, superficial ulceration, bleeding and formation of a pseudomembrane on ulcerated area. Pseudomembrane consists of fibrin, leukocytes, cell debris, necrotic mucous membrane and bacteria. Then granulation tissue fills the ulcer and scar tissue is formed.

Bacillary dysentery has short incubation period (1 to 7 days). There is frequent passage of loose motion containing blood and mucus with griping pain and tenesmus. *Shigella dysenteriae* type I may cause complications like arthritis, toxic neuritis, conjunctivitis, parotitis, intussusception and myocarditis.

Laboratory Diagnosis

Collection of specimen: Stools are collected under aseptic precaution and examined as under:

Microscopic examination: Wet cover slip preparation shows large number of pus cells with degenerated nuclei, RBC and macrophages. Bacterial flora is considerably diminished.

A loopful of pus or blood tinged mucus from freshly passed fecal sample is cultured on MacConkey and DCA. Selenite broth is used as enrichment medium. After 12 to 18 hours of incubation colorless colonies (non-lactose fermenter) appear on MacConkey medium. These are tested for motility and biochemical reactions. Non-motile organism which is urease, citrate, KCN and H_2S negative, indole and MR positive suggestive of Shigella. Identification is confirmed by slide agglutination with polyvalent and monovalent antisera.

An ECO RI generated 17 Kb fragment of *Shigella flexneri* serotype 5 virulence plasmid may identify specifically all *Shigella* species. This DNA hybridization technique may be useful in the identification of isolates of *Shigella* which fail to agglutinate with reference to *Shigella* antisera.

Serology: The fluorescent antibody technique has been employed for direct identification of shigellae in feces. It is of no value in diagnosis.

Treatment: Drugs like tetracycline or chloramphenicol are effective in *Shigella* infection. Ampicillin is bactericidal for this bacteria. Treatment with antibiotic should be continued for 5 to 7 days. Oral live vaccine using streptomycin dependent strains in polyvalent preparation have given highly significant protection against clinical disease. However, protection conferred was serotype specific and required 3 to 4 doses but immunity lasted for only 6 to 12 months. Single booster dose give prolonged protection for another year. A thymine requiring and temperature sensitive double mutant has been fully characterized and its lack of virulence tested using experimental animals while new attempts are being made to introduce a gene from *Escherichia coli* thus reducing the chances of reverting to pathogenicity and using it as vaccine. Transfer by conjugation of virulent strains of *Shigella sonnei* (produce surface antigen 1) to mutant of *Salmonella typhi*-Ty 21 a is another attempt towards preparation of vaccine. The new strain 1 Gal E protects mice against *Shigella sonnei*.

SALMONELLA

Genus *Salmonella* is found in the intestine of man, animals and birds. Sometimes food (egg and meat) may be contaminated with this organism. It may cause enteric fever, gastroenteritis and septicemia.

Morphology: It is Gram-negative rods, 2 to 4 μ × 0.6 μ in size, motile (except *Salmonella gallinarum* and *Salmonella pullorum*). They are non-capsulated and non-sporing but may have fimbriae.

Cultural character: They are aerobic and facultative anaerobic, optimum temperature for their growth is 37°C and pH is 6 to 8.

Broth: It shows uniform turbidity after overnight culture. There is no pellicle formation.

Blood agar: Colonies are large 2 to 3 mm in diameter, circular low convex, translucent, smooth and non-hemolytic.

MacConkey's media: It is non-lactose fermenter and colorless.

Desoxycholate citrate media: These colonies are non-lactose fermenter (colorless).

Wilson and Blair bismuth sulfite medium: Jet black colonies with metallic sheen due to H_2S formation may appear.

Selenite F and tetrathionate: These broth are commonly used as enrichment media.

Biochemical reactions: It ferments glucose, mannitol and maltose forming acid and gas except *Salmonella typhi* which produces only acid and no gas. It does not produce indole but is MR positive, VP negative and citrate may be positive. Urea is not hydrolyzed and H_2S is produced.

Resistance: It may be killed:
a. By heating at 60°C for 15 to 20 minutes,
b. Pasteurization,
c. Boiling, and
d. Chlorination.

It is sensitive to chloramphenicol. It can survive in ice, snow and water for months together. It is resistant to brilliant green, malachite green, bile salts, tetrathionate and selenium salts.

Antigenic structure: Following antigens are found:

Somatic antigen (O): It is phospholipid protein polysaccharide complex. It can withstand boiling, alcohol and acid treatment. O agglutination takes place more slowly. It is less immunogenic. Hence, titer of O antibody after infection or immunization is lower than that of H antigen. About 65 antigenic factors have been identified and each species contains several factors.

Flagellar antigen (H): It is heat labile protein. It is destroyed by boiling, alcohol but not by formaldehyde. It is strongly immunogenic. The flagellar antigen is of dual nature occurring in one of two phases. Phase I is designated as *a,b,c,— z1, z20,* etc. and is species specific. Phase II is non-specific and is shared by several unrelated species of *Salmonella*. It is designated as 1, 2, 3 or complex of *e, n* and *x*.

Vi antigen: It is surface and heat labile antigen. Bacilli inagglutinable with O antiserum becomes agglutinable after boiling or heating at 60°C for 1 hour. It is virulent to mice and Vi antibody may provide protection. The persistence of Vi antibody indicates carrier state. It is present in *S. typhi, S. paratyphi C* and *S. dublin*. It may also be present in citrobacter.

Salmonella classification: Asper modern toxonomical techniques all members of genus Salmonella belongs to two species as under:
1. *Salmonella enteric*
2. *Salmonella bongori*

Salmonella Enteric

❖ Corresponds to former subgenus I
❖ It is further classified into 6 subspecies as under
  ■ Enterica
  ■ Salmae
  ■ Arigonae
  ■ Diarizonae

- Houtenae
- Indica

❖ *Salmonella enteric* subspecies enteric includes the typhoid, paratyphoid bacilli and many other serotypes responsible for human disease.

❖ As per this taxonomy the appropriate name suggested for typhoid bacillus is *Salmonella enteric*, subspecies enteric serotype typhi, serotype name ought to be given in Roman only.

Antigenic classification: On the basis of somatic antigen, *Salmonella* can be divided into 65 serogroups. Each group is designated as A, B, C, D, etc., e.g., members of group A have 1, 2, 12, group B have 1, 4, 5, 12, group C 6, 7 or 6, 8 and group D have 1, 9, 12, 0 factors. Species among each sub-group are recognized by specific flagellar antigen (phase I and phase II).

Antigenic Variation

1. *S → R variation:* The smooth to rough variation is associated with change in colony morphology and loss of O antigen and virulence. SÄR variation is induced by prolonged incubation of broth culture. It can be prevented by maintaining cultures on Dorset egg media, in cold or lyophilization.

2. *H → O variation:* It is associated with loss of flagellar antigen. This is reversible change. Flagella are inhibited in media containing phenol (1 : 800). Flagella reappear when strain is subcultured in media without phenol.

3. *Phase variation:* The flagellar antigen of *Salmonella* may occur in one of two phases. Phase I antigen is more specific as it is shared by few species only. Phase II antigen is widely shared and is non-specific. Strains that have both phases are called diphasic. *S. typhi* occurs in one phase and called monophasic. A culture in one phase may be converted into other phase by passing through Craigie's tube containing homologous phase antiserum incorporated in agar **(Fig. 27.4)**.

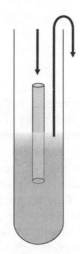

Fig. 27.4: Craigie's tube.

4. *V → W variation:* *S. typhi* carries surface antigen (Vi) which is agglutinable with Vi antiserum (V form). After repeated culture Vi antigen is lost and is inagglutinable with Vi antiserum (W form). Intermediate phase when it is agglutinable with both Vi and O antiserum is called VW forms.

Bacteriophage: Some serotypes of Salmonella strain indistinguishable biochemically and serologically may be subdivided into phage types. It is based on their susceptibility to lysis by different races of bacteriophage. Likewise *S. typhi* having Vi antigen may be divided into 106 phages types designated by letter numbers. Type A is sensitive to all Vi phages. The types predominant all over the world are E-1, A, B-2, C-1, C-2 and F-1. Paratype-B has 53 phage types and *S. typhimu rium* has 232 phage types with 30 phages.

Biotyping: On the basis of 15 biochemical properties uptill now 24 primary and 200 full biotypes are recognized of *Salmonella typhimurium*.

Plasmid typing: Quite a large number of plasmids are present in various Salmonella. They can be separated on the basis of molecular weight by electrophoresis and plasmid profile. This technique is comparable with phage typing.

Pathogenesis: It may produce 3 types of lesions:

a. Enteric fever.
b. Food poisoning.
c. Septicemia.

Enteric fever: It is caused by *S. typhi* (70 to 85% in India), *S. paratyphi A* (15 to 21%) and *S. paratyphi B*. Infection is through ingestion. The bacilli may enter the body through lymphoid of pharynx. In the gut organisms attach themselves with epithelial cells of intestinal villi and penetrate lamina propria and submucosa. They are phagocytosed by polymorph or macrophages. They enter mesenteric lymph node to multiply there. Then they enter thoracic duct and subsequently bloodstream.

As a result there is bacteremia and organism are seeded in liver, gallbladder, spleen, bone marrow, lymph node, lung and kidney, etc. In these organs further multiplication occurs. Then there is bacteremia and hence onset of clinical symptoms. The bacilli invade tissue, e.g., Payer's patches and lymphoid follicles of small intestine. The intestinal lesion ulcerates and hemorrhage or perforation may occur **(Fig. 27.5)**.

The organism liberate endotoxin which produces toxic symptoms like headache, anorexia, continuous fever and congestion of mucous membrane. Incubation period is 10 to 14 days. The typical features are step ladder pyrexia, palpable spleen and rose spots that fade on pressure and they appear in 2nd to 3rd week of infection.

S. paratyphi A and *S. paratyphi B* may cause paratyphoid fever resembling enteric fever.

Septicemia: It is frequently caused by *S. cholerae suis*. It produces chills and spiked fever. Local lesions occur in various parts of body producing osteomyelitis, pneumonia, pulmonary abscess and meningitis, etc. The bowel is not invaded and fecal culture is negative.

Food poisoning: It is by ingestion of contaminated food, e.g., meat and egg. Food poisoning is caused by *S. typhimurium, S. enteritides, S. newport,* etc. Incubation period is 12 to 48 hours. There is fever, vomiting, diarrhea (mucus and blood in stool). There may be ulceration of intestinal mucosa. There is no bacteremia.

Laboratory Diagnosis

1. *Hematological investigations:*
   a. Total leukocyte count in typhoid fever shows leucopenia. The count may be 3000 to 8000 per cu mm.

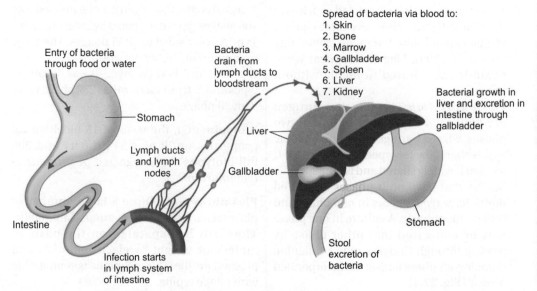

Fig. 27.5: Typhoid fever pathogenesis.

b. *Differential leukocyte count:* There may be lymphocytosis and monocytosis.

2. *Bacteriological investigations:* Organism may be isolated from blood, urine, feces, persistent discharge and in some cases from cerebrospinal fluids.

a. *Blood culture:* 5 to 10 mL blood of a patient is collected aseptically and is transferred into blood culture bottles containing 100 mL of bile broth. After 24 to 48 hours' incubation of bottle at 37°C, they are subcultured on blood agar and MacConkey, on which bacilli grow as non-lactose fermenting, Gram-negative and motile organism.

b. *Clot culture:* Blood clot is cultured in 15 mL bile broth bottle (0.5% bile salts). It is more frequently positive.

c. *Fecal culture:* It is positive throughout. Repeated cultures are required for successful isolation of organism. Fecal culture is useful more in cases who are on chloramphenicol.

Successful culture depends on use of enrichment and selective media. Fecal samples are plated directly on MacConkey, DCA and Wilson and Blair media. On MacConkey and DCA we find pale colonies. On Wilson and Blair we find black colonies with metallic sheen. *S. paratyphi A* produce green colonies.

For enrichment, specimen are inoculated into one tube each of selenite F and tetrathionate broth. It needs 12 to 18 hours' incubation before subculture.

Bile culture: It is important for detection of carriers and in later stages of disease. Bile aspirated by duodenal tube is processed like fecal specimen.

Urine culture: It is less useful than blood and feces. Culture is positive in 2nd and 3rd week. Clean voided urine is centrifuged and sediments are inoculated into enrichment and selective media.

Other material: Bone marrow culture is positive in most cases. Other specimens like rose spots, pus from lesion, CSF and sputum may be used for culture. At autopsy culture may be obtained from gallbladder, liver, spleen and mesenteric lymph nodes.

Serological test (Widal test): *Salmonella* antibody appears at the end of first week, Widal test is used for this purpose. This is a test to measure H and O antibodies in the sera of patient. Two types of tubes are used:

a. Narrow tube with conical bottom (Dreyer's tube) for H agglutination.

b. Short round bottomed tube (Felix tube) for O agglutination.

Serial two fold dilution of patient serum (1/10, 1/20, 1/40 and so on) are mixed with equal volume of antigen (TO, TH, AO and AH). At 37°C incubation is done for 4 hours and then rack is kept at 4°C overnight. H agglutination leads to formation of cotton wooly clump and O agglutination is seen as matted, granular irregular disk like pattern at the bottom of tube **(Fig. 27.6)**.

Interpretation of Widal Test

1. Agglutination appears by the end of first week. The titer increases steadily till 4th week after which it declines.

2. Demonstration of rising titer of antibody by testing two or more samples are more meaningful.

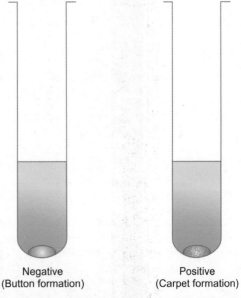

Negative
(Button formation)

Positive
(Carpet formation)

Fig. 27.6: Widal test (negative and positive tubes).

Table 27.1: Biochemical reactions of the main genera of enterobacteriaceae.

Genus	Motility	Glucose (Gas)	Lactose (Acid)	Sucrose (Acid)	Mannitol	Indole	Methyl Red	Voges Proskauer	Citrate	PPA	Urease	H$_2$S	KCN
Escherichia coli	+	+	+	d*	+	+	+	-	-	-	-	-	-
Shigella	-	-	- (except Sh. sonnei)	-	- (except Sh. dysenteriae)	+	+	-	-	-	-	+	-
Klebsiella	-	+	+	+	+	-	-	+	+	-	+	-	-
Enterobacter	+	+	+	+	+	-	-	+	+	-	-	-	+
Serratia	+	d*	d*	+	+	-	-	+	+	-	-	-	+
Hafnia	+	+	-	d*	+	-	-	d*	+	-	-	+	+
Salmonella	+	+	-	-	d*	+	+	-	+	-	-	d*	-
Citrobacter	+	+	+	d*	+	-	+	-	+	-	d*	+	+
Proteus	+	+	-	+ (except P. morganii)	- (except P. rettgeri)	d*	d*	-	d*	+	+	d*	+
Providencia	+	+	-	+	d*	+	+	-	+	+	-	-	+
Edwardsiella	+	+	-	-	-	+	-	-	-	-	-	+	-

d* = Different result in different strains

3. In single test 1/100 titer of O and 1/200 or more titer of H is significant.
4. In immunization, antibody against both *S. typhi* and *S. paratyphi* will be there whereas in infection antibody will be seen only against infecting organism.
5. Immunized person or patients who have had prior infection may develop anamnestic response during unrelated fever. In anamnestic response there is temporary rise in H titer only, whereas in enteric it is sustained.
6. Bacterial suspension should be free from fimbria otherwise false-positive result occurs.
7. Treated case may show poor agglutination response.

Tracing of typhoid carrier: Sewer swab technique is quite helpful in tracing of carriers. This is done by following the gauze pads, kept in sewers and positive for *Salmonella typhi* cultures, backwards from the main drain, ultimately lead to localization of the house of the carrier. However, typhoid carrier may be detected as follows:

1. Widal test may show raised antibody titers.
2. Vi agglutination test is positive in a titer of 1/10 or more.
3. Several stool cultures may help in the isolation of causative organism.
4. Organism may be cultured from bile obtained after duodenal intubation.

Treatment: Antibiotics like ciprofloxacilin chloramphenicol, furazolidine and ampicillin are effective. Trimethoprim sulfamethaxazole and amoxycillin are also used in the treatment. The treatment of the carrier is cholecystectomy.

Specific prophylaxis consists of TAB vaccine containing *S. typhi* 1000 million and *S. paratyphi A* and *B* 750 million each per ml of heat killed bacteria and preserved in 0.5% phenol. It is given in two doses of 0.5 mL subcutaneously at an interval of 4 to 6 weeks. However, encouraging results are noted with live vaccine (streptomycin dependent strain) and killed vaccine given as enteric coated tablets.

Nowadays Vi antigen parenteral is being evaluated. Recently oral vaccine prepared from attenuated strain of *S. typhi* designated as Ty 21a is gaining popularity. It contains capsules of about 1 billion live lyophilized *S. typhi* mutant Ty 21a strain organisms. The Ty 21a vaccine strain is a mutant developed by genetic manipulation lacking UDP galactose-4-epimerase, an enzyme responsible for incorporation of galactose into cell wall lipopolysaccharide. In the absence of exogenous galactose, the mutant grows as rough non-immunogenic strain devoid of antigen. When the ambient environment as in intestine contains galactose, immunogenic cell wall components could be produced through galactose-1 phosphate but owing to lack of epimerase, intermediate products of galactose metabolism continuously accumulate into bacterial cell wall and cause cell lysis. The restored biosynthesis of cell wall polysaccharide accounts for immune effect, while subsequent bacteriolysis accounts for the *in vivo* avirulence of the vaccine. The vaccine strain is no longer isolated from the stools a few days later after giving final (3rd dose) and there is no evidence of spread to contacts. For primary immunization a total of 3 oral doses are given at 2 days' interval. Protection stays for 3 years. It gives humoral (IgA) and cellular response in intestinal tract. Other strains being evaluated are Mutant Ty (Vi+ and Vi–) and genetically modified *S. typhimurium* axotropic mutant strain.

On the basis of biochemical reactions main genera of enterobacteriaceae can be differentiated **(Table 27.1)**.

They are mostly saprophytes being found in water, soil and wherever decomposing matter is found. They are frequently involved as secondary invaders causing suppurative and inflammatory lesions. Pathogenic member is *Pseudomonas aeruginosa*.

PSEUDOMONAS AERUGINOSA (PSEUDOMONAS PYOCYANEA)

Morphology: It is slender, Gram-negative bacilli of 0.5 μ × 3.5 μ size, actively motile by polar flagellum. It is non-capsulated.

Cultural character: It is aerobic growing on simple nutrient media with optimum temperature of 37°C.

Peptone water: After 18 to 24 hours' incubation it forms dense turbidity and surface pellicle. Bluish green pigment due to water soluble pyocyanin is seen.

Nutrient agar: It produces large, opaque, irregular colonies of butyrous consistency. It gives musty or earthy smell or fruity odor due to production of aminoacetophenone from tryptophane. It produces water soluble pigment pyocyanin which diffuses in medium. Pigments are of following types:
a. Pyocyanin (bluish green)
b. Fluorescein (yellowish green)
c. Proverdin (green)
d. Pyorubin (red)
e. Pyomelanin (black).
   Some strain may be non-pigmented.

Blood agar: It shows beta type hemolysis.

MacConkey: It produces non-lactose fermenting colonies.

Cetrimide agar: It is selective medium.

Antigenic Structure

i. Somatic antigens are 17 designated as 01 to 017. They divide the strains of *Pseudomonas aeruginosa* into 17 serogroups. Serogroup 06 and 011 are responsible for nosocomial infection.
ii. Flagellar antigens are two in number. Flagellar antigen I is uniform while flagellar antigen II is complex one with 5 to 7 factors.
iii. Common fimbreal antigens are 4 in number. They are unstable.
iv. Plasma membrane contains 4 protein antigens of which FI, and H1 and H2 have been characterized.

Typing methods: It is obligatory to type the strain for epidemiological knowledge as under:
A. *Bacteriocin typing:* It is also called pyocin typing. Three types of pyocins are recognized and they are R, F and S. The pyocin producing strains are resistant to their own pyocins but are sensitive to pyocins secreted by other strains. There are 13 indicator strains designated as 1 to 8 and A to E. There are 105 types recognized and identified. It is most popular method used for typing *Pseudomonas aeruginosa*.

B. *Phage typing:* It is tedious and difficult to go for bacteriophage typing.
C. *Serotyping:* Depending upon O to H antigen 17 serotypes of *Pseudomonas aeruginosa* are identified. Although it is reliable but it is done in reference laboratories.
D. *Molecular method:* It is most reliable method practiced for typing. Here restriction endonuclease with pulsed field gel electrophoresis is used for typing.

Biochemical reactions: Glucose is used oxidatively forming acid only. Nitrate are reduced to nitrites and nitrogen. Catalase and oxidase are positive.

Resistance: Heating at 56°C kills the organisms. It is resistant to common antiseptic and disinfectants. It is resistant to most of antibiotics. However, it is sensitive to polymyxin B, colistin, gentamicin and carbencillin, netilmicin, etc.

TOXINS AND ENZYMES PRODUCED BY PSEUDOMONAS

Toxins and enzymes have significant share to increase the virulence of *Pseudomonas* and they are as under:
1. *Extracellular products:* Pyocyanin inhibits mitochondrial enzymes in tissues. Thus, it causes disruption of aviary movements on ciliated nasal epithelium. This is the reason of these organisms being colonized in nasal mucosa.
2. *Extracellular enzymes and hemolysin:* Local lesion may be caused because of the activities of alkaline protease, lactase, hemolysin and lipase.
3. *Exotoxin:* Exotoxin is of two type A and B. Exotoxin A is a polypeptide and it inhibits protein synthesis.
4. *Endotoxin:* It is lipopolysaccharide. It has pyrogenic action and many other activities.

Pathogenesis: *Pseudomonas aeruginosa* is one of the most troublesome agents causing nosocomial infections. It is commonly encountered in secondary infection of wound, burns and chronic ulcers of skin. The bacterium attaches to and colonizes the mucous membranes of skin, invades locally and produces systemic infection. These processes are promoted by pili, enzymes and toxins. Besides these, lipopolysaccharide plays a direct role in causing fever, shock, oliguria, leukocytosis, leukopenia, disseminated intravascular coagulation and adult respiratory distress syndrome.

It has been described as one of the agents responsible for infantile diarrhea. Strains isolated from diarrhea produce heat stable enterotoxin and give positive rabbit ileal loop reaction.

Urinary tract infection may persist for longer time and may give rise to septicemia. Lesions of eye, otitis media, pulmonary empyema, brain abscess and meningitis may occur.

Laboratory Diagnosis

1. *Specimens:* Pus, exudate, sputum and swabs from conjunctiva are examined. Purulent discharge is usually greenish blue in color having sweetish odor.
2. *Culture:* On nutrient agar media characteristic greenish blue colonies appear. It may be confirmed by biochemical tests.

Treatment: Gentamicin, Polymyxin B and Carbencillin or Ticarcillin are effective in *Pseudomonas aeruginosa* infection. Clinical infection with this organism may not be treated with one antibiotic. One of the penicillins like mezlocillin may be used with an aminoglycoside (Gentamicin, amikacin or tobramycin). Ciprofloxacine is also found effective. Lipopolysaccharides vaccine may be administered to high risk patients which may provide some protection against *Pseudomonas sepsis* 10 days later. Such vaccine is instituted in cases of leukemia, burn, cystic fibrosis and immunosuppression.

Vibrio

General characters: They are thin, curved, comma-shaped Gram-negative, rigid and actively motile (polar flagellum) bacilli. They are non-lactose fermenting, growing at alkaline pH, produce indole and are oxidase positive. They ferment glucose with the production of acid only. Most important *pathogenic* members in man are:

1. *Vibrio cholerae.*
2. Vibrio El Tor.
3. Non-agglutinable vibrio (NAV).
4. *Vibrio parahemolyticus* (**Fig. 29.1**).

Classification of Vibrio

1. Nonhalophilic vibrio (Grow in media without sodium salt NaCl)
   a. *Vibrio cholera* (01 classical and E1 tor biotypes)
   b. Non 01 *Vibrio cholera* (Noncholera vibrio or no agglutinating vibrio)
2. Halophilic vibrio (Grow in media containing sodium salt NaCl)
   a. *Vibrio parahemolyticus*
   b. *Vibrio alginolyticus*
   c. *Vibrio vulnificus*
   d. *Vibrio mimicus*

▮VIBRIO CHOLERAE

Morphology: It is short, curved, comma-shaped about 1.5 μ × 0.2 to 0.4 μ in size and Gram-negative bacilli. It may occur singly or as "S" shaped semicircular pairs (**Fig. 29.2**). It is actively motile with a single flagellum. It shows darting type of motility.

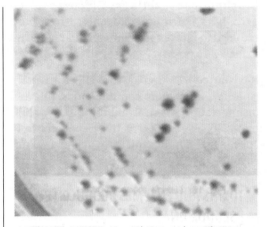

Fig. 29.1: TCBS agar *Vibrio parahemolyticus.*

Cultural characters: It is strongly aerobic. Growth occurs in alkaline pH (7.5 to 9.6) between 22 and 40°C (optimum 37°C). It grows well in ordinary media.

Alkaline peptone water: Rapid growth in about 6 hours is with formation of thick surface pellicle. Turbidity and powdery deposits on prolonged incubation may be present.

Nutrient agar: Colonies are moist, translucent, round 1 to 2 mm in size with bluish tinge in transmitted light. The growth has distinctive odor.

MacConkey's agar: Colonies are colorless.

Blood agar: Colonies show zone of green coloration around them which later become clear due to hemodigestion.

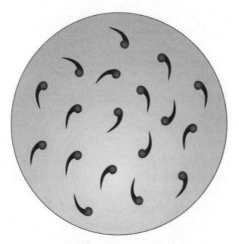

Fig. 29.2: *Vibrio cholerae.*

Special Media

For cultivation of *Vibrio cholerae:*
a. *Holding or transport media:*
   i. *Venkat Raman (VR) medium:* It contains 5 gm peptone and 20 gm crude sea salt per liter distilled water adjusting pH 8.5 to 8.8. In this medium, vibrio remain viable for weeks but do not multiply.
   ii. *Cary-Blair medium:* It is a buffered solution of sodium chloride, sodium thioglycolate, disodium phosphate and calcium chloride at pH 8.4.
b. *Enrichment media:*
   i. Alkaline peptone water pH 8.6.
   ii. Monsur's taurocholate-tellurite peptone water (pH 9.2).
c. *Plating media:*
   i. Alkaline bile salt agar pH 8.2 (BSA).
   ii. Monsur's gelatin-taurocholate trypticase-tellurite agar (GTTA).
   iii. *TCBS medium:* It contains thiosulphate, citrate bromothymol blue and sucrose. It is widely used.

Biochemical tests: Acid without gas is produced from glucose, sucrose, maltose and mannitol. Oxidase is positive, indole may be produced, nitrate reduction positive, liquefies gelatin and urease negative. Cholera red reaction is tested by adding few drops of H_2SO_4 to 24 hour growth in peptone water.

With *Vibrio cholerae* red pink color is produced due to formation of nitrosoindole.

Resistance: It is killed by heat at 55°C in 15 minutes. It is destroyed by drying. The acidity of gastric juice at once kills them. It is susceptible to streptomycin, chloramphenicol and tetracycline.

Classification: Heirberg (1934) classified vibrios into 6 groups on the basis of fermentation of mannose, sucrose, arabinose. Subsequently two more groups are added. *Vibrio cholerae* belongs to group I.

Antigenic structure: *Vibrio cholerae* contains somatic (O) and flagellar (H) antigen.
a. *O antigen:* It is heat stable and type specific. About 60 groups are identified. *Vibrio cholerae* and El Tor vibrio belong to subgroup I. *Vibrio cholerae* are antigenically divided into Inaba, Ogawa and Hikojima on the basis of O antigenic factors they contain. Inaba contains AC, Hikojima ABC and Ogawa AB.
b. Flagellar antigen (H) is nonspecific, heat labile and is common to cholera and cholera like organisms.

Phage types: The strain of cholera is identified as 5 types. All true *Vibrio cholerae* are sensitive.

Toxin: Like other organisms it produces endotoxin. It also produces heat labile enterotoxin called choleragen which is an exotoxin with molecular weight of 80,000. It consists of subunits A (molecular weight 28000) and B (molecular weight 52000). Ganglioside GM_1 serves as mucosal receptor for subunit B which facilitate the entry of subunit A into the cell whereas subunit A activates adenyl cyclase resulting prolonged hypersecretion of water and electrolytes leading to severe dehydration, shock, acidosis and death. The genes for *Vibrio cholerae* enterotoxin are on bacterial chromosomes.

Pathogenesis: Cholera occurs only in humans. Non-agglutinable vibrios are potential pathogens able to cause symptoms similar to cholera. The disease is transmitted from mild and convalescent cases by contaminated water, milk, fruit, vegetable, etc. Flies may disseminate organisms from feces to food. Cholera is endemic in India, China, Japan and Indonesia. Immunity after infection is short-living. Gastric acidity seems an important defense against cholera. Ingestion of at least 10^{10} organisms is necessary to demonstrate some evidence of infection. However, neutralizing the acidity of the stomach lowered the number 10^4 organisms.

The action of enterotoxin (exotoxin) seems to be mediated by adenosine—3', 5' cyclic monophosphate. Addition of enterotoxin (cAMP) to the mucosal surface of isolated ileal mucosa stimulates active secretion of chloride and inhibits absorption of sodium. As a matter of fact, the enterotoxin increases the level of cAMP in mucosal epithelial cells by activating the enzyme adenyl cyclase which converts ATP into cAMP.

Cholera causes an acute gastroenteritis. Incubation period is 24 hours to 5 days. Cholerae vibrio after getting establishment in the intestine, multiplies producing exotoxin get absorbed onto epithelial gangliosides which cause outpouring of fluid into the lumen. It may produce mucinases and endotoxin. Stools are rice water containing mucus flakes, epithelial cells and vibrios. As a result there is tremendous fluid loss, dehydration and hypochloremia.

Laboratory Diagnosis

Hematological Investigations

It is not diagnostically significant in early stages. However, there may be increase of packed cell volume upto 65 to 85%, hemoglobulin contents are increased from 15 to 25 gm% and there may be polycythemia (count may be more than 7 million per cu mm).

Bacteriological Investigations

a. *Specimen:* Feces may be collected with a spoon in a sterile container free from antiseptic. If there are chances of delay, transport media or holding media may be used (VR media). One to three gm stools are emulsified in 10 to 15 mL (VR media). In case of rectal swab, trypticase taurocholate tellurite broth (pH 9.2) or alkaline peptone water is used. If media is not available strips of blotting paper soaked in watery stool may be sent to laboratory.

b. *Smear examination:* Hanging drop preparation shows darting type motility. Gram-staining shows them to be Gram-negative and comma-shaped.

c. *Culture:* Specimen is inoculated in Monsur's medium. A tube of alkaline peptone water is inoculated simultaneously with fecal matter. After 6 to 8 hours Gram's stain shows curved Gram-negative bacilli with darting type motility. Sub-inoculation in Monsur's medium is done. The colonies in this medium are tested for biochemical reactions. It shows oxidase positive, nitrate reduction positive, fermen-tation of glucose, sucrose, mannose and arabinose, cholera red reaction positive, indole positive and slide agglutination with O group polyvalent or monospecific sera differentiates it into Ogawa, Inaba and Hikojima types.

Serology: It is of little use in the diagnosis of cholera. It may be helpful in assessing the incidence of cholera in an area. Indirect hemag-glutination, vibriocidal test and antitoxin assay are popular agglutination tests. Among them complement dependent vibriocidal antibody test is most useful.

Treatment: Generally adequate fluid and electrolytes replacement comprises the treatment. However, oral tetracycline is useful in reducing the period of vibrio excretion and need for parenteral fluid.

Vaccine is used for control of cholera infection. Killed cholera vaccine containing killed suspension (12000 million *V. cholerae* per ml) containing equal number of Ogawa and Inaba serotypes is used nowadays which gives 40 to 60% protection lasting for about one year. The other vaccine preparations are procholer-agenoid with killed Ogawa and Inaba, whole cholera vaccine with adjuvant like aluminium, liposomes or muramyle dipeptide, and live mutant vaccine strain (streptomycin resistant), B subunit toxoid (80 to 85% protection), etc. The candidate live oral cholera vaccine that is currently of greatest interest is *V. cholerae* 01 strain CVD-103-HgR. CVD-103-HgR is reported to elicit significantly higher serum vibriocidal antibody titer in person of blood group O. El Tor type vaccine offers protection about 90 to 100% which lasts for 3 years.

Vibrio El Tor

Originally, it was isolated from pilgrims at the tor quarantine station on the Sinai peninsula. It was the cause of epidemics of cholera in South East Asia. An association between the risk of cholera and ABO blood groups was confirmed and appeared to be specific to the El Tor biotype. The likelihood of developing severe cholera is related to the ABO blood groups and is least common in people with blood group O. Differentiation between classical cholera and El Tor vibrio is as follows:

Test	Classical cholera	El Tor vibrio
• Hemolysis	—	+
• Voges Proskauer	—	+
• Chick erythrocyte agglutination	—	+
• Polymyxin B sensitivity	+	—
• Group IV phage susceptibilities	+	—

Vibrio Cholerae 139

The characteristics of *Vibrio cholerae* 139 isolates are as follows:
1. Gram-negative curved bacilli.
2. Shows darting motility.
3. Not immobilized by antiserum to *Vibrio cholerae* O1.
4. On TCBS medium yellow colored colonies appear.
5. Oxidase test is positive.
6. Fermentation of glucose, sucrose and mannose without formation of gas.
7. Indole test is positive.

8. Hemolysis of sheep erythrocytes.
9. Resistant to polymyxin B (50 IU).
10. Agglutination of chicken erythrocytes.
11. Agglutination with O139 antiserum.
12. Resistant to furoxone and sensitive to amoxicillin, cotrimoxazole, nalidixic acid, cefotaxime, tetracycline, etc.

Widespread incidence of new strain of *Vibrio cholerae* is reported in 1992 and 1993 in India (Tamil Nadu and West Bengal) and Bangladesh. This strain is identified as non-01 type 0139. Toxin produced by this strain can trigger off diarrhea. This strain may lead to another pandemic.

Non-agglutinable Vibrios (NAV)

It may produce cholera-like disease. Morphologically and biochemically it resembles *Vibrio cholerae*. It is non-agglutinable with O antiserum of *Vibrio cholerae*.

Vibrio parahemolyticus: It is enteropathogenic halophilic organism (requires 7 to 8% NaCl) isolated from Japan and India (Kolkata). It causes food poisoning. It can grow in presence of 7 to 8% sodium chloride in peptone water **(Fig. 29.1)**.

Vibrio mimicus: This is newly recognized vibrio species that has been implicated in causing gastroenteritis.

Following consumption of raw oysters resulted in cholera like illness in Dacca (Bangladesh) as reported in 1976. Clinical spectrum, epidemiology and pathogenic significance of it is not clear.

Vibrio fluvialis: This is a newly designated species formerly referred to as enteric group EF-6 or group F vibrio organisms.

Aeromonas and Plesiomonas

Aeromonas hydrophilia causes red leg disease in frog. It is reported from cases of diarrhea and from pyogenic lesion of man. *Plesiomonas shigelloides* are reported from diarrheal diseases. Both of them are oxidase positive, polar flagellated and Gram-negative rods. They may be differentiated on the basis of biochemical tests especially utilization of amino acids.

They are small non-motile, Gram-negative coccobacilli. They cause brucellosis, which is zoonosis (transmitted from animal to man). The disease in man (undulent, fever, Malta fever) is characterized by an acute septicemia phase followed by chronic stage that may extend over years together and may involve many tissues.

GRAM-NEGATIVE COCCOBACILLI

These may belong to following genera:

Hemophilus: They are Gram-negative, non-motile coccobacilli which require X and or V factor for their growth. Some *Haemophilus* species are capable of causing severe respiratory tract infection, meningitis, arthritis, subacute endocarditis, etc.

Bordetella: These small coccobacilli may be motile or non-motile and may cause whooping cough. They do not require X and V factor for their growth.

Pasturella: These are Gram-negative ovoid bacilli which ferment sugar without gas production. The original genus of *Pasturella* has been subdivided into *Pasturella*, *Yersinia*, and *Francisella*.

Brucella: These small Gram-negative coccobacilli are non-motile. Three main species, i.e., *Brucella melitensis* (from goat), *Brucella abortus* (from cattles) and *Brucella suis* (from pigs) affect man. *Brucella abortus* has 9 biotypes while *Brucella melitensis* and *Brucella suis* each have 3 biotypes.

Classification

Three species of *Brucella* have been identified as follows:

a. *Brucella melitensis* is pathogen of goat and sheep. First of all it was isolated from spleen of patient of Malta fever.

b. *Brucella abortus* is responsible for abortion in cows and buffaloes. Its infection is very common.

c. *Brucella suis* is natural parasite of pigs. Its infection is very infrequent.

Morphology: It is short rod, 0.5 to 0.7 μ × 0.6 to 1.5 μ in size, coccobacilli arranged singly or in chains. It is non-motile, capsulated (mucoid and smooth variants), non-sporing, non-acid fast and Gram-negative bacilli.

Cultural characters: It is strict aerobes. The optimum temperature is 37°C and pH 6.6 to 7.4. Addition of 10% CO_2 improves the growth of *Br. abortus* and *Br. melitensis*. Some strains are cultivated on defined media of 18 amino acids, vitamins, salts and glucose. Growth is slow and scanty:

a. In liquid media (broth) growth is uniform. In old culture there may be powdery deposits.

b. *Nutrient agar:* Colonies are small, moist, translucent and glistening with butyrous consistency.

c. *Liver infusion agar:* After 48 to 72 hours, colonies of above description appear.

d. *MacConkey medium:* After 7 days' incubation 0.1 to 1 mm diameter, convex, amorphous, and yellowish colonies appear.

Biochemical reactions: It is catalase positive, oxidase positive and urease positive. Nitrates are reduced to nitrites. No carbohydrate is fermented. Basic fuchsin and thionine are the dyes which can be used to differentiate various species. *B. abortus* and *B. melitensis* show growth in basic fuchsin 1:50000 whereas *B. suis* shows growth in the presence of thionine 1: 250000.

Resistance: It is killed by pasteurization of milk. It is killed by 1% phenol in 15 minutes. It survives in soil and manure for many weeks. It is sensitive to direct sunlight, acid and buttermilk. It is susceptible to chlorotetracycline, oxytetracycline, chloramphenicol, streptomycin, neomycin, etc.

Antigenic structure: Somatic antigen has two components A and M. *Brucella abortus* contains 20 times as much A as M and *Brucella melitensis* about 20 times M as A. *Brucella suis* has intermediate antigenic pattern. The absorbed monospecific sera is used for identification of particular antigen. Antigenic cross reaction occurs between brucella and *Vibrio cholerae*. In addition, a superficial L antigen has been demonstrated that resembles the Vi antigen of salmonellae.

Phage typing: One of the strain phage is Tb. This (Tb) is specific as it lysis strains having character of *Brucella abortus*. Hence, this phage is of great value in identification and classification of brucella.

Pathogenicity: All the three species are pathogenic for man. *Brucella melitensis* is most pathogenic, *Brucella abortus* is least and *Brucella suis* is intermediate. Brucella can produce following types of infections:

a. *Latent infection:* Infection is serological positive but there is no clinical evidence.
b. *Acute brucellosis:* It is also called undulent fever. Incubation period is 4 to 30 days. It is mostly due to *Brucella melitensis*. There is prolonged bacteremia, irregular fever, muscular and articular pain, asthmatic attacks, nocturnal sweating, nervous irritability and chills.
c. *Subacute brucellosis:* It may follow acute brucellosis. Blood culture is less frequently positive. Skin test is positive.
d. *Chronic brucellosis* is usually non-bacteremic. Blood culture is rarely positive. Skin test and agglutination are strongly positive. There is lassitude sweating and joint pain. Illness lasts for years together.

Laboratory Diagnosis

A. *Hematological investigations:*
   a. Total leukocyte counts may show leukocytosis particularly in early acute phase of disease.
   b. Differential leukocyte count may show lymphocytosis.

B. *Bacteriological investigations:*
   a. *Blood culture:* It is most definite method for diagnosis of brucellosis. About 10 ml patient blood is inoculated into a bottle of trypticasesoy broth, tryptose broth or thionine tryptose agar or liver infusion broth, at 37°C in presence of 5 to 10% CO_2. Subinoculations are made on solid media every 3 to 5 days till 4 to 8 weeks. Castenada's method of blood culture **(Fig. 30.1)** is recommended as it minimizes. The chances of contamination of material and risk of infection to laboratory worker. Here both liquid and solid media are available in the same bottle. For subculture, bottle is tilted so that broth flows over the surface of slant. Bottle is incubated in upright position.

   Colonies appear on slant. It is positive in 30 to 50% of cases. Culture may be obtained from CSF, lymph node, bone marrows, urine, abscess, etc.
   b. *Serological methods:*
      i. *Agglutination test:* It is positive about a week after onset of infection. It is more reliable means of diagnosis. Titer of

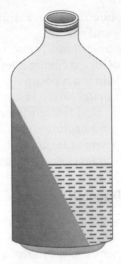

Fig. 30.1: Castenada's blood culture bottle.

1 : 100 or more in presence of clinical symptoms indicates active infection. Individuals immunized with cholera vaccine may develop agglutinin titers to brucellae. Here equal volumes of serial dilution of patient serum and standardized antigen (killed suspension of standard strain of *Brucella abortus*) are mixed and incubated at 37°C for 48 hours. Prozone phenomenon is common in brucellosis (1/640 titer). It means agglutination test negative in low serum dilutions although test is positive in higher dilutions. It may be because of presence of blocking antibodies identified as IgA, that interfere with agglutination by IgG and IgM. However, these blocking antibodies appear during subacute stage of infection and tend to persist for many years independently of activity of infection. Blocking antibodies may be detected by the Coombs' antiglobulin method. Radioimmunoassay and ELISA tests can readily distinguish acute from chronic brucellosis and also acute exacerbation of chronic illness. These tests are gradually replacing the standard tube agglutination test. The use of a specific phage is helpful for the identification of *Brucella abortus.*

ii. *2-Mercaptoethanol test:* The addition of 2-mercaptoethanol destroys IgM and leaves IgG for agglutination reaction. The test is not as sensitive as the standard agglutination test but the results correlate better with chronic active disease.

iii. *Complement fixation test:* It is more useful in chronic cases. It detects IgG antibodies.

iv. Indirect immunofluorescence test is specific and sensitive method for detecting antibodies.

v. *Indirect hemagglutination:* It is also very sensitive method.

vi. *Skin test:* It is useful for the diagnosis of chronic cases. It is called brucellin test and also Burn test. A positive reaction with 2 to 6 cm induration means past or present infection. It is nonspecific test.

vii. Some rapid methods for the detection of brucellosis are:
1. Rapid plate agglutination.
2. Rose Bengal card test.
Antibodies are detected by:
1. Milk ring test.
2. Whey agglutination test.

Treatment: Administration of tetracycline alone or with streptomycin for a period of not less than 3 weeks is quite effective. Response is good in acute cases and not in chronic cases.

A vaccine prepared from *Brucella abortus* strain 19 BA has been employed for human immunization in Russia. However, it has not been used elsewhere.

Haemophilus

They are small (coccobacilli), nonmotile, Gram-negative bacilli that are parasitic on man or animals. They are characterized by their requirement of one or both of two accessory factors (X and V) present in blood.

Species	Growth-factor		Hemolysis
	X	V	
H. influenzae	+	+	–
H. aegypticus	+	+	–
H. suis	+	+	–
H. hemolyticus	+	+	+
H. ducreyi	+	–	–
H. aphrophilus	+	–	–
H. parainfluenzae	–	+	±
H. vaginalis (Gardnerella vaginalis)	±	–	±

Haemophilus Influenzae

Morphology: It is small (1.5 × 0.3 μ), Gram-negative, nonmotile, nonsporing bacillus showing pleomorphism.

Culture characters: They have fastidious growth requirement. X factor present in blood is essential for growth and is heat stable iron prophyrin hematin. X factor is necessary for the synthesis of catalase and other enzymes necessary for aerobic respiration. The other factor is V factor which is a codehydrogenase present in many tissues. It is labile, present in red blood cells and other plant and animal cells. It is synthesized by some fungi and bacteria (*Staphylococcus aureus*). V factor

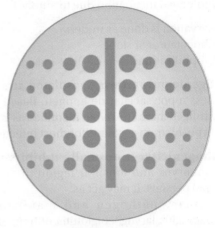

Fig. 31.1: Satellitism.

appears to act as hydrogen acceptor in the metabolism of cell.

It is aerobic and grows best at 37°C and pH 7.8.

Blood agar: Growth is scanty as V factor (inside RBC) is not available. So growth is better if source of V factor is provided. *Staphylococcus aureus* is streaked across a blood agar plate on which specimen of *Hemophilus influenzae* has been inoculated. After 37°C overnight incubation we will find colonies of *Haemophilus influenzae* large and well-developed alongside the streak of *Staphylococcus aureus* and smaller colonies farther away. This phenomena is called satellitism **(Fig. 31.1)**.

Other media used are chocolate agar, Leventhal (mixture of blood and nutrient broth), and Fildes agar media (adding peptic digest of blood to nutrient agar).

Biochemical reaction: Fermentation reactions are irregular and nitrates are reduced to nitrites. It is bile soluble. Capsulated strain produces indole. Otherwise biochemical reactions are of least use for identification of organism.

Resistance: They are destroyed by:
1. 55°C for 30 minutes.
2. Refrigeration (0 to 4°C).
3. Drying.
4. Disinfectants.
5. Prolonged incubation due to autolysis.

Preservation is done as under:
a. Chocolate agar slopes.
b. Lyophilization.

Antigenic properties: Capsulated strains possess a polysaccharide antigen. Based on this antigen there are 6 types identified as '*a*' to '*f*'. Type '*b*' strain accounts for most infection.

Pathogenicity: It normally inhibits the nasopharynx and tonsillar region in many normal persons. It may act as:
a. Primary pathogen and may cause meningitis, laryngoepiglottitis, otitis media, pneumonia, arthritis, endocarditis and pericarditis.
b. In second group, the bacillus causes secondary or superadded infection usually respiratory (chronic bronchitis, bronchiectasis, etc.)

Laboratory Diagnosis

a. *Hematological investigations:*
    i. Total leukocyte count shows leukocytosis in pulmonary infection.
    ii. Differential leukocyte count shows increase in neutrophil and in severe infection there may be leukopenia with neutropenia.
b. *Bacteriological investigations:*

Specimen: Sputum, nasopharyngeal swab and cerebrospinal fluid are used for culture.

CSF examination in case of meningitis shows turbidity with increase in cell count 100 to 800 cells/cu mm (polymorphs predominate).

Smear examination: It shows small clumps of fine pleomorphic Gram-negative bacilli. Charac-teristically they do not stain well.

Culture: Material may be inoculated on chocolate agar, blood agar and Levinthal's media. Penicillin may be incorporated in the medium to inhibit the growth of other organisms.

Treatment: *H. influenzae* is susceptible to sulfonamides, chloramphenicol, ampicillin, trimethoprim-sulfamethoxazole and other antibiotics. In resistant cases clarithromycin, amoxicillin-clavulanate and rifampicin (especially carriers) are quite effective. Immunization with capsular polysaccharides is now being considered for mothers who lack antibody. However, available PRP is not adequate vaccine for infants under age 2 years. Hib conjugate vaccine (PRP-T) (Polyribosy iribitol phosphate tetanus) in infants and children is a great success indeed. In addition to eliciting protective antibody, vaccines prevent disease by reducing pharyngeal colonization with Hib. All children should be immunized with Hib vaccine, first dose between 2 and 6 months of age, next dose at 12 to 15 months of age.

Haemophilus Aegypticus

It is worldwide in distribution and may cause contagious form of conjunctivitis (red eye). It is common in tropics and subtropics.

Haemophilus Suis

It is isolated regularly from pigs suffering from influenza. It is not pathogenic for man. Capsulated strain requires X and V factor while noncapsulated strain requires only X factor.

Haemophilus Hemolyticus

It is commensal of upper respiratory tract. It requires both X and V factors. It is nonpathogenic.

Haemophilus Ducreyi

It is short ovoid bacillus which has tendency to occur in short chains or end to end pairs. It may cause chancroid or soft sore which is venereal disease characterized by tender, non-indurated, irregular ulcer on genitalia.

The culture of *Haemophilus ducreyi* remains the definitive method to diagnose chancroid. Other new techniques are being evaluated, e.g., enzyme immunoassay, dot immunobinding assay, immunofluorescence, DNA probes, etc.

Haemophilus Aphrophilus

This requires only X factor. Growth is enhanced by 5 to 10% CO_2. It may cause bacterial endo-carditis and brain abscesses.

Haemophilus Parainfluenzae

It requires only V factor for growth. It is commensal of upper respiratory tract and is reported to cause subacute bacterial endocarditis.

Haemophilus Vaginalis (Gardnerella vaginalis)

This is associated with vaginitis and cervicitis (leukorrhea). Since X and V factors are not necessary for growth so it is excluded from genus *Haemophilus* and now named as *Gardnerella vaginalis*. They are small 1 to 3 μ × 0.3 to 0.6 μ in size, Gram-negative, nonsporing, noncapsulated pleomorphic bacilli. They can be cultured on blood agar or chocolate agar media. They may cause non-specific vaginitis and cervicitis. Vaginal discharge emits a fishy odor. Gram-stain shows clue cells (vaginal epithelial cells covered with many tiny Gram-negative rods). The fish odor of vaginal discharge is due to presence of amine. Amines get intensified by mixing with a drop of potassium hydroxide and is called amine test. It is treated using metronidazole.

General characters: They are elongated, motile, flexible bacteria which are twisted spirally round the long axis. Characteristically, there are varying number of fine fibrils between cell wall and cytoplasmic membrane of bacterial cell. The spiral shape and serpentine motility of cell depends on the integrity of these filament. Spirochaetes do not possess flagella but are motile. There are three types of motility:

a. Flexion and extension.
b. Corkscrew-like rotatory movement.
c. Translatory.

Spirochaetes belong to the order spiro-chaetales which is divided into two:

a. Spirochaetaceae (saprophytes).
b. Treponemataceae (human pathogen). It consists of 3 genera **(Fig. 32.1)**:
   i. Borrelia.
   ii. Leptospira.
   iii. Treponema.

BORRELIA

It is large motile, refractive with irregular, wide and open coils. It is 0.3 to 0.7 μ wide and 10 to 30 μ long and is Gram-negative. Borrelia of medical importance are:

1. *Borrelia recurrentis* (relapsing fever).
2. *Borrelia vincentii* (fusospirochaetosis).

Borrelia Recurrentis

Morphology: It is irregular, spiral with one or both ends pointed. It is 8 to 20 μ × 0.2 to 0.4 μ in size. It possesses 5 to 8 loose spiral coils. It is actively motile. It stains best with Giemsa and Leishman's stain.

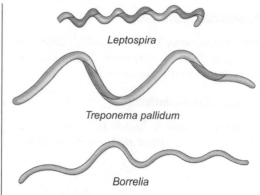

Fig. 32.1: Treponemataceae.

Cultural characters: Its culture is difficult. Culture is successfully done in ascitic fluid containing rabbit kidney (Noguchi's medium). Growth occurs on chorioallantoic membrane of chick embryo.

Pathogenicity: It causes relapsing fever. Incubation period is 2 to 10 days. It is sudden in onset. Borrelia are abundant in the patient's blood during this period. The fever subsides in 3 to 5 days. After an afebrile period of 9 to 10 days borrelia are not demonstrable in patient blood. The disease subsides after 3 to 10 relapses.

Splenomegaly, jaundice and hemorrhagic lesions in kidney, intestine and meningitis may occur.

Laboratory Diagnosis

Hematological investigations: During fever there is leukocytosis and during afebrile period there is leukopenia. There may be anemia, lymphocytosis and increased serum bilirubin. There may be reduction in platelets.

Bacteriological Investigations

Specimen: Blood is collected during rise of fever.

Smear examination: Thin and thick blood smears are made. They are stained with Leishman's stain or Giemsa stain or diluted carbol fuchsin. Smear is looked for large loosely coiled spirochaetes.

Organisms may be demonstrated by dark field examination of drop of centrifuged blood from buffy coat. However, phase contrast microscopy is considered the method of choice.

Animal inoculation: It is more successful method. About 1 to 2 mL of blood from patient is inoculated into white mice intraperitoneally and within 2 days organisms can be demonstrated from the peripheral blood film of animal. As a routine, smear prepared from blood, collected from tail vein, is examined daily for 2 days.

Serological tests: Cultivation of borrelias and demonstration of antibodies are difficult as well as unreliable to be used for diagnosis. Relapsing fever patient may develop false Wasserman positive reaction.

Treatment: Penicillin, tetracycline and strepto- mycin are safe and effective as well.

Borrelia vincentii

It is motile spirochaete about 4 to 20 μ long and 0.2 to 0.6 μ wide having 3 to 8 coils of variable size. It is Gram-negative and is obligatory anaerobic. It is normally a mouth commensal. Under predisposing condition like malnutrition, etc. it may cause gingivostomatitis or oropharyngitis (Vincent angina).

Borrelia vincentii is found generally in symbiotic association with *Fusobacterium fusiform.* This symbiotic infection is called fusospirochaetosis. Fusospirochaetal infection may cause choleraic diarrhea or dysentery but it requires confirmation. Diagnosis may be made by demonstrating spirochaetes and fusiform bacilli in stained smear of exudate from lesion (Fig. 32.2).

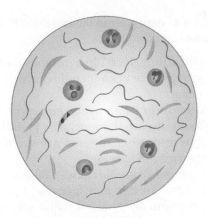

Fig. 32.2: Smear from Vincent's angina.

LYME DISEASE

This is named after the town of Lyme, Connecticut. Clinical presentation is annular skin lesion (erythema chronicum migrans). There is associated headache, stiff neck, fever, myalgia, arthralgia or lymphadenopathy. After few weeks to few months, patients may develop neurological symptoms and arthritis which may recur for several years. It is probably the deposition of antigen antibody complexes which is responsible for the recurrent arthritis or neurological manifestations which may occur in few patients. This disease typically occurs in summer. This disease is reported from USA, Europe and Australia.

The disease is transmitted by vector, a small ixodid tick, often *Ixodes dammini,* which carry spirochaetes, i.e. *Borrelia burgdorferi.* The patients develop IgM antibodies to this spirochaete 3 to 6 weeks after the onset of disease. The serum levels of IgM correlates with disease activity.

Tetracycline, or penicillin if administered initially in the acute stage of disease, prompt recovery occurs with no chance of complication like arthritis, etc.

LEPTOSPIRA

It is actively motile and delicate spirochaete. It possesses number of closely wound spiral and characteristic hooked end. It is very thin and is seen under dark ground illumination. It does not take stain readily.

Classification: Over 100 serotypes and 18 sero-groups have been identified which can infect man.

i. *Leptospira icterohemorrhagica* causes Weil's disease (hemorrhagic jaundice). Rats and other rodents are the main reservoirs of infection.

ii. *Leptospira canicola* causes canicola fever in man. In this meningeal symptoms predominate. The reservoirs are dogs, pigs and jackals. Infection in man occurs by invasion through skin abrasion.

iii. *Leptospira hebdomadis* is responsible for seven day fever of east. Organism is natural parasite of field mouse.

iv. *Leptospira autumnatis* causes Akiyami disease in Japan.

v. *Leptospira pyrogen* causes febrile illness among field workers of Indonesia. The reservoirs of infection are certain species of rats.

vi. *Leptospira australis* and *Zanoni* cause cane fever in North Queensland. Certain species of rat are the carrier of organism.

vii. *Leptospira pamona* causes seven day fever among dairy farmers in North Queensland. Pigs act as reservoir.

viii. *Leptospira grippotyphosa* causes swamp fever in agriculturists or workers of Asia, Africa, Israel and USA.

ix. *Lepotospira bataviae* causes leptospirosis in rice field workers of Italy and South East Asia.

x. *Leptospira segroe* has been isolated from human infection in island of Segroe (Denmark). Rodents carry this organism.

Leptospira Icterohemorrhagica

Morphology: It is 7 to 17 μ long and 0.1 μ broad. Coils are many, small and closely set. The ends are characteristically hooked. It is actively motile by rotatory movements. It may be stained with Giemsa's stain or silver impregnation methods of Levaditi and Fontana.

Cultural characteristics: It can be cultured on media enriched with rabbit serum. It is aerobic, microaerophilic with optimum temperature of growth being 25° to 30°C and optimum pH 7.2 to 7.5. It may be grown on chorioallantoic membrane of chick embryo. Culture may be obtained by inoculating the material intraperitoneally in guinea pig and culture the heart blood ten minutes later.

Resistance: It is susceptible to heat (60°C in 10 seconds) and acidic pH (< 6.8). Salt water has deleterious effect. Bile destroys them rapidly. It dies within 3 minutes in water containing 1 ppm chlorine. It is moderately sensitive to penicillin, streptomycin and tetracycline.

Pathogenicity

Weil's disease is very acute epidemic infection characterized by jaundice, hemorrhage from mucous membrane, fever, enlargement of spleen and nephritis. Wild rat is important reservoir. Human infection may result from water or food contamination with leptospirae. Less frequently organism may enter through abrasions in skin. Incubation period is 1 to 8 weeks. It is found in bloodstream and distributed throughout the body. Later they settle in organs like liver and kidney. Central nervous system is frequently involved causing meningitis.

The involvement of kidney in animal is chronic and results in passing large number of organism in urine. Human urine may contain leptospira in 2nd and 3rd week of disease.

Agglutinating, complement fixing and lytic antibodies appear and remain in detectable amount for several years.

Laboratory Diagnosis
Hematological Investigations

i. *TLC* in early cases shows moderate degree of leukocytosis.

ii. *DLC* shows increase in polymorphonuclear cells in early febrile stage.

iii. *ESR* is raised.

iv. *Serum bilirubin* and *blood urea* are raised.

Bacteriological Investigations

Collection of specimen: Blood is collected during first week and urine after second week of illness. Urine specimen should be examined fresh. Serum of patient is examined for antibodies which are always present from 2nd week onwards.

Examination of blood, urine and CSF: It is done by dark ground microscopy.

Culture: The leptospirae can be cultured in Bijou bottles containing Stuart or Korthof's medium. About 3 to 4 drops of patient's blood are mixed in 3 mL of fluid culture medium. Bottles are incubated at 30°C for two days to two weeks. Samples from culture are examined every third day for presence of leptospira under dark ground illumination.

Animal inoculation: Blood or urine may be inoculated intraperitoneally in about 6 weeks' old guinea pig. After 3 days peritoneal fluid is examined daily for the evidence of leptospira under dark ground illumination and when it is detected cardiac blood is withdrawn for culture purpose.

Serological Test

i. **Microscopic agglutination test:** Dilution of patient serum and culture suspension are incubated at 32°C for 3 hours and then at room temperature for 1 hour before reading the test. Microscopic agglutination test with formalinized antigen is safer and little inferior to live antigen test. A titer of 1/80 is suggestive and 1/100 conclusive of infection.

ii. **Indirect fluorescent antibody test** has been recently used widely.

iii. **Complement fixation test** is neither specific nor sensitive as compared to agglutination test. Complement fixation antibodies disappear soon after recovery and so demonstration of antibody is an indication of recent infection.

Treatment: Penicillin and tetracycline are useful.

▌TREPONEMA

They are very fine, spiral, slender with pointed or rounded ends. Pathogenic treponemes may cause following diseases in man:

a. *Treponema pallidum* is the causative agent of venereal syphilis.
b. *Treponema pertenue* may cause yaws.
c. *Treponema caratium* may cause pinta.
d. *Treponema vincentii* is found in association with fusiformis in Vincent angina.

Treponema Pallidum

Morphology: It is 6 to 8 μ in length, 0.2 μ in diameter with tapering ends. The body is coiled in 8 to 15 regular, rigid, sharp spirals. It is actively motile showing rotation around long axis, backward and forward movements and flexion of whole body. It is feebly refractile and so not stained with ordinary staining techniques. It ordinarily reproduces by transverse fission, and divided organisms may adhere to one another for some time. However, its morphology and motility can be seen under dark ground illumination.

It stains rose red with Giemsa stain. It may be stained with Levaditta, and Fontana method.

Culture: It has not been cultured in artificial media or in tissue culture. Pathogenic strain (Nichol's strain) may be maintained in the testis of rabbit. However, saprophytic strain (Reiter) may be cultured on a defined medium of 11 amino acids, vitamins salts and minerals. Serum albumin also supports its growth.

Resistance: It is inactivated by drying or by heat (41 to 42°C). It is killed in 1 to 3 days at room temperature and in 1 hour at 4°C. It may be stored when frozen at –70°C with 10% glycerol or in nitrogen (30°C) for 10 to 15 years.

Antigenic structure: Treponemal infection induces three types of antibodies:

1. The first type of antibody reacts in nonspecific serological tests like VDRL, Kahn, Wassermann.
2. It is protein antigen present in *Treponema pallidum* and nonpathogenic strain Reiter treponema. It is group antigen.
3. The third antigen is perhaps polysaccharide in nature and is species specific. It may be demonstrated by *Treponema pallidum* immobilization test.

Pathogenicity

A. *Congenital syphilis:* A pregnant syphilitic woman can transmit *Treponema pallidum* to the fetus through placenta beginning about the tenth week of gestation. Some of the infected fetuses die and miscarriages result while others are stillborn at term. Some are born live but develop the signs of congenital syphilis in childhood, e.g., interstitial keratitis, Hutchinson's teeth, saddle nose, periostitis and many central nervous system anomalies. However, adequate treatment of mother during pregnancy prevents congenital syphilis.
B. *Acquired syphilis:* Natural infection in man is usually acquired by sexual contact. The organism enters through microabrasions on the skin or mucosa of genitalia. The incubation period is 10 to 90 days. The clinical picture falls into 3 stages: *primary, secondary, tertiary.*

Primary lesion: It is painless, avascular circumscribed, indurated superficially ulcerated lesion. It is called hard chancre. Chancre is covered by thick exudate which is rich in spirochaetes. Regional lymph nodes are swollen, discrete, rubbery and nontender. Chancre heals up in 10 to 40 days leaving thin scar.

Secondary lesion: It occurs in 2 to 6 months after primary lesion. Then lesion of secondary stage develops with papular skin rashes, mucous patches in oropharynx and condylomata at mucocutaneous junction. Patient is highly infectious during secondary stage. There may be eye and meningeal involvement. Twenty-five percent patients ultimately undergo spontaneous healing in 4 to 5 years' time. Twenty-five percent infection remains latent. In rest 50% cases tertiary lesions develop after a latent period of 1 to 33 years.

Tertiary syphilis: It consists of cardiovascular lesions consisting of aneurysm, chronic granulomata and meningovascular manifestations. Only few spirochaetes are present and this stage represents delayed hypersensitivity.

Laboratory Diagnosis

Hematological investigations: There is leukocytosis. In early stage there is increase in polymorphs whereas in chronic cases there is lymphocytosis.

Bacteriological Investigations

Primary stage: The specimen should be collected with care. The lesion is cleaned with a gauze soaked in warm saline. Gentle pressure is applied to the base of lesion and exudate is collected. Wet films are prepared and covered with coverslips. They are examined under dark ground microscope.

Dark ground microscope is very useful. Repeated examination should be done in negative cases. Fluorescent antibody test or smear of exudate gives more positive rate.

Secondary Stage

a. *Dark ground microscopy:* Serous exudate from skin eruption or specimen collected from mucous patches and condylomata are examined as discussed above.
b. *Serological test:*
   1. *Standard test for syphilis (STS):* Alcoholic extract of ox heart tissue in which added lecithin and cholesterol is used as antigen. The test employed are Wassermann, Kahn, Venereal Diseases Research Laboratory (VDRL).

Wassermann reaction: It is complement fixation test. Patient serum is inactivated at 56°C for ½ hour to destroy complement. It is then incubated with cardiolipin (liquid extract of beef heart) and guinea pig complement. Now sheep erythrocytes and antisheep erythrocyte serum is added to mixture. If hemolysis occurs it means complement was not used up as no antigen antibody reaction occurs. It means test is negative and patient is not suffering from syphilis. If no hemolysis it means antigen antibody reaction occurs and complement is used up. It occurs in positive test when patient is suffering from syphilis.

Kahn's test: Carefully measured 0.15 mL of inactivated serum is taken in 3 tubes containing 0.05, 0.025, 0.0125 mL freshly prepared antigen. They are shaken on Kahn's shaker at 280 oscillation/minute. Normal saline solution is added. Floccules appear in positive test.

VDRL test: It is most widely used as it is simple and rapid test requiring very small quantity of serum. 0.05 ml inactivated serum is taken in special slide with ring (14 mm diameter). One drop of antigen is added with a syringe delivering 60 drops in 1 mL. Slide is rotated at 120 revolutions per minute for four minutes. It is studied under microscope. Uniformly distributed needles show negative results (nonreactive). Presence of clumps means reactive serum. In reactive serum further dilution is done to obtain reactive titer.

VDRL has one disadvantage as it gives false biological reaction in conditions like leprosy, malaria, relapsing fevers, infectious mono nucleosis, hepatitis, tropical eosinophilia, systemic lupus erythematosus, rheumatoid arthritis, bloodless menstruation, vaccination and pregnancy, etc. Positive VDRL tests revert to negative 6 to 24 months after effective treatment of early syphilis.

A positive STS (Wassermann reaction or VDRL) with negative Kahn test is always nonspecific.

Rapid plasma reagin test (RPR): In this test finely divided carbon, i.e. charcoal particles and choline may be added to VDRL antigens. There is no need to read the results with the microscope, because results can be seen with naked eyes. The advantages of RPR test are as follows:

1. There is no need to heat the test serum.
2. Test may be performed on plastic or paper cards.
3. Blood from patient may be obtained by finger prick only.
4. Test is so easy and simple that it may be used for field study.
5. This test may be performed using either serum or plasma.

Uses of nontreponemal tests: Nontreponemal tests may become positive after pimary lesion. They are positive in over 70 percent primary and around 98 percent in secondary syphilis. Highlights of nontreponemal tests are:

1. A four-fold or more rise in titer occurs during evolution of primary syphilis.
2. A titer of over 32 is observed in secondary syphilis.
3. An increase in reagin titer with time may indicate congenital syphilis.
4. If there is decline in reagin titer after antibiotic treatment of syphilis in early stage indicates effective treatment. Hence, nontreponemal tests may be used to monitor effective antibacterial therapy.

A new serological test: To conduct this test a VDRL antigen may be used to coat the wells of microtiter plate. Antibodies to cardiolipid present in the serum of patient get attached to the antigen in the well. These antibodies may be detected using antihuman IgG labeled with peroxidase enzyme. This test can be sensitive to the extent of over 96 percent in untreated syphilis. This test is based on enzyme immunoassay.

   2. *Treponemal test:*

     A. *Reiter's protein complement fixation test* (RPCF): Principle is same as Wassermann reaction but antigen is an extract of *Reiter treponema*. It is least sensitive in early syphilis but is more sensitive in late or latent syphilis. It is more specific than standard tests for syphilis.

B. Tests using *Treponema pallidum* as antigen:

Tests using live T. pallidum

Treponema pallidum immobilization (TPI), in which test serum is incubated with suspension of live treponema and complement. If antibodies are present treponema will be immobilized. Test is positive if more than 50% of treponema are immobilized. It is the most specific test available for syphilis.

Tests using Killed T. pallidum

i. *Treponema pallidum agglutination test (TPA):* Nicholas strain inactivated with formaline is used. This test is not specific as false positive reactions occurs and test is technically difficult.

ii. *Treponema pallidum immune adherence (TPIA):* If a suspension of treponema is mixed with test serum, complement and heparinized whole blood from normal man after incubation treponema will be found to be adhered to erythrocytes in the presence of antibody. In the absence of antibody *Treponema pallidum* adherence will not occur. It is not widely used.

iii. *Fluorescent treponema antibody (FTA):* This is indirect immunofluorescent test. Nicholas strain of *Treponema pallidum* is smeared on slide (can be stored in deep freeze for months together). Patient's serum is allowed to act on smear. This is treated with antihuman gammaglobulin fluorescence conjugate. Excess of unfixed conjugate is washed off. The slide is examined under ultraviolet microscope. If the test is positive treponema are seen as fluorescent objects.

This test is modified and called FTA-ABS test. Test serum is absorbed with extract of Reiter's treponema which remove group reactive antibody first. This is as specific as TPI test.

Tests using T. pallidum extract

Treponema pallidum hemagglutination test (TPHA) in which tanned sheep erythrocytes are sensitized with extract of *Treponema pallidum*. This test can be made more sensitive and specific if test serum is absorbed with extract of Reiter's treponema which remove group reactive antibodies. It is reported to be specific like *Treponema pallidum* immobilization test (TPI).

Hemagglutination Treponema test for syphilis (HATTS) and microhemagglutination *Treponema pallidum* (MHA-TP) are automated version of FTA-ABS test. Main advantages of HATTS and MHA-TP are:

❖ Simple technique
❖ Economical
❖ Have good quality control

However, HATTS and MHA-TP lack sensitivity for diagnosing primary syphilis.

Tertiary stage: The serological tests are same as in secondary stage.

Treatment: Penicillin, chloramphenicol, erythromycin and tetracyclines are useful.

Diagnosis of congenital syphilis: Prenatal diagnosis can be established by demonstrating maternal antibodies against syphilis organism. Confirmation of diagnosis in infants is made by demonstrating *Treponema pallidum* in skin or CSF by virtue of detection of corresponding antibodies using serological tests like microhemagglutination assay for antibodies *Treponema pallidum* (MHA-TP) and FTA-ABS.

Treponema pertenue

It causes chronic nonvenereal disease called Yaws. It is less common in India. The organism is indistinguishable from *Treponema pallidum* morphologically and antigenically. The primary lesion is extragenital papules which form ulcerating granuloma. Like syphilis secondary and tertiary manifestations follow. Destructive lesions of bones are common. Cardiovascular and neurological manifestations are quite rare.

Infection is by direct contact. There appears some cross immunity between syphilis and yaw.

Treponema carateum

It causes *pinta,* a skin disease in which papule appears which does not ulcerate and become lichenoid or psoriform patch.

Secondary lesion shows hyperpigmentation and hypopigmentation.

It is not antigenically related to *Treponema pallidum* and hence partial cross immunity between syphilis and pinta exists.

Nonpathogenic treponema: *Treponema micro-dentum* and *Treponema macrodentum* occur in mouth. The former is shorter with shallow coils and later is large, thicker, regular coil and very actively motile.

Treponema refrigens is found in genital tract of syphilitic and nonsyphilitic genital lesion. It has wavy middle and more regular and deeply curved extremities with pointed end.

Virology

SECTION OUTLINE

- ❖ General Characteristics of Viruses
- ❖ Classification of Viruses
- ❖ DNA Viruses
- ❖ RNA Viruses
- ❖ Severe Acute Respiratory Syndrome
- ❖ Avian Influenza (Bird Flu)
- ❖ Acquired Immune Deficiency Syndrome

SECTION 5

General Characteristics of Viruses

Viruses are unicellular, ultramicroscopic particles containing either RNA or DNA, which reproduce inside living cells, pass through filters that retain bacteria and are covered by a protein coat.

The general properties of viruses are (**Table 33.1**):

i. Do not possess cellular organization.
ii. Contain one type of nucleic acid, either RNA or DNA but never both.
iii. Lack enzymes necessary for protein and nucleic acid synthesis and so depend upon synthetic machinery of host cells.
iv. They multiply by complex process and not by binary fission.
v. They are unaffected by antibiotics.
vi. They are sensitive to interferon.

Rivers' postulates: At the time Koch's postulates were formulated true viral pathogens were unknown. In 1937, TM River created a similar group of rules to establish causative role of viruses in disease Rivers' postulates are as follows:

1. The viral agent must be found in the host's body fluid at the time of the disease or in the cells showing lesions.

2. The viral agent obtained from the infected host must produce specific disease in a suitable healthy animals or plant or provide evidence of infection in the form of antibodies against the viral agent. It is important to note all host material used for inoculation must be free of any bacteria or other microorganisms.

3. Similar material from such newly infected animals or plants must in turn be capable of transmitting the disease in question to other hosts.

Morphology

Size: Viruses vary widely in size. The largest among them is pox virus measuring about 300 nm. The smallest viruses is foot and mouth disease virus measuring 20 nm.

The methods of estimating the size of virus particles are:

i. Collodion membrane filter of graded porosity.
ii. Ultracentrifugation.
iii. Electron microscope.

Table 33.1: Properties of viruses in comparison to prokaryotes

	Cellular organization	Growth in inanimate media	Binary fission	Both RNA and DNA	Ribo-somes	Sensitivity to antibiotics	Sensitivity to interferon
Bacteria	+	+	+	+	+	+	–
Mycoplasma	+	+	+	+	+	+	–
Rickettsiae	+	+	+	+	+	+	–
Chlamydiae	+	+	+	+	+	+	–
Virus	–	–	–	–	–	–	+

Shapes: Some viruses have characteristic shape, e.g., rabies virus has bullet shape, pox viruses are brick-shaped, tobacco mosaic virus is rod-shaped, bacteriophage has head and tail, like sperm, influenza or polio viruses are spheroidal and so on.

Structure and symmetry: Viruses have central core of nucleic acid which is either RNA or DNA but never both. This central core of nucleic acid is covered by protein coat called capsid. The capsid itself is composed of number of subunits called capsomere (**Fig. 33.1**). The capsomere may be arranged as follows:

i. Around coiled nucleic acid which is known as helical arrangement.
ii. As cubes around spheroidal nucleic acid known as icosahedral arrangement.
iii. Some viruses do not fit either helical or icosahedral symmetry due to complexity of these structure, e.g., pox virus, bacteriophage, etc.

Virion may be enveloped or nonenveloped. The envelope is derived from host cell membrane when virus is released by budding. Envelope is lipoprotein in nature.

Protein subunits may be seen as projecting spikes on the surface of the envelope. These are called peplomers. A virus may have more than one type of peplomer, e.g., influenza virus has two peplomers:

i. Triangular spike, i.e., hemagglutinin.
ii. Mushroom-shaped, i.e., neuraminidase.

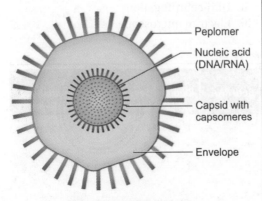

Fig. 33.1: Structure of virus

Reaction to Physical and Chemical Agents

i. *Heat and cold:* Viruses are mostly destroyed by heating at 60°C for 30 minutes except hepatitis virus, adeno-associated virus, scrapie virus. Viruses may be preserved by storage at –20 to –70°C in deep freezer (except poliovirus).
ii. *pH:* They are usually stable at pH 5 to 9.
iii. *Ether susceptibility:* Arbo, myxo and herpes viruses are destroyed by ether whereas entero, reo and adeno are resistant to the action of ether.
iv. *Radiation:* UV light, X-rays and *heavy particles* inactivate viruses, the UV rays dimerizes the pyrimidine bases of nucleic acid strand and gamma rays cause lethal break in the genome.
v. *Vital dyes:* Toluidine blue, neutral red and acridine orange penetrate virus particles. These dyes unite with nucleic acid making viruses susceptible to inactivation by visible light.
vi. *Glycerol:* Viruses remain viable in 50% glycerol whereas bacteria die.
vii. *Stabilization by salt:* Magnesium chloride, magnesium sulfate stabilize some of the viruses so that they are not inactivated by heating at 50°C in one hour.
viii. *Disinfectants:* Lysol, dettol, are ineffective against viruses. Higher concentration of chlorine, iodine may kill viruses. Dilute formaldehydes and beta propiolactone, hydrochloric acid, $KMnO_4$, H_2O_2 are most useful disinfectants against virus.
ix. *Antiviral agents:* I-methylisatin β-thio-semi-carbazone are used against small pox, amantidine against influenza, rubella and respiratory syncytial virus.

Viral Multiplication (Fig. 33.2)

Virus depends on the synthetic machinery of host cell for replication because it lacks biosynthetic enzymes. The sequence of events are as follows:

1. *Adsorption:* The virus is adsorbed at a particular site on the host cell which is

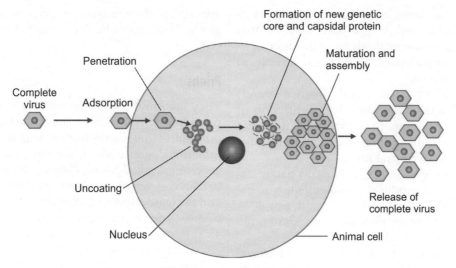

Fig. 33.2: Viral multiplication

called receptor. In case of poliovirus the receptor is lipoprotein present on the surface of primate. The host cell receptor for influenza virus are glycoproteins present on the surface of respiratory epithelium. Adsorption or attachment is specific and is mediated by binding of virion surface structure known as legands, to receptors on cell surface. In HIV surface, glycoprotein (gp120) acts as a legand and it binds to the CD4 60 kD glycoprotein on the surface of mature T lymphocyte.

2. *Penetration:* Virus particles may be engulfed by animal cell by the mechanism called viropexia. Viropexia is like phagocytosis. In case of enveloped virus, viral envelope may fuse with plasma membrane and release nucleocapsid into the cytoplasm.

3. *Uncoating:* This is a process by which the virus lose its outer layer and capsid. In some cases, uncoating is effected by lysozomal enzyme of host cell. For example, in pox virus, uncoating occurs in two steps. Outer coating is removed by lysozyme present in phagocytic vacuole of host cell. This is the first step. In second step, internal core of virus (nucleic acid and internal protein) is released into cytoplasm and is effected by viral uncoating enzyme. Thus, DNA is released.

4. *Biosynthesis:* There is synthesis of viral nucleic acid and capsid protein. There is synthesis of regulator protein which shuts down the normal cellular metabolism and direct sequential production of viral component. DNA viruses synthesize their components in host cell nucleus except pox virus which synthesize their components in cytoplasm. Likewise RNA viruses synthesize their components in cytoplasm of host cell except orthomyxoviruses, paramyxovirus and leukoviruses. Biosynthesis consists of following steps:
   i. Transcription of messenger RNA from viral nucleic acid.
   ii. Translation of mRNA into early proteins. They initiate and maintain the synthesis of virus component and shut down the host protein and nucleic acid synthesis.
   iii. Replication of viral nucleic acid.
   iv. Synthesis of late proteins, which are the components of daughter virion capsids.

Transcription: Mechanism of transcription and nucleic acid synthesis differs in different types of viruses:

a. In single stranded (SS) nucleic acid, comple-mentary strand is first synthesized producing double stranded (DS) replicative forms.

b. Double stranded (DS) viral DNA acts as template and for its replication RNA virus uses various methods for replication:
  i. In poliovirus, SS RNA acts directly on mRNA.
  ii. SS RNA parenteral (positive strand) acts as template for production of complementary strands (negative strand) which act as template for progeny viral RNA.
  iii. In SS RNA (e.g. influenza) parenteral RNA produces complementary negative strands which act both as mRNA and as template for synthesis of progeny viral RNA.
  iv. Oncogenic RNA viruses (leukovirus) exhibit unique replicative cycle. The virus genome is SS RNA which is converted into RNA-DNA hybrid by viral enzyme reverse transcriptase (RNA directed DNA polymerase) from its hybrid DS DNA is synthesized which is integrated into host cell genome (provirus). Provirus acts as template for the synthesis of progeny viral RNA.
      This integration of provirus with host cell genome may cause transformation of the cell and development of neoplasm.
5. *Maturation:* Assembly of daughter virion follows synthesis of viral nucleic acid and proteins. It may take place in nucleus (herpes, adeno) or cytoplasm (picorna, pox). Enveloped virus gets envelope from the cell membrane of the host during a process of budding. Nonenveloped viruses are present intracellu-larly as fully developed virion.
6. *Release:* In bacterial viruses release take place by lysis of infected bacterium. In animal, viruses release occur without lysis (myxo). Some viruses like polio may cause cell lysis during their release.
   Cycle of replication:
   a. Fifteen to thirty hours in animal virus.
   b. Fifteen to thirty minutes in bacterial phage.
   Eclipse phase is the time from stage of penetration of virus into host cell till appearance of mature daughter viruses. In this phase, virus cannot be demonstrated in host cell.

Prions

They are small proteinaceous infectious particles which resist inactivation by procedures that modify nucleic acid. In short infectious agents which lack nucleic acid genome are called prions. They are about 5 nm in diameter, resistant to heat, ultraviolet rays and nuclease. However, they are sensitive to proteases. Some features of prions are:
1. They cause diseases which are confined to central nervous system.
2. The diseases caused by prions have prolonged incubation period.
3. The diseases due to prions show slow, progressive and fatal course.
4. Prion diseases may show spongiform encephalopathy and vacuolation of neurons.

Immune response: Prions do not cause an inflammatory response. They do not induce the formation of interferons. There is no antibody response against prions. Obviously, it is not possible to screen people for exposure to prions by demonstrating antibodies.
   Prion diseases are often called spongiform encephalopathies because of the postmortem appearance of the brain large vacuoles in the cortex and cerebellum. Specific examples of prion diseases in mammals include:

Scrapie	Sheep
TME (Transmissible mink encephalopathy)	Mink
CWD (Chronic wasting disease)	Muldeer, Elk
BSE (Bovine spongiform encephalopathy)	Cows

Humans are susceptible to several prion diseases too some of which are:

CJD	Creutzfeld-Jacob disease
GSS	Gerstmann-Straussler-Scheinker syndrome
Kuru	Alper's syndrome

Humans might be infected by prions by two ways as follows:
1. Acquired infection through diet and following medical procedures like surgery, growth hormones injections, corneal transplants, etc.
2. Apparent hereditary mendelian transmission where it is autosomal and dominant trait.

Thus, prion diseases are distinct in the sense that they are both infectious as well as hereditary.

Characters of Prions

❖ Resistant to chemicals, radiation and heat.
❖ Proteinaceous and filterable.
❖ Do not produce inflammatory reaction in host.
❖ Do not produce antibody in host.
❖ Abnormal fibers and plaques may be formed in the brain of host by prions.
❖ Difficult to treat.

Cultivation Viruses

Since, they are obligate intracellular parasites and cannot grow on inanimate culture medium, 3 methods are used for their cultivation:
a. Animals inoculation.
b. Chick embryo.
c. Tissue culture.
a. **Animal inoculation**: It is one of the oldest methods for the cultivation of viruses. The poliomyelitis virus after intraspinal or intracerebral inoculation in monkeys causes typical paralytic disease and so isolation of viruses. Suckling mice is susceptible to Coxsackie viruses with manifestation of severe myositis and paralysis. Smallpox virus may be inoculated in the scarfied skin or cornea of rabbit. Brain tissue of rabied dog when inoculated intracerebrally in mice or rabbit develop encephalitis.

Growth of virus in animals may be known by the disease, visible classical lesions or death. Sometimes immunity in experimental animal may interfere with the growth of viruses in that animal. It is not out of place to mention the other utility of animal inoculation, i.e., to study pathogenesis, immune response, and epidemiology.

b. **Chick embryo**: They are better than animal inoculation because of following reasons:
   i. They are clean and bacteriologically sterile.
   ii. They do not have immune mechanism like animals to counteract virus infection.
   iii. They do not need feeding and caging.
   iv. Chick embryo offers several sites for cultivation of viruses, i.e., chorioallantoic membrane (CAM) for variola or vaccinia and herpes viruses, allantoic cavity provides rich yield of influenza and some paramyxo-viruses, amniotic sac may be used for the isolation of influenza virus and yolk sac for the cultivation of chlamydiae, rickettsiae and some viruses (**Table 33.2**). Allantoic inoculation may be used for growing influenza virus for vaccine purposes. Yellow fever (17 D strain) and rabies (flury strain) are other vaccines produced from chick embryo (**Fig. 33.3**).

Disadvantages of Egg Inoculation
1. Eggs may be contaminated with mycoplasma and latent fowl viruses which may interfere with the growth of other viruses.
2. The susceptibility of chick embryo is limited to a few viruses only.
3. Even slight amount of bacterial contamination in the inoculum may kill the embryo.

c. **Tissue culture**: Tissue culture of human or animal cells are frequently used for the cultivation of viruses. There are mainly three types of tissue culture:
   i. *Organ culture,* e.g., tracheal ring organ culture is employed for the isolation of coronavirus.
   ii. *Explant culture:* Minced tissue may be grown as explant embedded in plasma clots. This is not useful in virology. In the past, adenoid tissue explant culture were used for adenovirus.

Table 33.2: Growth of viruses in chick embryo

Route of inoculation	Virus	Lesion on CAM	Hemagglutination
Chorioallantoic	Poxviruses	+	–
Membrane (CAM)	Herpes simplex	+	–
	Herpes virus B	+	–
Amniotic cavity	Influenza virus	–	+
	Mumps virus	–	+
Allantoic cavity	New castle disease	–	+
	Influenza	–	+
	Mumps	–	+
Yolk sac	JE virus, West Nile virus	+	–
	Nile virus	+	–

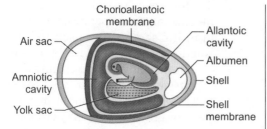

Fig. 33.3: Structure of chick embryo

iii. *Cell culture:* This is very popular and useful technique routinely used for cultivation of viruses. From tissue, fragments cells are dispersed by proteolytic enzymes like trypsin and mechanical shake. After washing the cells, they are suspended in growth medium and distributed in petridishes, test tubes or bottles. The cells adhere to glass surface and grow out to form a monolayer sheet and can be seen *in situ* under low power.

Cell Cultures in Use

Primary Cell Cultures

❖ Rhesus monkey kidney cell culture
❖ Human amnion cell culture
❖ Chick embryo fibroblast cell culture

Diploid Cell Strains

❖ WI-38 (Human embryonic lung cell strain)
❖ HL-8 (Rhesus embryo cell strain)

Continuous Cell Lines

❖ HeLa (Human carcinoma of cervix cell line)
❖ HEP-2 (Human epithelioma of larynx cell line)
❖ Vero (Vervet monkey kidney cell line)
❖ McCoy (Human synovial carcinoma cell line)
❖ KB (Human carcinoma of nasopharynx cell line)

There are three types of cell cultures **(Table 33.3):**

a. **Primary cell cultures:** When normal cells freshly taken from body grown for the first time, they are called primary cell culture. They can be maintained in serial culture. They are useful for isolation and cultivation of viruses for vaccine production, e.g., rhesus monkey kidney cell culture, human amnion cell culture, chick embryo fibroblast culture, etc.

b. **Diploid cell strains:** They are capable of 100 divisions in culture. They are useful for the isolation of fastidious pathogens and also for the production of viral vaccines. Examples are human embryonic lung cell strain (WI-38) and rhesus embryo cell strain (HL-8).

c. **Continuous cell lines:** They are single type of cells mainly derived from cancer cells. These also can be grown in successive generation by transferring them from one test tube to another without change in

Table 33.3: Isolation of viruses from cell lines

Cell line	Virus isolation
Primary	
African green monkey	HSV, RSV, mumps, rubella
Chick embryo fibroblast	Rabies, poxviruses
Diploid Cell	
Human fetal lung	Rabies, adeno, CMV
(WI-38, MRC-5)	
Continuous	
HeLa	Polio, pox, reo RSV
HEp-2	Adeno, RSV
MDCK	Influenza
RD	Polio, enteroviruses
Vero	Polio, rabies, measles

character of cells. These are used only for the isolation of virus. Vaccine preparation on these cells is not safe for human use, e.g., HeLa (human carcinoma of cervix cell line).

Other examples of continuous cell lines are:

KB (human carcinoma of nasopharynx cell line), HEP-2 (human epithelioma of larynx cell line), McCoy (human synovial carcinoma cell line), BAK 21 (baby hamster kidney cell line) and Detroit-6 (sternal marrow cell line).

Detection of virus growth on cell cultures: Viruses multiplying in tissue culture manifest their presence by producing:

1. Changes in the cells called cytopathogenic effects (CPE), e.g., measle virus produces syncytium formation and SV_{40} produces prominent cytoplasmic vacuolation.
2. When viruses grow in cell culture, cell metabolism is inhibited and there is no acid production. In normal cell culture because of active metabolism there is active acid production. Phenol red (indicator) can detect the presence of acid formation by changing its color into yellow.
3. *Hemadsorption:* When influenza and para-influenza viruses grow in cell culture their presence may be detected by addition of guinea pig erythrocytes to the culture. If the viruses are multiplying in culture, erythro-cytes will adsorb on the surface of cell.

4. *Interference:* Growth of first virus will always check infection by the second virus by interference.
5. *Transformation:* Oncogenic or tumor producing viruses cause cell transformation and loss of contact inhibition.
6. Fluorescent antibody straining is also a method of detecting viral multiplication.
7. Hemagglutination test may be performed by using tissue culture fluid, e.g., ortho-myxoviruses and paramyxoviruses.

INCLUSION BODIES

During multiplication of virus in host cells, virus specific structures are produced and they are called inclusion bodies. Sometimes, they may become larger than the individual virus particles. They have distinct size, shape, location and staining properties. The size of inclusion bodies may be from 1 to 30 μ. They are rounded, oval, pyriform or irregular in shape. They can be demonstrated under light microscope. Acidophilic inclusion bodies can be seen as pink structure when stained with Giemsa, or eosin methylene blue stain. Some viruses produce basophilic inclusion bodies. Inclusion bodies are believed to be the site of development of viruses.

Vaccinia infected cells show small multiple intracytoplasmic inclusion (Guarnieri's bodies) **(Table 33.4)**. Large intracytoplasmic inclusions (Bollinger's bodies) are seen in fowlpox. Again Molluscum bodies are intracytoplasmic, quite large about 30 μ and seen in *Molluscum contagiosum*. Negri bodies are intracytoplasmic seen in rabies virus infection.

Intranuclear bodies are Cowdry type A (seen in herpes, yellow fever virus) in granular form and variable in size. On the other hand, Cowdry type B are circumscribed and multiple. They are found in adeno- and poliovirus.

Inclusion bodies which are both intranuclear and intracytoplasmic are encountered in measles virus.

Laboratory Diagnosis

The appropriate specimen is collected, preserved and transported using proper techniques along with clinical information.

Table 33.4: Cell membrane receptors for viruses

Viruses	Receptors membrane
Influenza	Sialic acid on glycoproteins including glycoprotein A molecule
Rabies	Acetylcholine receptors
HIV	CD 4 molecule on T cells
Epstein Barr	C3d receptor on B cells
Vaccinia	Epidermal growth factor receptor
Reovirus	Beta-adrenergic hormone receptor
Rhinovirus	Intercellular adhesion molecule

The following approach is used for diagnosis of viral disease:

Microscopic Examination

Viruses can be demonstrated and identified by direct microscopic examination of clinical specimens. The various procedures involved include:

Light microscopy: It can reveal characteristics such as inclusion bodies (e.g. Negri bodies) or multinucleated giant cells. Tzanck smear showing herpes virus induced multinucleated giant cells in vesicular skin lesions can be easily observed under light microscopy.

Electron microscopy: It is clinically being used for viruses that are difficult to culture. Rotavirus and hepatitis A virus in feces are increasingly being detected by electron microscopy.

Immunoelectron microscopy: Addition of specific antibody to the specimen enhances the sensitivity of electron microscopy. The added antibody aggregates with the virus particle thereby making its demonstration easier.

Fluorescent microscopy: Direct or indirect fluorescent antibody technique is useful for detection of viruses or viral antigens in clinical specimens. Some of the common viruses detected by fluorescent microscopy include rabies virus, paramyxovirus, orthomyxovirus, adenovirus and herpes virus.

Identification in Cell Culture

The viruses can be grown by inoculation into animals, eggs or cell cultures. The presence of a virus in the clinical specimen can be detected by observing a "cytopathic effect" in cell culture, hemadsorption etc. A definitive diagnosis of the virus in cell culture is made using known antibody by tests like complement fixation, hemagglutination inhibition and neutralization of the cytopathic effects. Other procedures that can be used are ELISA, fluorescent antibody, radioimmunoassay and immunoelectron microscopy.

Detection of Viral Antigens

ELISA, radioimmunoassay and latex agglutination may be useful for detecting viral antigens.

Detection of Viral Nucleic Acids

The detection of viral DNA or RNA is increasingly becoming the "gold standard" in viral diagnosis. Labeled nucleic acid probes are highly specific with rapid results. Polymerase chain reaction (PCR) technique allows rapid amplification of target DNA sequence so that it can be readily identified using labeled probes in a hybridization assay. The detection of HIV-1, HIV-2, human papillomavirus, hepatitis B virus, hepatitis C virus, enterovirus and Epstein-Barr virus has been simplified using the above technique.

Serology

A rise in antibody titer against the virus during the course of viral infection is a definitive evidence of its etiology. However, an antibody titer in a single specimen does not distinguish between a previous infection and a current one. Paired serum samples, collected during the acute and convalescent phases are required. Presence of IgM specific antibodies is meaningful in certain viral infections. The antibody titer can be determined by the immunological tests mentioned above. Other nonspecific serologic tests include heterophil antibody test (Monospot) used for diagnosis of infectious mononucleosis.

Classification of Viruses

INTRODUCTION

Rapid progress in the field of virology with new information enforces the review and revision of virus nomenclature. Seven or eight schemes of classification for viruses have been produced in the past.

Till 1950 little was known about the viruses. Viruses may affect animals, insects, plants and bacteria. Attempt was made to group or classify the viruses on the basis of their affinity to different systems or organs of the body, e.g.,

1. Those producing skin lesion (smallpox, chickenpox, measles).
2. Those affecting nervous system (polio, rabies).
3. Respiratory tract involving viruses (influenza, common cold).
4. Viruses causing visceral lesions (yellow fever, hepatitis).

It was also suggested that viruses should be classified based on epidemiological criteria. Some of the examples are as under:

1. Enteric virus:
   a. Picornavirus.
   b. Adenovirus.
   c. Reovirus.
   d. Hepatitis virus.
2. Respiratory:
   a. Orthomyxovirus.
   b. Paramyxovirus.
   c. Coronavirus.
   d. Rhinovirus.
   e. Adenovirus.
   f. Reovirus.
3. Arbo (arthropod borne):
   a. Togavirus.
   b. Bunyavirus.
   c. Rhabdovirus.
   d. Orbovirus.

It is not out of place to enumerate the criteria that have been used in forming groups of animal viruses:

1. Type of nucleic acid.
2. Chemical composition (Table 34.1).
3. Susceptibility to physical and chemical changes.
4. Size measurement.
5. Design and construction.
6. Antigenic characters.

Nowadays viruses are classified into two groups depending on the type of nucleic acid they possess; those containing RNA are called ribovirus and those containing DNA are deoxyriboviruses (Fig. 34.1). They may be further classified on the basis of following characters:

   i. Strands of nucleic acid.
   ii. Symmetry of nucleocapsid.
   iii. Presence of envelope.
   iv. Number of capsomers.

Further discussion is based on above mentioned characters. Deoxyribose (DNA) viruses are at present placed in five groups and ribovirus (RNA) into nine groups.

Major Groups of DNA Viruses (Fig. 34.1)

1. *Poxvirus:* They are large brick-shaped particle 230 to 300 nm × 200 to 250 nm,

Table 34.1: Chemical composition of viruses.

Family	Configuration	Molecular weight (Dalton)	Protein (Polypeptide)	Transcription
DNA:				
Parvo	SS	2	3	–
Papova	DS	3–5	6	–
Adeno	DS	20–25	9	–
Herpetic	DS	100	12–27	–
Pox	DS	160	730	+
RNA:				
Picorna	SS	2–3	4	–
Toga	SS	4	3	–
Bunya	SS	6	3	+
Arena	SS	6	?	?
Corona	SS	9	16	+
Retro	SS	10–12	7–8	+
Ortho	SS	5	7	+
Paramyxo	SS	7	6	+
Rhabdo	SS	4	7	+
Reo	DS	15	7	+

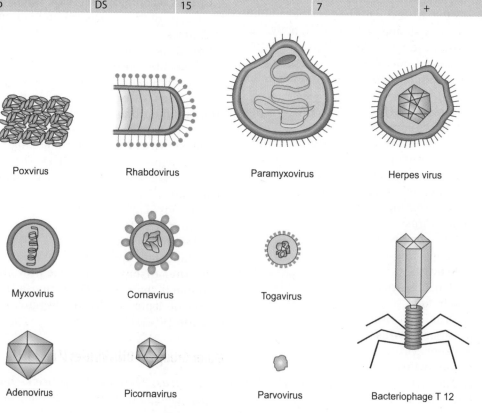

Poxvirus   Rhabdovirus   Paramyxovirus   Herpes virus

Myxovirus   Cornavirus   Togavirus

Adenovirus   Picornavirus   Parvovirus   Bacteriophage T 12

Fig. 34.1: Different types of viruses.

visible by light microscope. They may cause smallpox, vaccinia, molluscum contagiosum, cowpox and milker nodes. Examples of poxvirus are variola, vaccinia, molluscum contagiosum, avian pox, etc.

2. *Herpes virus:* They are enveloped and icosahedral. They multiply within nucleus. They are covered by ether sensitive envelope. They may cause vesicular skin lesions, encephalitis, chickenpox, etc. Examples are *Herpes simplex virus*, varicella zoster virus, cytomegalovirus, etc.

3. *Adenovirus:* They multiply in nucleus. They are ether resistant. They may cause latent infection of lymphoid tissue, mild respiratory diseases, conjunctivitis, keratitis, etc. Example is adenovirus, etc.

4. *Papova virus:* They are icosahedral, multiply in nucleus and are ether stable. They may

cause human warts, papillomata (PA) of rabbits, dogs, etc. polyoma (PO) in mice. Some viruses act as vacuolating agents (VA), e.g., SV40. All are potentially oncogenic. Examples are papilloma virus, polyoma virus, SV40, etc.

5. *Parvovirus:* They are very small 18 to 22 nm in diameter and are ether resistant, e.g., minute virus of mice, Kilhamirat virus (RVM) and adenosatellite virus.

Major Groups of RNA Viruses (Table 34.2)

1. *Orthomyxoviruses:* They are spherical or filamentous, enveloped with lipoprotein, studded with neuraminidase and hemagglutinin subunits. They may cause epidemics and endemics of influenza, etc. Examples are influenza viruses type A, B and C, etc.

Table 34.2: Morphology of virus.

Family	Shape	Diameter	Environment	Symmetry (nm)	No. of capsomers
DNA					
Parvovidae	Spherical	20	–	Icosa	32
Papilloma					
Papova					
Polyoma	Spherical	45–55	–	Icosa	72
Adeno	Spherical	70–80	–	Icosa	252
Herpetic	Spherical	150	+	Icosa	162
Pox	Brick	100 × 240 × 300	–	Icosa	–
RNA					
Picornavidae	Spherical	20–30	–	Icosa	? 60
Toga	Spherical	40–60	+	Icosa	?
Bunya	Spherical	90–100	+	Helical	–
Arena	Spherical	85–120	+	Helical	–
Corona	Spherical	80–120	+	Helical	–
Retro	Spherical	100–120	+	Helical	–
Orth	Spherical of filamentous	80–120	+	Helical	–
Paramyxo	Spherical of filamentous	100–200	+	Helical	–
Rhabdo	Bullet	70–180	+	Helical	–
Reo	Spherical	50–80	–	Icosa	?

2. *Paramyxovirus:* They are similar to myxovirus but are larger and more pleomorphic. They may cause respiratory infections, bad cold, measles, mumps, etc. Examples are parainfluenza virus 1 to 4, measles virus, distemper virus, rinder-pest virus, mumps virus, Newcastle virus, etc.

3. *Rhabdovirus:* They are large enveloped, bullet-shaped and ether sensitive. They may cause rabies in mammals and vesicular stomatitis in cattle, etc. Examples are rabies virus, vesicular stomatitis virus, etc.

4. *Togavirus:* They are icosahedral and enveloped by lipid. They require arthropod vectors and may cause meningoencephalitis, lympha denopathy, bleeding and purpuric rashes, yellow fever, etc. Examples are yellow fever, sindbis and dengue viruses.

5. *Arenavirus:* They are enveloped and ether sensitive causing benign meningitis and encephalitis, e.g., lymphocytic choriomeningitis virus, etc.

6. *Reovirus:* They are ether resistant, naked icosahedral with double stranded RNA causing mild respiratory and enteric diseases.

7. *Picornavirus:* They are small icosahedral, ether and acid resistant causing neuronal damage with paralysis (polio 1 and 3), aseptic meningitis, etc., e.g., polio virus, echovirus, coxsackie virus, rhinovirus, etc.

8. *Leukovirus:* They induce malignant transformation of cells with formation of new antigens and enzymes with loss of contact inhibition, e.g., leukemia, sarcoma in fowls and mice, e.g., Rous sarcoma, murine leukemia, murine mammary tumor virus, etc.

9. *Coronavirus:* They are elliptical or spherical and ether sensitive causing cold and acute respiratory infection, mouse hepatitis, etc. Examples are human, murine and avian virus.

DNA Viruses

POXVIRUS

They are the largest and most complex viruses of vertebrates. They are DNA viruses. Pox viridae family is divided into following groups on the bases of antigenic reactions and morphological differences:

Group I (Viruses of Mammals)

1. Variola
2. Vaccinia
3. Cowpox
4. Ectromelia
5. Rabbitpox
6. Monkeypox

Group II (Viruses of Birds)

1. Fowlpox
2. Turkeypox

Group III (Tumor Producing)

1. Myxoma
2. Fibroma

Group IV (Miscellaneous)

1. Contagious pustular dermatitis
2. Milker nodule
3. Bovine pustular stomatitis.

Morphology

It is brick-shaped measuring 300 × 200 × 100 nm. It consists of central biconcave DNA core. It is covered by: (a) inner coat adhered to nucleoprotein, and (b) outer irregular layer. On either side of nucleoid is oval structure called lateral body **(Fig. 35.1)**.

In dry state virus may remain infective at room temperature for one year. In moist state virus can be destroyed at 60°C in 10 minutes. Acid may destroy the virus in hour time (pH 3 to 5). They are susceptible to ultraviolet light, formalin and oxidizing agents.

Antigenic Properties

There are about 8 antigens demonstrated by precipitations in gel. Some of them are:
1. *LS antigen:* It has 2 components: heat labile (L) and heat stable (S). Antibodies to L-S antigen is not protective in any way. They are responsible for flocculation, precipitation and complement fixation reaction.
2. *Agglutinogen:* This is responsible for agglutination with specific antiserum.

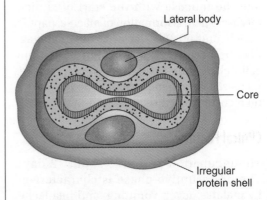

Fig. 35.1: Structure of poxvirus.

3. *Nucleoprotein antigen* (NP): It is responsible for neutralization of infectivity and acquired immunity. However, NP antigen is common to poxviruses.
4. *Hemagglutinin:* It is lipoprotein complex with a molecular weight of 100,000 to 200,000. It is heat stable and does not exhibit receptor destroying activity. Antibodies to this antigen are not protective.
5. Protective antigen has been isolated during early stage of virus replication. Their role in immunity has not been proved so far.

Cultivation: They can be cultivated on chick embryo (11 to 13 days old), tissue culture (monkey kidney, He La and chick embryo cell), animals (monkey, calves, sheep and rabbit).

SMALLPOX (VARIOLA MAJOR)

It is infectious disease manifested as skin lesion (single crop) which are macular to start with and subsequently may pass through papular, vesicular and pustular stages in 10 to 12 days. There may be systemic involvement.

Pathogenesis

Variola viruses may enter through mucosa of upper respiratory tract. Virus may propagate in regional lymph nodes. They are transported through bloodstream to reticuloendothelial cells. There virus multiplication occurs. From here viruses are again thrown into bloodstream and then they settle at skin and the mucosa with the start of clinical disease. There is formation of macule, papule, vesicle and pustule. Fever at pustular stage may be because of absorption of necrotic cell debris from skin. Since smallpox gives increased degree of protection hence there is no recurrence of disease.

Clinical Features

The incubation period is about 12 days. The pre-eruptive phase is characterized by malaise, fever, vomiting, and headache. After 2 to 3 days skin rashes start appearing.

Single crop of eruptions appears on the 3rd to 5th days of onset of illness. The lesion first appears on the buccal mucosa (exanthem) which may develop into macule, papule and vesicle. Vesicle is associated with virus shedding through oropharyngeal secretions (infective stage). There may be conjunctivitis. Corneal exanthems may become the cause of blindness.

Scab starts forming after 12 days and crusts start separating after 3 to 6 week of the onset of disease leaving behind scars. In pre-eruption phase the disease is noninfective but virus can be isolated from blood up to 2nd day of fever. From 6 to 9 days saliva becomes infective, may be because of ulceration of lesions in mouth. In vesicular stage first broken skin lesion and later dried scabs appear.

Laboratory Diagnosis

It is significant especially in nonendemic areas or in areas from where disease has been eliminated. A case identified as smallpox must be informed to health authorities so that proper measures could be undertaken promptly. It becomes still more important when smallpox is declared eradicated from all over the world.

Collection of Specimen

A special kit has been designed by WHO for collection of specimen containing:
1. Hagedorn needle.
2. Clean and sterile slides.
3. Clean pasteur pipettes.
4. A labeled screw capped container.
5. A double container of metal or wood for dispatching samples to the concerned laboratory.

We can collect specimen like maculopapular, pustular, crusting stage lesions. In special cases blood may be collected in pre-eruptive stage.

Demonstration of Virus

1. By light microscope by demonstrating Guarnieri bodies **(Fig. 35.2)**.

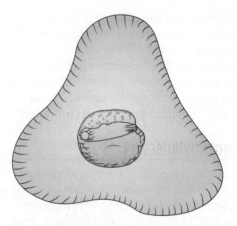

Fig. 35.2: Guarnieri bodies.

2. By electron microscope.
3. Viral antigen may be demonstrated by serological techniques like complement fixation, hemagglutination, immunofluorescent and convenient and routinely used precipitation in gel (PIG).
4. Isolation of viruses from throat, washing, skin lesions and blood. Specimen may be cultured on chorioallantoic membrane of chick embryo.

Demonstration of Antibody

Retrospective diagnosis may be made by demonstration of antibodies rise by testing paired sera. In smallpox convalescent's PIG test is useful for the retrospective diagnosis of smallpox.

Prophylaxis

Some of the preventive measures include immunization and chemoprophylaxis.

Vaccination

There are three strains available for vaccine production:
a. Elstree (Lister Institute)
b. EM63 (Moscow)
c. New York Board of Health strain.

Commercial vaccine may be prepared by inoculating vaccinia virus on scarified skin of calves, sheep and buffalo. Alternatively virus may be cultured in bovine cells or CAM of chicken embryo. Vaccine thus prepared is stored and dispensed in liquid form or in freeze-dried form.

Method of Vaccination

It consists of introducing intradermally sufficient live vaccinia viruses. Recommended sites are outer aspect of upper arm at the insertions of deltoid muscles. The methods includes multiple puncture with bifurcated needle and multiple pressure with a sharp needle.

Response of Vaccination

There are 3 types of response:
1. *Primary reaction:* This is manifested 3 to 4 days after inoculation as papule which rapidly becomes vesicle and it enlarges with secondary erythema. On 8th to 9th day center is depressed with turbid contents. It is also associated with axillary lymphadenopathy and fever.

   On 10th day pustule dries up and scab is formed which separates in a week's time. Immunity appears after 10th day and persists for years.
2. *Accelerated reaction (vaccinole):* It occurs in case of limited residual immunity from previous vaccination. It is more rapid than primary reactions. Vesiculation appears with maximum intensity between 3 and 7 days after vaccination. It enhances waning immunity.
3. *Immediate reaction:* It occurs in immune cases. It is most marked on 2nd to 3rd day as papule. It is hypersensitivity response. Immediate response neither indicates level of immunity nor it leads to immunity.

Complication of Primary Vaccination

1. Post-vaccinal encephalitis may occur which may be due to activation of latent infection, neuroallergy, and interaction of vaccinia virus. Encephalitis may occur 10

to 12 days after vaccination. The mortality is about 50%.

2. Vaccinia gangrenosa in which primary lesion fails to heal and extend slowly with loss of tissue. Fresh vesicles may appear with ulceration of nasopharynx. This is associated with abnormality of immune response and is usually fatal.

3. Abortion may occur due to intrauterine infection of fetus. Hence, it is contraindicated in pregnant women.

Since 1977, when last case was reported in Somalia, smallpox has been eradicated worldwide, hence vaccination is unjustified in view of its several complications.

MOLLUSCUM CONTAGIOSUM

It is human disease with multiple discrete nodule 2 mm size, limited to epidermis and occurs anywhere in the body except palm and sole. Each lesion at its top carries small opening having white core. The incubation period is 19 to 50 days. Transmission is through abrasion and swimming pool. It is very uncommon and involves children and adults. Its transmission in animals is not successful.

Cowpox: It occurs in cattle as ulcer of teats and contiguous part of udder. Lesions appear also in the hands of man. It produces hemorrhage in chorioallantoic membrane of chick embryo and rabbit skin. Vaccinations with vaccinia virus protects human beings.

Milker nodules: It occurs in hands of man from lesions of teats and udder. Warty, nonulcerating nodules on hand and arm are caused by poxvirus of ORF subgroup. Regional lymph nodes are enlarged. Immunity in man does not last long and second attack may occur after few years.

ORF: Infection of man occurs with virus of contagious pustular dermatitis of sheep. There is single lesion of hand, forearm or face, a slowly developing papule which become flat and vesicular and ultimately heals without scarring. The disease occurs by handling of sheep. There is no infection to man.

Yaba and tanapox: Yaba is benign tumor under natural condition in monkeys of African countries. Laboratory worker handling these animals may develop similar lesions.

Tanapox is isolated from solitary skin lesion in Kenyans. Patient looks quite ill. Perhaps, it is derived from monkey by insect transmission.

ADENOVIRUSES

It is nonenveloped DNA virus with diameter 70 to 90 nm and are spherical. It has icosahedral symmetry. It is relatively stable between 4° and 36°C and can be stored in frozen state. It is heat labile destroyed at 56°C within minutes. It resists ether and bile salts.

It is host specific. Human adenoviruses grow only in tissue cultures of human origin, e.g., human amnion, HeLa or HEp. Cytopathogenic changes include rounding of cell and aggregations into grape-like clusters. Intranuclear inclusion may be demonstrated by staining (**Fig. 35.3**). Human adenovirus may produce undifferentiated sarcoma in 30 to 90 days when inoculated in newborn hamster.

Adenovirus can be classified into two subgroups based on their ability to agglutinate rat and monkey erythrocytes. Around 33 serotypes are identified of adenovirus infecting man. They cause self-limited infection of respiratory tract, eye and may be intestine.

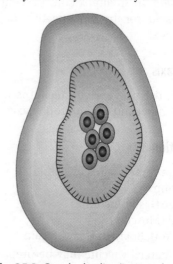

Fig. 35.3: Cowdry bodies (intranuclear).

It may cause pharyngitis and tonsillitis (types 1 to 5), pneumonia (types 4 and 7), acute respiratory disease (types 4, 7 and 21), pharyngoconjunctival fever (types 3 and 7), epidemic keratoconjunctivitis (type 8), acute follicular conjunctivitis (types 3 and 7a), intestinal lesions causing gastroenteritis and obesity (type 36). They may cause oncogenesis in hamster (types 12, 18 and 31).

Laboratory diagnosis may be established by isolating virus from throat, eye or feces. The specimen may be inoculated on A 549 cell line (American type culture collection USA) tissue cultures like HeLa, HEP-2, and then noting the cytopathic effects. Serological techniques like complement fixation, hemagglutination, hemagglutination inhibition and neutralization are useful.

a. *Adenovirus SV40*: Monkey kidney tissue culture, used in identification of adenovirus, may be contaminated with SV40 virus. They do not produce cytopathic effect on rhesus monkey kidney. Hence, both the viruses replicate and produce mature viral particles. In the process we may get viral particle containing genome of SV40 and capsid of adenovirus, which may be called hybrid virus.

b. *Adeno associated virus:* It is defective virus because it does not replicate in the absence of adenovirus. It is nonpathogenic and anti-genically different from adenovirus. It is DNA virus about 20 nm. It is also known as adeno-satellite virus.

HERPES VIRUS (FIG. 35.4)

It is double stranded DNA viruses about 100 to 150 nm in size, lipid enveloped and sensitive to ether and chloroform. It replicates in the nucleus of host cell. It produces intranuclear eosinophilic inclusion bodies. It does not possess common antigen. Examples are:
1. Herpes simplex types 1 and 2.
2. Varicella.
3. Herpes zoster.
4. Cytomegalovirus.
5. EB virus.

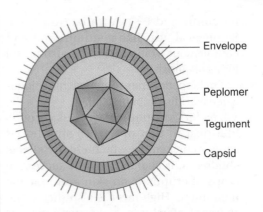

Fig. 35.4: Morphology of herpes virus.

1. *Herpes simplex:* It may produce mild vesicular eruption in skin or mucous membrane. It has two types; type 1 strain causes infection of mouth, eyes, central nervous system, etc. and type 2 strain causes infection of genitals. Type 1 and type 2 may be differentiated antigenically also.

It may be cultured on chorioallantoic membrane producing typical white, shining, non-necrotic pocks. Pocks are less than 0.75 mm in type 1 and more than 1 mm in type 2 strain. They can also be grown on rabbit kidney, HeLa, HEp-2 or human amnion tissue culture. They may produce experimental infection in animals like rabbit, mice, etc.

It is one of the most common infection of man. Only man is the natural host and may produce illness like herpes labialis, eczema herpeticum, keratoconjunctivitis, and meningoencephalitis. The herpes type 2 is venereal infection and produce genital herpes and neonate herpes. The virus may remain latent for years perhaps in sensory nerve ganglia and get reactivated.

Laboratory diagnosis is established by isolation of virus from infected material which may be inoculated on chorioallantoic membrane of chick embryo where we get typical pocks. They may also be isolated in rabbit kidney and human amnion tissue culture where typical intranuclear inclusion bodies appear. The isolate may be confirmed by neutralization tests. Serological tests like neutralization and complement fixation tests are also useful for its diagnosis.

For herpetic keratoconjunctivitis, 5-iodo-2 deoxyuridine is beneficial.

2. *Varicella:* Morphology of this virus is identical to that of herpes simplex. It causes chickenpox which chiefly affects children. It is characterized by successive crops of eruptions on skin and mucous membrane. High fever is also there. The source of infection is chickenpox patient or herpes zoster patient. There are no animal reservoirs. Portal of entry is respiratory tract. Incubation period is 7 to 23 days. Chickenpox is usually uneventful disease with complete recovery. Sometimes complications may occur like secondary bacterial infection, e.g., rash, encephalitis and pneumonia. One attack confers life-long immunity.

The virus does not grow on animal and chick embryo, but may multiply in human embryonic tissue culture producing intranuclear inclusion bodies (Cowdry type A). Laboratory diagnosis may be established by examining smear from vesicle. Giemsa stain shows multinucleated giant cells and intranuclear eosinophilic inclusion bodies. Virus may be isolated on human tissue culture. If vesicle fluid is examined under electron microscope we may see typical particles of herpes virus. Serological techniques like agar gel precipitation test, complement fixation and neutralization tests may be useful. A fluorescent antibody technique is also helpful for detection of varicella antigen.

Following varicella vaccines (given at 15 months of age) are available:

i. Takahashi live attenuated vaccine (not used because of oncogenicity and possibility of herpes zoster in later life).

ii. Formalin killed vaccine.

iii. Live attenuated OKA (varicella strain) vaccine after prolonged field trial is found quite effective. It is indicated for prevention of chickenpox in immuno-compromised children including those with hematological cancers or solid tumor. This vaccine is being evaluated for routine immunization of healthy children.

iv. Development of subunit or recombinant vaccine may eliminate the risk of herpes zoster.

Convalescent sera from herpes zoster patients contain much more levels of antibody than serum from varicella convalescents. Hence, the administration of this sera may confer protection to contacts of chickenpox patients.

3. *Herpes zoster:* It is the disease of old age still it may occur at any age even newborn are not spared. The disease is characterized by appearance of skin eruptions over the distribution of sensory nerves.

The portal of entry is unknown but in some cases varicella virus becomes neurotropic and is localized in nerve cells. From here infection spreads along posterior nerve root fibers with formation of vesicles in the segment of skin supplied by that particular nerve. The rash is usually unilateral. The commonest sites are areas innervated by spinal cord segments T3 to L2 and trigeminal nerve mostly ophthalmic branch. The rash disappears in 2 weeks but pain and paresthesia may persist for months together. In some cases lower motor neuron paralysis with meningoencephalitis and generalized zoster may occur.

Laboratory diagnosis is like that of varicella infection. Varicella and zoster viruses appear identical antigenically. It appears that the same virus in children during primary infection produces varicella (generalized infection) and when adults are involved they develop zoster (localized infection).

4. *Cytomegaloviruses:* They are indistinguishable from other viruses

of herpes group. They may infect man, monkey, guinea pig, etc. Characteristically they cause enlargement of infected cell with acidophilic or basophilic intranuclear inclusion body. Human strains are antigenically heterogeneous. They can be grown on human fibroblast cultures. Since cytopathic effects are slow in appearance they require prolonged incubation.

It may cause subclinical localized infection of salivary glands, kidney and rarely generalized disease in infants. The infection can be transmitted by urine, saliva droplets via respiratory route and through placenta from infected mother to fetus. The generalized infection is associated with hepatospleno-megaly, jaundice, thrombocytopenic purpura, hemolytic anemia and microcephaly. Apart from this there may be chorioretinitis and cerebral calcification. Sometimes syndrome resembling infectious mononucleosis may occur. It may lead to insidious hepatitis or pneumonia.

Laboratory diagnosis is established by isolating the virus from throat swab, urine and various affected organs. This material is inoculated on human fibroblast tissue culture and after 1 to 6 weeks characteristic cytopathic effects appear with presence of inclusion body. Serological diagnosis like complement fixation and neutralization may be helpful. Histological study of various organs may show large swollen cell with inclusion bodies (intranuclear) suggesting cytomegalovirus infection.

5. *Epstein Barr virus:* It is indistinguishable from other viruses of herpes group. It has the affinity for lymphoblastoid cells. There is now strong evidence that infectious mononucleosis is caused by Epstein Barr virus (EB virus).

To establish diagnosis blood examination shows leukopenia in early stages followed by leukocytosis. The abnormal mononuclear cell with basophilic vacuolated cytoplasm and kidney-shaped nucleus with fenestrated chromatin is seen. By electron microscope examination EB virus may be identified. Serological tests like Paul Bunnel, complement fixation, immunofluorescence and gel diffusion may be useful.

Human Herpes Virus Type 6

❖ First isolated in 1986 from peripheral blood leukocytes from patients of lympho proliferative disorders. Reported to be wide spread in UK, Japan, USA, etc.
❖ Although previously called B-lymphotropic virus, now identified as primarily T-lymphotropic.
❖ Two genetically distinct variants are recognized and are HHV-6A and HHV-6B.
❖ HHV-6 frequently develops during infancy.
❖ HHV-6 can cause exanthem subitum, febrile seizures without rash during infancy, etc.
❖ In older age HHV-6B has been associated with mononucleosis syndromes, focal encephalitis, pneumonitis, disseminated disease.
❖ HHV-6A has not been associated with disease.
❖ Virus is transmitted through saliva and probably by genital secretion.
❖ There is no established treatment or vaccine available for this virus.

Human Herpes Virus Type 7

❖ Isolated in 1990 from T-lymphocytes of healthy man from peripheral blood.
❖ The virus was subsequently isolated from other persons too.
❖ Virus is acquired during childhood and present in saliva of healthy persons.
❖ Some cases of exanthem subitum may be associated with this virus.

Human Herpes Virus Type 8

❖ Unique herpes virus like DNA sequence reported in 1994-95 in tissue derived from Kaposi's sarcoma and body cavity based on lymphoma in AIDS patients.

❖ HHV-8 isolation in cell culture may define its role in disease.
❖ They are partially homologous to the DNA of Epstein Barr virus, herpes virus samiri of squirrel monkeys.
❖ These herpes virus like DNA sequences have also been reported from Kaposi's sarcoma tissues sarcoma from non-AIDS patients, in a subgroup of AIDS related B-cell body cavity based lymphoma, and in brain tumor some proliferative skin lesions of organ transplant recipients.

❖ These DNA sequences have also been seen in semen of both AIDS and non-AIDS patients.

Initially discovered by molecular biology techniques in Kaposi's sarcoma, this new herpes virus has been isolated in Kaposi's sarcoma using cell cultures. This virus is associated with 3 conditions, i.e., Kaposi's disease, B-cell lymphoma and Castleman's disease.

RNA Viruses

PICORNAVIRUSES A

They are very small, 20 to 30 nm in size, non-enveloped and resistant to ether. Picornavirus group of medical importance includes:
A. Enteroviruses
B. Rhinoviruses

Enteroviruses

From the medical point of view important viruses of this group are polio, echo and coxsackie viruses. Enteroviruses are stable, and resistant to bile and ether. They remain unharmed in water and sewage for quite a long time. They are described as under:

a. *Poliovirus:* They are 30 nm diameter with capsomere arranged in icosahedral symmetry and are spherical. They are resistant to ether, chloroform and bile. They survive in low pH and low temperature. They are killed by formaldehyde, cholinination and lyophilization. By neutralization poliovirus strains are classified into types I, II and III. Type I is the most common and is responsible for epidemic. Natural infection occurs only in man.

The virus enters body by ingestion or inhalation. The virus multiplies in lymphatic tissue of alimentary canal (from tonsils to Peyer's patches) entering regional lymph nodes and then viruses are carried to bloodstream. From here viruses are taken to spinal cord and brain. They destroy neurons with degeneration of Nissl body. Lesions are mostly in anterior horn of spinal cord. Sometimes we may find extensive lesions

like encephalitis. The incubation period is about 10 days with range from 4 days to 4 weeks.

Laboratory diagnosis is made by isolation of viruses from throat (early stage) and feces (throughout the course of disease). After processing specimen is inoculated into tissue culture and virus growth is indicated by cytopathic effects in 2 to 3 days. Identification of virus should be interpreted along with clinical picture. Serodiagnosis is not of much use, still complement fixation and neutralization test may be valuable.

Immunization is achieved by using vaccine. Salk killed polio vaccine is formalin inactivated consisting of 3 types of polioviruses. It gives 80 to 90% protection against paralytic poliomyelitis. Killed vaccination is given by injection. On the other hand, Sabin live polio vaccine is also available and is prepared by growing the attenuated strain in monkey kidney cells. Live vaccine is easy to administer as it is given orally, much more economical, single dose gives lifelong immunity and gives local immunity in the intestine.

b. *Coxsackieviruses:* They are called coxsackievirus as first of all they were isolated from patients coming from the village of coxsackie in New York. They are classified into group A and B. By neutralization method group A viruses are divided into 24 types. Characteristically the viruses have the ability to infect suckling mice and not the adult mice. All group B viruses grow on monkey kidney tissue culture and some group A viruses grow in HeLa cells.

They may cause vesicular pharyngitis (group A), aseptic meningitis (groups A and B), minor respiratory infections (A21), Bronholm disease manifested as stitch-like pain in abdomen and chest (group B), myocarditis (group B) and pericarditis (group B).

The laboratory diagnosis may be made by isolating the viruses from lesion or feces by inoculation in suckling mice. Since there are several antigenic types so serodiagnosis is not feasible.

c. *Echoviruses:* Their description designation is enteric cytopathogenic human orphan viruses (ECHO viruses). They are classified into 33 serotypes. They infect man naturally. They are not pathogenic to laboratory animals.

They may produce fever with rash and aseptic meningitis (types 4, 6, 9 and 16). Laboratory diagnosis is by inoculating feces, throat swab or CSF on monkey kidney tissue culture and virus growth is detected by cytopathogenic changes.

Newer Enteroviruses (68 to 72)

Four types of viruses, i.e., 68, 70, 71, 72 associated with diseases of man as under:

    68 Pneumonia
    70 Acute hemorrhagic conjunctivitis
    71 Mumps
    72 Hepatitis A.

Rhinoviruses

They differ from enteroviruses in being more acid labile and heat stable. They have been classified into over 100 types and immunity is type specific. Depending upon growth in tissue culture, rhinoviruses are classified as H strains (grow only on human cells) and M strains (grow equally well on human as well as monkey cells). Because of too many serotypes (over 100) it is impossible to make ideal vaccine. However, antiviral chemotherapy may be helpful in bringing specific control.

ORTHOMYXOVIRUSES

It includes the enveloped RNA viruses capable of adsorbing on to mucoprotein receptor on erythrocytes. This results in hemagglutination. They are 80 to 120 nm in size and spherical in shape. Influenza virus represents this group.

INFLUENZA VIRUSES

They are responsible for infectious disease of respiratory tract occurring mostly in epidemic and pandemic forms. The classification of influenza virus into 3 (A, B and C) is based on the antigenic nature of ribonucleoprotein.

Influenza virus is spherical with diameter 80 to 120 nm. The virus has ribonucleoprotein in helical symmetry. Single stranded RNA genome is segmented and nucleocapsid is surrounded by envelope having virus coded protein layer and lipid layer derived from host cell. Attached to lipid layer are hemagglutinin spikes and neuraminidase peplomers **(Fig. 36.1)**. The virus is inactivated at 50°C for 30 minutes, ether, formaldehyde, phenol and salts of heavy metals.

The characteristic feature of influenza virus is its ability to undergo antigenic variation. Depending on degree antigenic variation may be classified as **(Table 36.1)**:

i. Antigenic shift (abrupt, drastic, disconti-nuous variation in antigenic structure causing major epidemic).

ii. Antigenic drift (gradual changes in antigenic structure regularly, resulting in periodical epidemic).

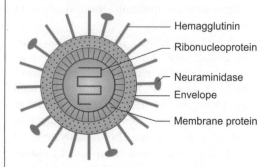

Fig. 36.1: Structure of influenza virus.

Table 36.1: Emergence of antigen subtypes of influenza A associated with pandemics or epidemic diseases.

1889–90	H2N8	Severe pandemic
1900–03	H3N8	Moderate epidemic
1918–19	H1N1 (formerly Hsw N1)	Severe pandemic
1933–35	H1N1 (formerly H0N1)	Mild epidemic
1946–47	H1N1	Mild epidemic
1957–58	H2N2	Severe pandemic
1968–69	H3N2	Moderate pandemic
1977–78	H1N1	Mild pandemic
1988–89	H1N1/H3N2	Have circulated either in alternating years or concurrently
2009	H1N1(Swine flu)	Pandemic April 2009

The virus grows in amniotic cavity and allantoic cavity of chick embryo. It is detected by appearance of hemagglutinin in allantoic and amniotic fluid. They are also grown in monkey kidney cells. Route of entry is respiratory tract. The viral neuraminidase facilitates infection by reducing the viscosity of mucus lining and exposing the cell surface receptor for virus adsorption. These cells are damaged and shed, laying bare the cells in trachea and branchi.

The incubation period is 1 to 3 days. The onset is abrupt with fever, headache, generalized myalgia and prominent respiratory symptoms. If no complication follows the disease resolves in 2 to 7 days. Complications include pneumonia due to bacterial superinfection, congestive heart failure and encephalitis. Reye's syndrome is associated with influenza B virus.

Diagnosis in the laboratory is established by demonstration of virus antigen (immunofluorescence) isolation of virus (chick embryo or monkey kidney cell culture), serology (complement fixation test, hemagglutination inhibition test) and radial immunodiffusion tests in agarose gel (screening test).

Influenza vaccine is in use. Vaccine may be prepared by growing virus in allantoic cavity and inactivating the virus with formalin. Because of presence of egg protein this vaccine may cause allergic reactions. This difficulty is removed by preparing subunit vaccines (virus treated with ether). The other vaccines in use are: (i) recombinant live vaccines obtained by hybridization between its mutants of established strain, (ii) new antigenic variant, a neuraminidase specific vaccine, and (iii) a live vaccine using temperature sensitive (TS) mutant, etc.

Antiviral drug amantidine hydrochloride which inhibits adsorption of virus to cell is useful in influenza infection. Combined yearly vaccination of persons at high risk, using the best mix of important antigens and administration of amantidine at time of stress, e.g., surgery or hospitalization, etc. is suggested.

PARAMYXOVIRUSES

They are larger and more pleomorphic than orthomyxoviruses. They possesses hemagglutinins, neuraminidases and hemolysin. They are antigenically stable. This group includes viruses like mumps, parainfluenza, respiratory syncytial and measles.

Mumps

It is responsible for acute infectious disease characterized by parotitis. The name mumps is derived from mumbling speech of patients.

The virus is spherical varying from 100 to 250 nm. The envelope has hemagglutinins, a neuraminidase and hemolysin. The virus can be grown on yolk sac or amniotic fluid of chick embryo, and human or monkey kidney cell culture. They are inactivated at room temperature, ultraviolet light or by chemicals like formaldehyde and ether. Two complement fixing antigens have been identified as soluble (S antigen) and viral (V antigen).

Infection may be by inhalation and through conjunctiva. Incubation period is 18 to 21 days.

Clinical symptoms start with sudden non-suppurative enlargement of parotid glands. Skin over the enlarged parotid glands may be stretched, red and hot. Viremia may be responsible for the involvement of other organs. Orchitis and viral meningoencephalitis are important complications of mumps. The pancreas, ovary, thyroid and breast may be involved. However, it is important and most common cause of aseptic meningitis.

Diagnosis is confirmed by isolation of virus from saliva, CSF or urine. For this purpose amniotic cavity of chick embryo or monkey or human kidney cell culture may be used. Serological test like complement fixation, hemagglutination inhibition and neutralization tests may be helpful. Skin test is not very useful but still it can be used to detect susceptible patient.

Mumps infection confers life long immunity. Normal human gamma globulin prepared from mumps convalescent serum appears useful for prophylaxis.

For active immunization killed vaccine (virus grown in allantoic cavity), Jeryl-Lynn strain (live attenuated vaccine) and now live vaccine is available which can be sprayed into mouth without any side effect.

Respiratory Syncytial Virus

Although these viruses resemble para-myxoviruses structurally but they do not have either hemagglutinin or neuraminidase. They are antigenically stable and grow on HeLa cells, HEp-2 and in monkey kidney cells. They are responsible for bronchiolitis and pneumonia. In adults, it may cause afebrile rhinitis and in aged persons it may cause exacerbation of bronchitis.

For diagnosis, nasal and pharyngeal secretion are inoculated in human (He La, HEp2) or monkey kidney cell culture. It takes 5 to 14 days' time. Rapid diagnosis may be made by immunofluorescent technique. Serological techniques like complement fixation and neutralization test may be useful. No vaccine is available at present.

Parainfluenza Viruses

They may produce febrile respiratory infections throughout the year. They possess hemagglutinin, neuraminidase and hemolysin. They grow well in human or monkey kidney cell culture. Growth in chick embryo is poor or absent. They are inactivated by heat and by ether. They are classified into four groups: Parainfluenza 1, Parainfluenza 2, Parainfluenza 3, Parainfluenza 4.

Parainfluenza viruses are responsible for about 10% respiratory infection in children. Types 1 and 2 cause croup which is a serious clinical disease. Type 3 causes lower respiratory infections and type 4 causes minor respiratory infections.

Measles

It is highly acute infectious disease characterized for generalized maculopapular rash proceeded by fever, cough, nasal and conjunctival catarrh, etc. **(Fig. 36.2)**.

The viruses possess hemagglutinin and no neuraminidase. They do not grow in eggs but may grow on human embryonic kidney or amnion cell cultures. The virus's core may be inactivated by heat, ultraviolet light, ether and formaldehyde. They are antigenically homogeneous.

Incubation period is 10 to 12 days. Infection manifests as fever and respiratory tract involvement. At this stage, Koplik's spots may be seen on buccal mucosa and 2 to 4 days later rash appears. Uneventful recovery

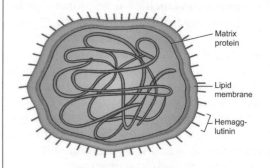

Matrix protein

Lipid membrane

Hemagglutinin

Fig. 36.2: Measles virus.

occurs in most of the patients. In small number of cases complications like croup or bronchitis, secondary bacterial infection, giant cell pneumonia and meningoencephalitis may occur. Very rarely we may have late complication like subacute sclerosing panencep-halitis (SSPE).

The diagnosis may be established by isolating the virus from nose, throat, conjunctiva, blood and urine. Primary human embryonic kidney and amnion cells are quite useful. Rapid diagnosis of virus growth is possible by immunofluorescence. However, smear can be prepared from nasal, pharyngeal and conjunctival secretion and examined microscopically after staining with Giemsa's method for presence of giant cells and inclusion bodies (Cowdry type A). Serological techniques like complement fixation test, neutralization, and hemagglutination inhibition may be useful for establishing diagnosis of measles.

Normal human gamma globulin if given within 6 days of exposure can prevent disease. A formalin inactivated vaccine against measles proved not of much use. Live attenuated vaccine is developed using Edmonston B strain. This vaccine can be given in combination with mumps and rubella vaccines (MMR). The other live attenuated vaccines are Schwartz and Mortin strain and Backham 31 strain.

Rubella Virus

It is an enveloped RNA virus causing rash and lymphadenopathy (posterior and suboccipital) in children. In adults, there is involvement of joint and purpura. Infection in early pregnancy may lead to developmental defects in fetus (embryopathy).

The virus is pleomorphic, spherical, 50 to 70 nm in diameter and enveloped. It has one type of antigen (hemagglutinin). It is heat labile and inactivated by ether and chloroform. Rubella virus can be grown in primary African green monkey kidney tissue cell lines (VERO, RK 13), human amnion and thyroid tissue culture. The presence of virus is detected by interference test.

It enters the body by inhalation and replication of virus occurs in cervical lymph nodes. After incubation period (2 to 8 weeks) viremia occurs which lasts till rash, fever and lymphadenopathy appears. Arthritis is common complication especially in females. If rubella occurs in early pregnancy the fetus may die otherwise congenital malformation is common in first trimester. The most common malformation produced by rubella are cardiac defect, cataract and deafness. The other features in babies of congenital rubella are hepatosplenomegaly, thrombocytopenic purpura, myocarditis and bone lesions.

Incidence of defects in rubella infection is closely linked to stage of pregnancy when the infection is acquired:

Stage of pregnancy	Incidence of defects
1 month	50%
2 months	25%
3 months	17%
4 months	11%
5 months	6%
6 months onwards	Very low

Rubella virus is found in all excretions of congenitally infected infants. That is the reason of infected babies constituting important source of infection to the staff in nurseries.

Diagnosis can be established by virus isolation from blood (early stage) and throat swabs. Growth on rabbit kidney or vero cell culture is detected by interference with Echo 11 virus. However, serological diagnosis is made by hemagglutination inhibition, neutralization, complement fixation, immunofluorescent of platelets and aggregation tests. Four-fold or more rise in convalescent serums is diagnostic. In congenital rubella diagnosis is made by demonstrating IgM.

Rubella infection gives lifelasting immunity as there is one antigenic type of virus. Prophylaxis is relevant only to women of childbearing age. The vaccines (live attenuated) available are Cendehill and HPV 77 (serial passage in tissue culture). They are administered subcutaneously. Drawback is that arthritis occurs after vaccination. To 336 and HPV 77 DES are other vaccines. New vaccine has come up (RA 27/3) which is administered intranasally conferring local immunity as well. The safe period of giving vaccine in young girls is 11 to 13 years and in women immediately after delivery.

RHABDOVIRUS

They are classified as rhabdovirus with bullet-like shape. They are enveloped RNA which multiply in cytoplasm of host cell and mature by budding from plasma membrane. The most important virus of this group is rabies virus.

Rabies Virus

They are bullet-shaped with one end blunt and other end pointed, 120 to 200 nm long with cylindrical diameter of 60 to 80 nm. The core contains RNA in helical symmetry. The virion is surrounded by lipoprotein envelop from which project hemagglutinin spikes (Fig. 36.3). They are killed by ultraviolet light, heating at 56°C for one hour and 60°C for 5 minutes, ether, strong acid, strong alkalies and trypsin. All strains are antigenically similar. They induce formation of fixing, neutralizing and hemagglutination inhibition antibodies.

Virus can grow almost in all warm blooded animals, suckling mice being better suited for virus isolation. They can also be grown on chick embryo, duck embryo, tissue cultures prepared from mouse or chick embryo (fibroblast), hamster kidney and human diploid tissue.

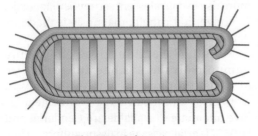

Fig. 36.3: Rabies virus.

Man is infected by the bite of rabid animals, e.g., dog. Saliva of the infective animal contains rabies virus which are deposited in wound conferred by the bite of animal. The viruses travel through nerve fibers to the spinal cord and brain. From central nervous system viruses spread to salivary glands and other tissues. Incubation period is from 1 to 3 months. Prodromal phase usually lasts for 2 to 4 days with manifestations as malaise, anorexia, nausea, vomiting, headache and fever. This stage is followed by sensory phase when patient feels peculiar sensation around wound and attempt to swallow results in painful spasm of muscles of deglutition. This phase is followed by excitory phase in which patient gets generalized convulsions and coma. Many a time death is preceded by paralysis.

It is more important to demonstrate virus in the rabid animal than in patients. However, in patients, demonstration of viral antigen from facial skin biopsy and in corneal smear may be done. Immunofluorescent may be employed for antemortem diagnosis whereas postmortem demonstration of inclusion body or virus antigen in the brain or isolation of virus by mouse inoculation are the standard procedures. For the diagnosis in animals suspected to die of rabies preferably severed head should be sent to laboratory. If possible brain of the animal may be removed and divided into two portion, one in 50% glycerol saline (biological test) and the other in Zenker's fixative (microscopic examination). Hippocampus major part of brain should be included as it contains abundant inclusion bodies. Impression smears are stained by Seller technique. The inclusion bodies (Negri bodies) are seen as intracytoplasmic, round and purplish pink structure (Fig. 36.4). By indirect immunofluorescence test using antirabies serum fluorescein conjugate, deposit of virus antigen may be demonstrated in infected cell long before Negri bodies appear. Ten percent suspension of brain is injected intracerebrally

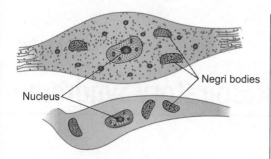

Fig. 36.4: Negri bodies.

into mice. Impression smears of brain show many Negri bodies. Isolation of virus from saliva of man or animal may be tried for this purpose by intramuscular injection to Syrian hamster because of its susceptibility.

Prophylactic measures of rabies consist of washing the wound with water and soap and then cauterizing it with carbolic acid or quartenary ammonium compounds. Currently, following antirabic vaccines are available:

a. Neural vaccines:
   i. Fermi vaccines not in use now.
   ii. Semple vaccine is widely used.
   iii. Sheep brain vaccine.
   iv. Inactivated vaccine is prepared from suckling mouse or rabbit. It carries little risk of neurological complication.

b. Live attenuated chick embryo vaccine is available in two forms:
   i. Low egg passage (LEP)
   ii. High egg passage (HEP)

c. Duck egg vaccine.

d. Tissue culture vaccines have low potency.

The recommended dosage schedule of semple vaccine for different classes is as below:

Class	Semple vaccine
Class I	
Licks on fresh cuts with saliva all over the body except head, face and neck, licks on intact mucosa of mouth, nose, and conjunctiva or bites scratches without bleeding and handling raw flesh of rabid animals.	2 mL for 7 days
Class II	
Licks on fresh cut or abrasions on fingers, unlacerated bites or scratches on the fingers (½ cm long) and bites or scratches on all parts of body except head, face, neck or finger which have drawn blood. Number of bites should not be more than five.	5 mL for 14 days
Class III	
Licks and bites or fresh cut or abrasions on head, face and neck, bites, (lacerated) on finger (more than 1 cm), bites causing laceration and drawing blood, more than 5 in number, all jackal and wolf bites and class II patient who has not received treatment within 14 days of injury	10 mL for 14 days

Severe Acute
Respiratory Syndrome

Towards the tail end of 2002 a new syndrome emerged in southern China. It was named as Severe Acute Respiratory Syndrome (SARS). The initial outbreak was in peak in April 2003. By June 2003 there had been 8,000 cases worldwide and 775 deaths.

SARS is caused by a novel coronavirus (CoV). It does not appear to be related with 3 known classes of coronavirus. It is hypothesized on the basis of available data that animal virus recently mutated and developed the ability to productively infect man. Groups 1 and 2 contain mammalian virus while Group 3 contains avian virus. SARS CoV defines 4th class of coronavirus and it exhibits following features:

1. It has 29,727 nucleotides in length.
2. It has 9 open reading frames that are not found in other coronavirus and may code for proteins that are unique to SARS virus.
3. It is large, enveloped having positive stranded (27 to 30 kb) and may cause respiratory and enteric diseases in man and animal.
4. Its genome is largest found in any RNA virus.
5. Human coronaviruses are found both in Group I (H Cov -229 E) and Group II (H CoV-OC 43) and are responsible for 30 percent mild respiratory tract infection **(Figs 37.1 and 37.2)**.

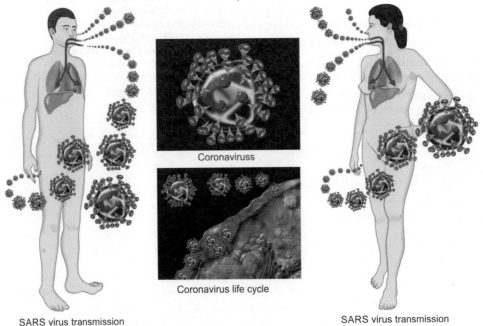

Coronaviruss

Coronavirus life cycle

SARS virus transmission

SARS virus transmission

Fig. 37.1: Severe acute respiratory syndrome (SARS).

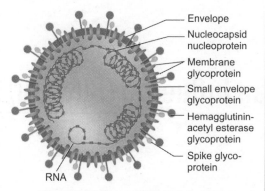

Fig. 37.2: SARS-associated coronavirus.

Envelope
Nucleocapsid nucleoprotein
Membrane glycoprotein
Small envelope glycoprotein
Hemagglutinin-acetyl esterase glycoprotein
Spike glyco-protein
RNA

CLINICAL PICTURE

SARS is transmitted by inhalation because the virus may be present in droplets aerosol of respiratory tract secretions of the patients. Incubation period of SARS is 5 to 7 days. Manifestations of SARS are as under:

1. Fever 38°C or more
2. Dry non-productive cough
3. Myalgia
4. Sore throat
5. Shortness of breath
6. Atypical pneumonia
7. Mortality and morbidity resembles 1918 influenza epidemic
8. Death may occur from progressive respiratory failure in 3 to 30% of cases.

LABORATORY DIAGNOSIS

1. Isolation of SARS CoV in monkey Vero E 6 cells in tissue culture.
2. Reduction in lymphocyte count.
3. Rise in aminotransferase activity which indicates damage to the liver.
4. Reverse transcription PCR using respiratory secretions.
5. Indirect immunofluorescent to demonstrate rising antibodies.

6. ELISA to detect rising titer of antibodies.
7. Chest radiograph.

MANAGEMENT

There is no consensus so far treatment for SARS is concerned. Only symptomatic treatment and quarantine of the patient seems to be feasible for the time being. The drug of particular interest and promising is the one which blocks the protease function. No vaccine has been developed. A major hurdle towards development of vaccine is antigenic shift.

HIGHLIGHTS OF COVID-19

❖ Its new version of Corona virus responsible of causing pandemic
❖ It spreads from person-to-person.
❖ COVID-19 symptoms range from mild to severe illness.
❖ One can infected by coming in close contact with COVID-19 patients, respiratory droplets when patients coughs, sneezes or talks and by touching surface or object that has virus on it and then by touching mouth, nose or eyes.
❖ Everyone is at risk of getting COVID-19 especially older, adults having-medical underlying conditions like diabetes, heart problems, kidney problems, etc.
❖ Preventive measures include stay at home, avoid close contacts with others, use mask, covering nose and mouth in public places.
❖ Wash hands with soap and water (for 20 seconds). 60% alcohol containing sanitizer must be used if soap and water is not available.
❖ Clean and disinfect touched surface frequently.
❖ Practice social distancing (6 feet).
❖ No specific treatment is available. Only symptomatic treatment may be given.
❖ Till now no vaccine is available.

Avian Influenza (Bird Flu)

Birds are especially important species because all known subtypes of influenza A viruses circulate among wild birds, which are considered the natural hosts for influenza A viruses. Influenza viruses that infect birds are called avian influenza viruses.

The causative agent is H5 N1 a subtype of influenza A virus. It generally affects bird population all over Asia. Outbreaks of avian influenza A (H5 N1) have been confirmed among poultry in Cambodia, China, Hong Kong, Indonesia, Japan, Laos, South Korea, Thailand and Vietnam. The virus H5 N1 was first isolated from birds in South Africa in 1961.

Influenza A viruses may be divided into subtypes on the basis of their surface proteins, i.e. hemagglutinin (HA) and neuraminidase (NA). There are 15 known H subtypes. Whereas all subtypes are found in birds, only 3 subtypes of HA (H1, H2 and H3) and two subtypes of NA (N1 and N2) are known to have circulated widely in man. This virus makes wild birds sick, but may make domesticated birds very sick and may kill them. Several instances are on records where human infections and outbreaks have occurred in last 8 years. There is possibility of different variations of H5 N1. Following information has been gathered about H5 N1:

1. All genes are of bird origin. Since virus has not acquired genes from human influenza virus so possibility of person to person spread is more likely.
2. There is possibility of different variations of H5 N1 virus which is in circulation at this time. Genetic sequencing of virus samples from South Korea and Vietnam suggest that viruses of these countries are different.

SPREAD OF INFECTION

Infected birds shed viruses in saliva, nasal secretions and feces. Bird to birds transmission is by contact with contaminated excretions. H5 N1 infection in man may be because of contact with infected poultry or contaminated surfaces. Of late human to human transmission has been reported.

SYMPTOMS

The symptoms in man include fever, cough, sore throat, muscle aches. Additionally there may be eye infection, pneumonia, acute respiratory distress and other severe life-threatening conditions.

PREVENTION AND TREATMENT

Prevention measures include killing of sick and exposed birds, isolation and treating the patients. Travellers to countries in Asia with H5 N1 outbreaks must avoid poultry farms and any surface contaminated with feces from poultry. Other preventive measures include wearing of mask and gloves, cleaning kitchen surfaces, cooking chicken till boiling temperature, controlling human traffic into poultries and reporting to authorities any unusual death or illness of chicken or other birds as well as illness of workers in poultry farms.

Antivirals drugs like oseltamivir and zanamavir are quite effective. Some strains however do show resistance to amantadine and rimantadine.

Chapter 39

Acquired Immune Deficiency Syndrome

▇ IMPORTANT EVENTS IN AIDS

1981 The first case of AIDS reported in USA.

1983 LAV, i.e,. HIV isolated.

1984 Serological tests developed to identify infected persons.

1985 Report of anti-HIV activity of suramin, ribavirus published.

1985 Report of *in vitro* anti-HIV activity of HPA 23, interferon alpha, foscarnet and zidovudine published.

1986 Clinical trials of zidovudine show efficacy in AIDS and advanced AIDS-related complex.

1987 Zidovudine (AZT)—licensed for clinical use in many countries. Large scale clinical trials of zidovudine and other agents began.

1991 Didanosine is licensed for use by USFDA in selected AIDS patients.

AIDS is a immunoregulatory disorder that is often fatal because it predisposes the person to severe opportunistic infections or possibly to neoplasms. It happens so because of depletion of helper T cells owing to infection by HIV (human immunodeficiency virus).

History

Acquired Immune Deficiency Syndrome (AIDS) was first recognized in USA in July 1981. In August 1981, AIDS was reported in intravenous users. In June 1982, clusters of AIDS patients appeared among homosexuals and later in hemophiliacs and blood transfusion associated patients. In January 1983, it was reported in heterosexual cases in female.

Isolation of etiological agent of AIDS was first reported in May 1983 by Luc Montagnier from Pasteur Institute, Paris. They isolated a retrovirus from a West African patient with generalized lymphadenopathy and they named it lymphadenopathy associated virus (LAV). In March 1984, Robert Gallo from National Institute of Health, Bethesda (USA) reported isolation of retrovirus and named it HTLV-3. In March 1985, ELISA test kit was approved by FDA. In May 1985, blood bank screening for HIV was introduced. In 1986, the virus was named HIV.

India started a serosurveillance among high risk groups in 1985 to know the magnitude of HIV infection. First case of HIV infection in India was reported in 1986 and that of HIV-2 in 1991.

Structure and Properties of HIV

It belongs to the Lentivirus subgroup of Retroviridae family. HIV is an RNA retrovirus. The unique morphologic feature of HIV is its cylindrical nucleoid in the mature virion. The diagnostic bar-shaped nucleoid may be seen in electron micrographs. Under electron microscope it exhibits the characteristic exotic flower appearance **(Fig. 39.1)**. Dr Rober C Gallo discovered HIV in 1984.

The virus contains the 3 genes required for a replicating retrovirus—gag, pol and env **(Fig. 39.2)**. The virus has outermost envelope rich in glycoproteins (gp41, gp120, gp160) and inner core with two component proteins (p18,

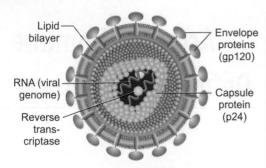

Fig. 39.1: Face of AIDS virus.

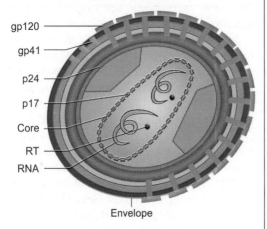

Fig. 39.2: Structure of HIV.

p24) while the enzyme reverse transcriptase capable of the retrograde transcription of viral RNA to viral DNA marks its special feature. The core proteins, the surface proteins and the regulatory proteins (p31, p66) are under the genetic control by the gag, env and the pol loci respectively. Amongst the three inbuilt control mechanisms the env locus is under frequent genetic alteration, leading to modification in the antigenic structure of the virus.

In addition following 5 genes code for polypeptides are identified as under:
* TAT (transactivation gene)
* REF (regulator of virus gene)—May be involved in regulation of HIV expression
* NEF (negative factor gene).
* VIF (viral infectivity factor gene)
* VPU in HIV-I—May weaken transcriptional activator.
* VPX in HIV-II—May be required for efficient budding.

HIV is T lymphotropic especially for helper T cells identified by monoclonal antibody OK T4 (Leu-3). Virus infection causes cytopathic effect including the formation of multinucleated giant cells followed by cell death. This explains the quantitative and functional depletion of T4 lymphocyte subset that is the hallmark of AIDS lymphodepletive terminal event. In the end stage, there is reduced T4 count (less than 60%), nonspecific proliferation of B lymphocytes producing functionally incompetent wasteful serum immunoglobulins (IG and IgA) and nonreactivity (energy) to recall antigens. The final outcome is total depletion of lymph node, impairment of the CMI making the patient susceptible to vast spectrum of opportunistic infection (bacterial, viral, fungal and parasitic).

Etiopathogenesis: HIV effects T4 lymphocytes through infected semen, the contaminated blood and blood products and rarely through saliva, urine and the fecal material.

Once the virus binds with CD4 receptor, the outermost cover is lost at the site of entry. The inner protein coat is being subsequently cast off and the bare enzyme RT transcribes viral RNA and DNA (provirus). Subsequent to its entry into host nucleus the viral DNA genome (provirus) integrates with host DNA genome. In the absence of immunological activation the T4 lymphocyte continues to survive with provirus and the subsequent integration in host DNA is halted leading to the latent HIV infection. What influences the viral replication or dormancy is unpredictable at this stage. The viral messenger RNA (mRNA) subsequent to its transcription redirects the host cytoplasmic machinery to synthesize the newer viral particles. The cell eventually dies and newly generated viruses bud out from dying cell, leading to lymphodepletive terminal events.

The end stage is characterized by reduced T4 count (60%), nonspecific unrestrained proliferation of B lymphocytes producing excessive functional incompetent wasteful immunoglobulins (IgG, IgA) and nonreactivity to recall antigens. The lymph node in the terminal stage may show a total depletion with the characteristic "burnt-out" picture. The final outcome is long-standing impairment of CMI making the affected person unusually susceptible to a vast spectrum of life-threatening opportunistic infection and malignancies of varying types.

Clinical picture: The incubation period seems to be long, ranging from 6 months to more than 2 years. AIDS occurs in homosexuals (75%) but bisexual males, heterosexuals, intravenous drug users and hemophiliacs treated with blood products or factor VIII are also at risk to get infected.

AIDS is characterized by pronounced suppression of immune system, the development of unusual neoplasms especially Kaposi's sarcoma or wide variety of severe opportunistic infections. Other symptoms include fatigue, malaise, unexplained weight loss, fever, shortness of breath, chronic diarrhea, white patches on tongue (hairy leukoplakia or oral candidiasis) and lymphadenopathy.

The most common complication of AIDS may be (*protozoal Toxoplasma gondii*, etc.), fungal, (*Pneumocystis carinii, Candida albicans, Cryptococcus neoformans, Histoplasma capsulatum*, etc.), bacterial (*Mycobacterium avium, Mycobacterium tuberculosis, Listeria monocytogenes, Salmonella, Nocardia asteroides*, etc.) and viruses (cytomegalovirus, herpes simplex, adenovirus, hepatitis-B, etc.).

HIV can infect other cell types including B lymphocytes and monocytes *in vivo* and a variety of human cell lines *in vitro*. Viruses can spread throughout the body, and are demonstrated in lymphoid cells, brain, thymus, spleen and testes. No animal models have been developed for AIDS.

Inactivation of HIV: 10 minutes' treatment at 37°C can inactivate this virus, with:

i. 10% household bleach
ii. 50% ethanol
iii. 35% isopropanol
iv. 1% NP40
v. 0.5% lysol
vi. 0.5% paraformaldehyde
vii. 0.3% H_2O_2

Besides extreme pH (pH 1.0 and 13.0), heating at 56°C for 10 minutes can inactivate HIV.

Global situation of AIDS: 23 million people all over the globe are now infected with HIV. 8500 people are infected with HIV each day and as per calculation it is ample clear that by 2000 AD every 6th or 7th person in world will be a victim of this infection. WHO data suggested 1.3 million adult AIDS cases in 193 countries with epicentre of epidemic shifting from Africa to Asian subcontinent. India has emerged quickly as the country with large number of people infected with AIDS virus. More than 3 million of India's 950 million people are estimated to be infected with HIV. Trailing India in the number of people infected are South Africa 1.8 million, Uganda 1.4 million, Nigeria 1.2 million, Kenya 1.1 million.

The first case of AIDS in India was registered in 1986. Since then, HIV prevalence has been reported in all states and union territories of India. By October 31, 1997, of a total of 3.20 million individual practising risk behaviors and suspected AIDS case who were screened for HIV infection, 67,311 were found to be seropositive. Up to May 31, 1998, the number of AIDS cases in India is reported as 6052, the largest number of cases are from Maharashtra

Table 39.1: Break-up of HIV-infected persons in India.

Category	% of total
• Heterosexually promiscuous	45.30
• Homosexuals	0.12
• Blood donors	19.33
• Patients on dialysis	0.38
• Antenatal mothers	0.42
• Recipient of blood/blood products	1.98
• Relatives of HIV patients	0.90
• Suspected AIDS related cases or AIDS cases	3.68
• Drug addicts (I/V)	18.03
• Miscellaneous	9.86

(2,955) followed by Tamil Nadu (1,424) and Manipur (301). The break-up of HIV cases in India is depicted in **Table 39.1**.

Laboratory Diagnosis

Direct Methods

i. *Cultivation of T lymphocytes:* T lymphocytes with normal lymphocytes are cultured on special cell lines (Hg, HUT78 U937) with interleukin II. Stimulation of T cell and demonstration of multinucleated giant cells is possible by 2 to 20 weeks. It is the classical method to confirm the HIV infection.

ii. *Detection of reverse transcriptase:* It is possible on virus grown cells by radio labeling.

iii. *Solid phase ELISA:* It is useful to detect HIV antigen.

iv. *Phase contrast microscopy:* It is helpful in assaying the prevention of reclustering of MT-4 cells.

v. *Electron microscopy:* Demonstration of fuzzy envelope of infected T4.

vi. *Animal study:* Reproduction of human lesions in nonhuman primates have a limited diagnostic importance.

Indirect Methods

Antibodies to HIV usually appear in 6 to 8 weeks after the exposure to virus. Following methods are simple, easy and quite useful to diagnose AIDS patients.

i. ELISA

ii. *Western blot assay:* The antigene fractions specific for HIV, initially resolved by SDS polyacrylamide gel are transferred on nitrosocellulose membrane by electroblotting. The antigenic profile on membrane contains P17, P24, P31, gp41, P55, P56, gp160 in the increasing order of molecular size. The later steps involve reaction with HRP labeled anti-IgG antibody and chromogen substrate reaction. The development of pink colored bands indicate the site of specific antigen antibody complex on the membrane.

However, IgM-Western blot assay test is slightly different from Western blot assay. In this test basic technique is identical, diaminobenzedine as a substrate and P24 as a positive control are two deviations. Besides resolution of brown components indicate the site of immune complex. Appearance of all the three gene products (env, gag and pol) are consistent with a classical HIV infection. Otherwise two env bands (gp41, gp120) show a positive pattern too.

The ELISA at times, particularly so in multiparous women gives rise to false-positive results because of antibodies crossreacting with T4 lymphocytes. This is rarely seen in Western blot technique **(Fig. 39.3)**.

iii. *Radioimmunoprecipitation assay:* This technique involves radioactive antigen.

iv. *Polymerase chain reaction:* The polymerase chain reaction (PCR) is a new and exciting technology. It is gaining widespread use in the diagnosis and management of genetic, oncologic, hematologic and infectious diseases. In this method, there is direct detection of disease specific sequences of either RNA or DNA from the tissue or body fluid of patient. It is quite sensitive.

This technique is widely used in HIV infection. In addition to quantitative PCR technique is useful in monitoring the efficacy of antiviral chemotherapy.

v. Dot blot hybridization.

vi. Agglutination tests using RBC/latex gelatin, colloidal gold, immuno dot/strip and PAT (particle agglutination tests).

vii. Detection of antibody to nef gene product (27 KD protein) along with p20 and gp120.

viii. *Fujerbio agglutination test:* In this test, antigen coated gelatin particles are agglutinated by antibody present in the serum of patient. It is quite simple and

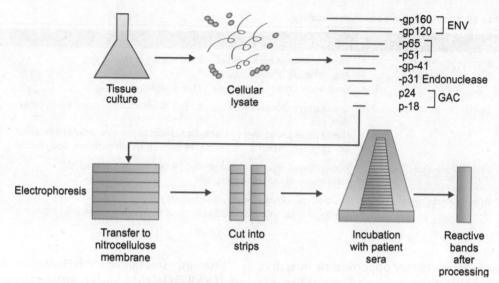

Fig. 39.3: Western blot technique.

convenient test. However, false-positive reactions do occur.

ix. *Karpas test:* In this test, HIV infected cells are fixed on teflon coated slide wells to which serum of the patient is added. After some time horse radish peroxidase labeled antihuman immunoglobulin is added. Later appropriate and corresponding substrate is added. Color develops if test is positive. No color develop if test is negative. It is easy to do and not expensive as slide immunoperoxidase test.

Other Investigations

Reduced T4 lymphocytes, reversal T4:T8 ratio, defective T cell plus NK cell cytotoxicity and anergy to tuberculosis indicate a basic T cell defect which possesses a definite role in the diagnosis of HIV infection.

WHO and National HIV testing policy recommends HIV testing for following purposes:
- Screening blood, organ and tissue for transplantation.
- Epidemiological surveillance.
- Diagnosis of symptomatic infection (AIDS).

- Early diagnosis of HIV infection among asymptomatic persons with only informed consent.

Laboratory tests for diagnosis of HIV infection are:
1. Screening test
   a. ELISA
   b. Rapid tests like
      - Latex agglutination
      - Dot blot test
   c. Simple tests
      - Particle agglutination test.
2. Supplement tests: These tests are required for validation of the positive results of screening tests. They include:
   - Western blot tests
   - Immunofluorescence test
3. Confirmatory tests
   - Virus isolation
   - Detection of p24 antigen by ELISA
   - Detection of viral nucleic acid may be detected by *in situ* hybridization and polymerase chain reaction.

Treatment: In a nutshell, thymus and bone marrow transplantation, interferon and interleukin therapy is useful in reconstituting basic T cell dysfunction. The antibiotics have a key

Table 39.2: Preventive measures in biosafety.

Steps	Preventive measures
1. Pre-use screening	• Avoid avoidable risky procedures like mixing, grinding etc. • Avoid the use of sharp objects • Keep away person with ulcerating or weeping skin lesions
2. Barrier precautions	• Use of gloves contact with blood, body fluids, mucous membrane, broken skin, etc. • Use of mask protective eye wear face shield to prevent droplet infections • Use of gowns, aprons, long shoes to prevent splash of blood, body fluids
3. In use precaution	• Prevention of injuries by sharp objects, i.e., needles, scalpel, etc. • Needles need not to be recapped.
4. After use precaution	• Drop all used instrument in disinfectant jar. • Placing the jar with disinfectant as close as possible to the working place.

role in taking care of opportunistic infection. Many HIV drugs are found useful like AZI and suramine (block the action of reverse transcriptase). Inactivation of the virus with monoclonal antibodies is another approach to combat against HIV infection. Phosphonoformate, 'Posearnet', are other anti-HIV drugs reported recently.

Now it is beyond doubt that zidovudin benefits disappear within a year because HIV mutates into new forms that are resistant to this drug. Hence, a new AIDS therapy devised by Yung Kang Chaw is advocated. It consists of administration of 3 drugs, i.e., zidovudine (AZT), dideoxyinosine (DDI) and either nevirapine or pyridinone.

Vaccine against HIV infection: DNA recombinant vaccine with yeast and vaccinia virus, the synthetic peptides are few candidates. Unfortunately, due to genetic alterations vaccine trials are ineffective.

Recent report on the trial of fusion inhibitor *Enfuvirtide* is encouraging. This new drug prevents the entry of HIV 1 into the target cells of the host. It also prevents fusion of HIV transmembrane (gp41) glycoprotein with the CD 4 receptor of the host cell.

Currently treatment for HIV comprised of HAART (Highly active antiretroviral therapy). Here two nucleoside analog reverse transcriptase inhibitors or NRTI plus either protease inhibitor or a nonnucleoside reverse transcriptase inhibitor (NNRTI).

Strategies of HIV Testing in India

Strategy I: Blood Donation

Serum is subjected once to ELISA, Rapid, Simple tests for HIV. If negative, serum is considered free of HIV. In case it is positive, sample is taken as HIV infected.

Strategy II: Surveillance and Diagnosis

Test serum sample is taken as negative for HIV if first ELISA test report is negative, and subjected to a second ELISA which utilizes a system different from first one.

Strategy III: Diagnosis

Here 3 ELISA kits are used. First ELISA is done with highest sensitivity, and second and third ELISA with highest specificity.

Preventive Measure in Biosafety

See **Table 39.2.**

Mycology

SECTION 6

Mycology

Fungi and yeasts constitute eumycetes. These eukaryotes lack chlorophyl pigments. They possess differentiated nuclei surrounded by nuclear membrane and reproduce either by budding or by forming spores. They have rigid chitinous cell walls. They lack differentiation of root, stem and leaves. Morphologically the fungi may be either simple, oval cells or long, tubular, septate hyphae showing true lateral branching.

The yeasts and fungi need organic compounds as nutrients. Their role in nature appears to be as scavanger, i.e., breaking down the complex carbohydrates and proteins of dead bodies of other organisms. Needless to mention that only a few of them are pathogenic. In many ways, fungi have been of service to man, as in the making of bread, fermented drinks, cheese, antibiotics, etc.

MORPHOLOGICAL CLASSIFICATION OF FUNGI

Fungi can be divided into four groups each of which have some human pathogenic species.

1. **Moulds:** They are filamentous and mycelial fungi. They grow as long filaments or hyphae which branch and interlace to form a meshwork or mycelium. They reproduce by forming various kinds of spores. The part of the mycelium which grows on and penetrates into the substrate, absorbing nutrients for growth is called vegetative mycelium. The part of mycelium which protrudes into the air is called aerial mycelium. On artificial medium they are seen as filamentous mould colony which may be dry and powdery. The pathogenic members are *Trychophyton, Microsporum* and *Epidermophyton*.

2. **Yeasts:** They are unicellular occurring as spherical or ellipsoidal cells. They reproduce by budding. On solid media they form moist, compact, creamy, mucoid colonies resembling those of staphylococci. *Cryptococcus neofor-mans* is the only important pathogens.

3. **Yeast like fungi:** They grow partly as yeasts and partly as long filamentous cells joined, end to end forming a pseudomycelium. On solid media moist creamy colored colonies are produced. *Candida albicans* is the example.

4. **Dimorphic fungi:** They grow in mycelial form at low temperature, i.e., 22°C or in soil whereas growth at 37°C or in animal body occurs in yeast form. The pathogenic members are *Histoplasma capsulatum, Sporotrichum, Blastomyces* and *Coccidioides immitis*.

SYSTEMATIC CLASSIFICATION

Based on sexual spore formation fungi are kept in four classes as described below:

1. **Phycomycetes:** They are fungi having non-septate hyphae. They form endogenous asexual spore (sporangiospore) contained within sac-like structure called sporangia. Sexual spores are also found and are of two varieties—oospore and zygospore.

2. **Ascomycetes:** They form sexual spores (ascospores) within a sac. This sac is called ascus. They include both yeasts and filamentous fungi. They form septate hyphae.
3. **Basidiomycetes:** They reproduce by means of sexual reproduction. Basidiospores are borne at the tip of basidium. These basidia are sometimes quite large leaf-like structure as in mushroom. They form septate hyphae.
4. **Fungi imperfecti:** They consist of group of fungi whose sexual phases have not been identified. Fungi of medical importance belong to this group, e.g., *Sporothrix schenckii*.

Laboratory Diagnosis

A presumptive clinical diagnosis of mycosis must be confirmed by a laboratory diagnosis methods. This includes the following:

Direct Microscopy

Potassium Hydroxide (KOH) Preparation

The specimen placed in a drop of 10% KOH on a slide covered with a coverslip can be observed under a microscope. Fungal chains of arthrospores and free arthrospores may be seen and their recognition permits a diagnosis of fungal infection. Budding yeast cells mixed with long filaments are indicative of a yeast-like fungus.

In case of doubt as to the nature of any fungus-like elements in the specimen, KOH is replaced by lactophenol blue, or clacflour stain.

Gram Stain

Gram positive yeasts such as those of *Candida* species can be observed by Gram stain.

India Ink Preparation

India *ink is helpful in demonstrating the capsule, e.g., Cryptococcus neoformans.*

Culture

Sabouraud's Dextrose Agar (SDA) is the most suitable medium as fungal growth is favored by a high sugar concentration and is relatively tolerant to acidity (pH 5.4). The agar is prepared as slopes in test tubes stoppered with cotton-wool as most of the fungi are aerobic. Chloramphenicol is incorporated in the culture medium to prevent contamination by bacteria. Similarly addition of cycloheximide (actidone) can suppress the contaminating fungi. The fungal growth can be identified by its color and morphology on visual examination and pigmentation on the reverse.

Microscopic examination is done to evaluate the morphology of hyphae, spores and other structures. Teased mounts are made in lactophenol blue and examined under a microscope. The morphology of various spores is characteristic of different fungi. Slide culture is useful for studying the exact morphology of the fungus.

Tissue Sections

Although many fungi can be seen with Hematoxylin and Eosin stain, special stains also used for fungi include Periodic acid Schiff stain (PAS), Gomori methenamine Silver stain (GMS), Mayer's mucicarmine stain and Gridley fungal stain.

Serology

Serological diagnosis of fungal infections usually lacks complete specificity because some of the pathogenic fungi have common antigens. Fractional separation of the active antigenic components of a fungus has not been achieved with complete success. However, serology may be useful in reaching a presumptive diagnosis.

Mycology is discussed in this section in following scheme: Superficial mycosis, subcutaneous mycosis, systemic mycosis, opportunistic fungus and miscellaneous others.

Superficial Mycosis

Pityriasis versicolor

Etiology: Pityrosporum orbiculare (*Malassezia furfur*)

Specimen: Scraping from skin lesion

Direct microscope examination: KOH preparation shows clusters of yeast-like cells and short branched hyphae.

Culture: Not cultured so far.

Other diagnostic tests: Examination under Wood's lamp shows fungus giving yellow fluorescence.

Clinical picture: Pityriasis versicolor is a superficial chronic fungus infection of the horny layer of the epidermis involving the trunk of the body. The normal skin pigmentation is altered resulting in a blotchy appearance. The infected areas are usually brownish. The lesions fluoresce a pale yellow under a Wood's light.

Treatment: Application of soap and water followed by application of sodium thiosulphate solution or 3% salicylic acid in 7% alcohol. Miconazole and clotrimazole are also effective.

Tinea nigra

Etiology: *Cladosporium mansonii (in Asia, Africa) Cladosporium werneckii.*

Specimen: Scrapings from skin lesions.

Direct microscopic examination: KOH preparation shows brownish branched septate hyphae and budding cells.

Culture: On Sabouraud's dextrose agar the colonies are moist, shiny, black yeast like after 3 weeks' incubation at 35°C.

Microscopic examination of above-mentioned colonies shows dark hyphae and budding cells which are single or two celled.

Clinical picture: Lesions are largely confined to the palms where they appear as irregular, flat darkly discolored areas (dark brown to black). This lesion is flat and not scaly.

Treatment: Three percent sulfur and 2% salicylic acid, tincture of iodine or weak Whitfield ointment may be beneficial.

Black Piedra

Etiology: Piedra hortai

Specimen: Infected hair with nodule

Direct microscopic examination: KOH preparation shows on hairshaft, dark brown, dichotomous branched hyphae. Septation in thickwalled hyphae give appearance of arthospores. Broken nodules show asci containing 2 to 8 ascospores.

Culture: On Sabouraud's dextrose agar after incubation at 25°C for 3 weeks, colonies grow as greenish black, elevated in center or flat, glaborous or smooth to cribriform.

Microscopic examination of these colonies shows dark, thickwalled hyphae, multiseptate with many chlamydospores. Rarely asci and ascospores like those seen in hair are spotted.

Clinical picture: Piedra hortai forms hard, dark nodules on the shaft of infected scalp hair.

Treatment: Clip or shave the infected area and apply antifungal agents like 1 : 2000 solution of bichloride of mercury, 3% sulfur ointment or benzoic and salicylic acid combination.

White Piedra

Etiology:Trichosporon cutaneum.

Specimen: Infected hair with nodule.

Direct microscopic examination: KOH preparation shows on hair shaft, transparent greenish brown mycelial mass. Hyphae are at right angle to shaft and segmented into oval cells. Rarely there is budding but no asci.

Culture: On Sabourand's, dextrose agar after incubation at 25°C for 3 weeks there appear rapidly growing, shiny colonies which are first cream colored and later on center heaped and colony wrinkled.

Microscopic examination of the colonies show transparent greenish brown mycelial mass which form round to rectangular cells. No asci are observed.

Clinical picture: There is involvement of scalp or beard hair. Soft, pale nodules appear on the shaft of the hair.

Treatment: Use of 1 : 2000 solution of bichloride of mercury, 3% sulfur ointment or benzoic acid and salicylic acid combination is quite beneficial.

Dermatophytoses: Ringworms, athlete's foot, jock itch and dermatomycosis are other names given to dermatophytoses.

Dermatophytoses refer to infection of skin, nails or hair that are caused by fungi classified as dermatophytes. It does not cause systemic disease and with only one minor exception *(Trichophyton verrucosum),* none of this group of fungi can grow at 37°C.

All fungi of dermatophytoses are discussed in three genera, i.e., *Microsporon, Trichophyton* and *Epidermophyton.*

MICROSPORUM

Microsporum gypseum: This fungus resides in soil (geophilic).

Direct microscopic examination: KOH preparation **(Figs. 40.1A and B)** of infected hair shows spores surrounding the hair (ectothrix infection).

Culture: On Sabouraud's dextrose agar the colonies are flat, light brown and very powdery in appearance at 25°C.

Microscopically it forms thin-walled, spindle-shaped spores which contain 4 to 6 septa **(Figs. 40.2 A and B)**.

Microsporum canis: This fungus is zoophilic and causes sporadic outbreaks of hair and skin infection. Erythema is common in lesions caused by this fungus.

Direct microscopic examination: KOH preparation of hair and skin shows spores.

Culture: On Sabouraud's dextrose agar the colonies are white and fluffy. Reverse side of the colony is pigmented as bright brownish yellow at 25°C.

Microscopically this fungus is characterized by the formation of large, thick-walled, spindle-shaped macroconidia which contain 8 to 12 septa **(Fig. 40.3)**.

Microsporum audouinii: It is anthropophilic and is the etiologic agent in most epidemics of ringworm of the scalp in children and rarely attacks animals.

Direct microscopic examination: KOH preparation shows spores.

Culture: On Sabouraud's dextrose agar forms white fluffy colonies after 1 to 2 weeks incubation at 25°C. The underside of the colony is pale yellow to light orange in color.

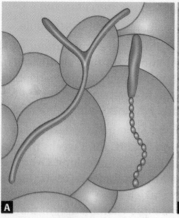
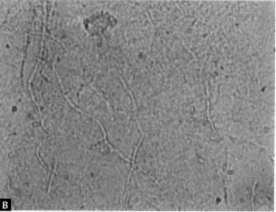

Figs. 40.1A and B: (A) Dermatophyte in KOH preparation of skin or nail showing branching hyphae and arthrospores (B) KOH wet mount showing branched septate hyphae with arthroconidia (40x).

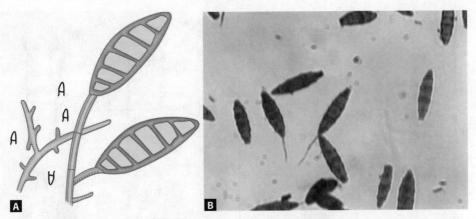

Figs. 40.2A and B: (A) *Microsporum gypseum* (B) LCB Mount of *Microsporum gypseum* showing macronidia with rat tail filaments (40x).

Microscopically there are thick-walled chlamydospores.

Trichophyton

Trichophyton rubrum

Direct microscopic examination: KOH preparation of tissue (skin and nails) shows branching septate hyphae or chain of arthrospores.

Culture: On Sabouraud's dextrose agar at 25°C for 1 to 4 weeks the growth is velvety with red pigment on reverse side of medium (**Figs. 40.4A and B**) and (**Fig. 40.7A**).

Microscopic examination of growth shows few long pencil shaped macroconidia. There are rarely cigar shaped macroconidia or spiral hyphae. The microconidia show bird on fence arrangement (**Fig. 40.5**)

Diseases Produced

1. *Tinea corporis*
2. *Tinea pedis*
3. *Tinea cruris*
4. *Tinea barbae*
5. *Tinea unguium*

Trichophyton Mentagrophytes

Direct microscopic examination: KOH preparation of hair shows spores surrounding the hair (ectothrix).

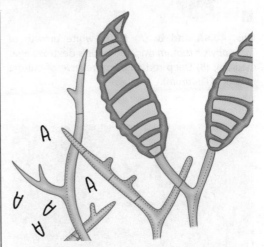

Fig. 40.3: *Microsporum canis.*

Culture: On Sabouraud's dextrose agar at 25°C for 1 to 4 weeks there appears white to tan colored, cottony or powdery colonies. Pigment is variable (**Fig. 40.7B**).

Microscopic examination of growth shows grape like clusters of microconidia. There are rarely cigar shaped macroconidia or spiral hyphae seen (**Figs. 40.5, 40.6 and 40.8**).

Diseases Produced

1. *Tinea corporis*
2. *Tinea pedis*
3. *Tinea cruris*
4. *Tinea barbae*
5. *Tinea unguium*

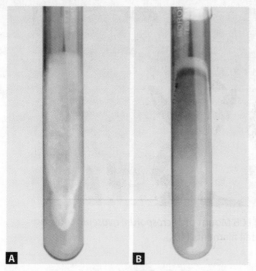

A   B

Figs. 40.4A and B: (A) Fluffy white growth of *Trichophyton rubrum* on Sabouraud's dextrose agar medium; (B) Deep red color on reverse of culture medium (*T. rubrum*).

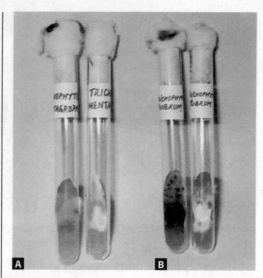

A   B

Figs. 40.7A and B: (A) Colony of *T. rubrum* (a) Reverse showing floccose pink white colonies (b) reverse showing red to tan pigment. (B) Colony of *T. mentagrophytes* (a) obverse showing powdery white colonies, (b) reverse showing yellow to brown pigment.

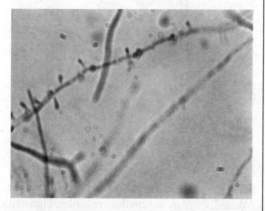

Fig. 40.5: LCB Mount of *T. rubrum* showing bird on fence arrangement of the microconidia (40x).

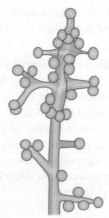

Fig. 40.8: *Trichophyton mentagrophytes.*

Trichophyton Tonsurans

Direct microscopic examination: KOH preparation of hair shows spores inside hair shaft (endothrix).

Culture: On Sabouraud's dextrose agar medium at 25°C for 1 to 4 weeks colonies **(Fig. 40.9)** appear which are cream or yellow colored with central furrows **[Fig. 40.9(4)]**.

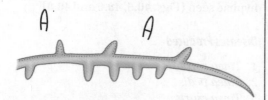

Fig. 40.6: *Trichophyton rubrum.*

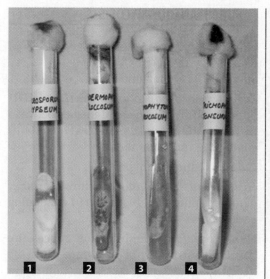

Fig. 40.9: Left to right: Culture tubes showing colonies of: (1) *M. gypseum;* (2) *E. floccosum;* (3) *T. verrucosum;* (4) *T. tonsurans.*

Microscopic examination of these colonies shows numerous microconidia (**Figs. 40.10A and B**). Rarely there is thick-walled irregular macroconidia.

Diseases produced: Tinea cruris.

Trichophyton Schoenleinii

Direct microscopic examination: KOH preparation of the hair shows endothrix invasion with hyphae and air spaces in the hair shafts.

Culture: On Sabouraud's dextrose agar, colonies are slow growing, waxy or suede-like with a deeply folded honey-comb-like thallus and some sub-surface growth. No macroconidia and microconidia are seen in routine cultures; however numerous chlamydoconidia may be present in older cultures. However, characteristic "nail head" hyphae also known as "favic chandeliers" may be observed.

Disease produced: Favus.

▮ EPIDERMOPHYTON

Epidermophyton floccosum: This fungus contains only one species and infects only man. It attacks skin and nails only.

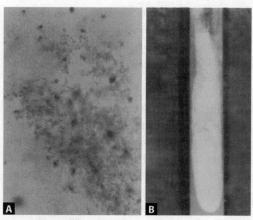

Figs. 40.10A and B: (A) Grape-like arrangement of microconidia of *Trichophyton;* (B) Powdery colonies of *Trichophyton mentagrophyte* on SDA medium.

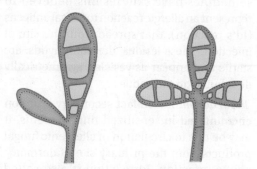

Fig. 40.11: *Epidermophyton floccosum.*

Direct microscopic picture: KOH preparation shows macrospores which are smooth-walled and contain 2 to 3 septa having blunt or rounded ends (**Fig. 40.11**).

Culture: On Sabouraud's dextrose agar colonies are yellow to greenish and are quite wrinkled and folded at 25°C. The colonies have very fine fuzzy texture almost like suede leather (**Fig. 40.9(2)**).

Microscopically one can find club-shaped macrospore usually formed singly or in clumps of 2 to 3. No microspores are formed.

Pathogenesis: The pathogenicity of dermatophytes is not understood. The fungus grows in the keratinized layer of the skin, throughout the thickness of nails and inside hair shaft, the keratin being attacked by extracellular enzymes. Usually hyphae do not penetrate into living tissue and mechanism by which these superficial infections stimulates inflammatory reactions is not clear. It could be a reaction to products of fungal metabolism or to fungal constituents.

As far as a variability of pathogenicity for different hosts, the dermatophytes vary in their ability to attack particular structures or areas of the body. *Microsporum audouinii* usually confines its attack to the hair of children under the age of puberty and no *Microsporum* species attacks nails. *Trichophyton* is a common cause of skin and nail infections but does not attack hair. *Epidermophyton* attacks skin and never the hair.

Immunology: Persons with dermatophytoses sometimes have skin lesions believed to represent an allergic reaction to fungal antigens (Id's reaction), that spread from the site of infection. These lesions, dermatophytids, are sterile and appear as vesicles, symmetrically distributed on the hands.

'Id's reaction: It is in fact secondary eruption encountered in sensitized tinea patients. It may be due to circulation of allergenic fungal products from the primary site of dermato-phytic infection. Id reaction is also called dermatophytid. Actually fungal products are absorbed from the skin resulting in itching. The lesions are sterile. There are two types of Id reaction:

1. Lichen scrofulosporum like reaction which is seen in tinea capitis in children. There are small grouped follicular lesions on the body. These lesions are symmetrical and central in distribution. They are seen mostly on limbs and face.
2. Pompholyx like lesion seen in patients having tinea pedis infection. Lesions appear on the sides and flexor aspects of fingers and palms. The lesion may be popular or vesicular, pompholyx like mostly bullous. It is because of type III type of hypersensitivity.

Treatment: Griseofulvin, clotrimazole and miconazole are effective drugs.

SUBCUTANEOUS MYCOSIS

Rhinosporodiasis

Etiology: Rhinosporidium seeberi

Specimen: Polyp material.

Direct microscopic examination: KOH preparation of polyp material crushed between two slides shows fungal spherules (10 to 200 µ) containing endospores.

Culture: Culture is not possible.

Histological examination: It shows number of fungal spherules (100 to 200 µ) containing endospores.

Clinical picture: The infection causes the development of polyp in the submucosa of the nose, mouth and other areas, like conjunctiva and occasionally the skin. Reports of this infection are mostly from India and Sri Lanka. Affected persons give a history of repeated bathing in polluted river and pond water. Natural infection with this fungus occurs in horses, mules and cows. There is no tendency of dissemination.

Treatment: Excision of polyp.

Chromoblastomycosis

Etiology

Fonsecaea pedrosoi
Fonsecaea compactum
Fonsecaea dermatitides
Phialophora verrucosa
Cladosporium carrioni **(Fig. 40.12)**.

Specimen: Scraping from skin lesions and skin biopsy tissue.

Direct microscopic examination: KOH pre-paration shows dark brown, round, thick-walled, fungal bodies with septae.

Culture: On Sabouraud's dextrose agar at 25°C for 1 to 3 weeks' incubation, black colored velvety growth appears. Microscopic examination is done for species identification.

Histological examination: It shows fungus which is seen as round or irregular dark brown bodies with septae **(Fig. 40.13)**.

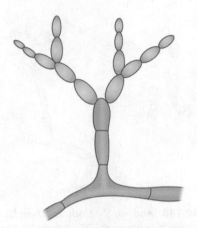

Fig. 40.12: *Cladosporium.*

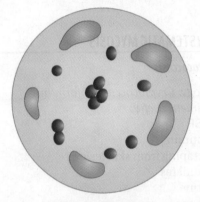

Fig. 40.13: Chromomycosis (pigmented fungal cells in giant cell).

Clinical picture: Chromoblastomycosis is a chronic warty dermatitis, usually of legs and feet caused by traumatic inoculation of one of the five closely related pigmented fungi which normally grow on wood. The lesions appear as warty, ulcerating and cauliflower-like growth.

Treatment: Early lesions may be excised. However, neither surgery nor medical treatment has been successful with late lesions.

Mycetoma

Etiology

A. Maduromycotic mycetoma (True fungi).
   1. *Madurella mycetomi*
   2. *Madurella grisea*
   3. *Phialophora jeanselmei*

4. *Alescheria boydii*
5. *Cephalosporium*

B. Actinomycotic mycetoma (Higher bacteria)
   1. *Nocardia asteroides*
   2. *Nocardia brasiliensis*
   3. *Actinomadura madurae*
   4. *A. pelletere*
   5. *Streptomyces somaliensis*

Specimen: Pus curretage material, biopsy from skin, and grains or granules of pus.

Gross and microscopic examination of granules: Granules are washed, separated and examined grossly first. White to yellow granules are seen in *A. boydii, Nocardia asteroids, Nocardia brasiliensis, A. madusae, Streptomyces somaliensis,* etc. Brown to black granules are seen in *M. mycetomi, M. grisea, P. jeanselmi, A. pelleteri,* etc.

Microscopic examination of maduromycotic mycetoma shows grains composing of broad hyphae which are often septate with chlamydospore. However, actinomycotic mycetoma grains are composed of very small less than 1 μ, Gram-positive bacteria-like filaments.

Culture: It is done on Sabouraud's dextrose agar with chloramphenicol and cyclohexamide at 25°C for 1 to 2 weeks incubation for maduromycotic mycetoma and only Sabouraud's dextrose agar without antibiotics for actinomycotic mycetoma. Each fungus is identified by its colonial characters and microscopic morphology.

Histological examination: H and E stained section shows granules or grain surrounded by eosinophilic material.

Clinical picture: The fully developed mycetoma is a chronic suppurative, granulomatous lesion with progressive destruction of contagious tissue and vascular dissemination (lymphatics and blood vessels). Skin and subcutaneous tissues are involved originally, but as the disease progresses fascia and bone become infected. The foot is the most infected part of the body. With the progress of disease, the foot becomes grossly deformed with multiple sinus formation and fistula tract which communicate with each other and with deep abscesses including ulcerated areas of the skin. Within suppurative foci the fungi or bacteria form characteristic grain which are composed of colonies embedded in and surrounded by an eosinophilic and homogenous material.

Treatment: It is very important to differentiate between actinomycotic (bacterial) and eumycotic (fungal) mycetoma. Actinomycotic mycetoma usually responds to antibiotics used for Gram-positive bacterial infections. For eumycotic mycetoma amputation of the infected extremity is done.

Sporotrichosis

Etiology:Sporotrichum schenckii

Specimen: Pus and skin biopsy

Direct microscopic examination: KOH preparation shows cigar shaped yeast cells. However, fungus is not demonstrable (**Fig. 40.14A**).

Culture: It is done on Sabouraud's dextrose agar at 25°C and 37°C incubation for 1 to 3 weeks. First cream white and later brown to black colonies which are rough and yeast like with wrinkled surface appear. At 37°C yeast colonies appear.

Microscopic examination of these colonies show delicate branching septate hyphae. On lateral branches of these hyphae there appear microconidia (2 to 5 μ) pyriform in shape and in clusters. However, microscopic examination of yeast colonies (37°C) shows flower-like cluster of oval to fusiform budding cells (1 to 3 μ × 3 to 10 μ) (**Fig. 40.14 B**).

Histological examination: H and E stained section shows asteroid bodies composed of central fungus cell with eosinophilic material radiating from it.

Methanamine silver stained section shows fungus as cigar-shaped yeast cells.

Other laboratory tests: Mice inoculated intra-testicular or intraperitoneal and then tissue examined for cigar-shaped bodies.

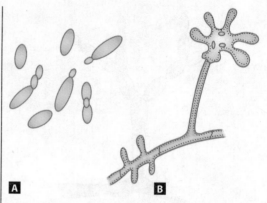

Figs. 40.14A and B: *Sporothrix schenckii.* (A) Blastospores in tissue or at 37°C culture; (B) Conidia formation in 20°C culture.

SYSTEMATIC MYCOSIS

Cryptococcosis

Etiology: Cryptococcus neoformans.
Specimens useful:
1. CSF
2. Sputum
3. Scraping from skin lesions
4. Exudates
5. Urine
6. Tissue (autopsy).

Direct microscopic examination: KOH preparation shows budding yeast cell whereas India ink preparation reveals capsulated yeast cells with budding.

Culture and identification: On Sabouraud's dextrose agar with chloramphenicol at 37°C and 25°C for 1 week, there appears smooth mucoid cream colored colonies. Microscopic examination of these colonies show encapsulated budding yeast cells.

Other identifying characters are hydrolysis of urea, brown colored colonies, and pathogenicity to mice.

Other laboratory tests
1. Precipitation
2. Complement fixation test
3. Latex agglutination test
4. Counter-current immunoelectrophoresis

5. Histological examination of H and E stained section shows budding yeast cells with little tissue reactions.

Pathogenesis: Inhalation of *Cryptococcus neoformans* is assumed to initiate pulmonary infection, with subsequent hematogenous spread to other viscera and the central nervous system. In the severe, chronic and disseminated form, brain, meninges, lungs, skin, bones, etc. are involved.

Treatment: Amphotericin B is particularly effective.

Candidiasis

Etiology: Candida albicans
Specimens:
1. Swabs or scraping from skin
2. Sputum
3. Exudates
4. Feces

Direct microscopic examinations: KOH preparation shows yeast cells with budding and pseudohyphae.

Gram-stained smear shows gram-positive yeast cells with budding and pseudohyphae.

Culture and identification: On Sabouraud's dextrose agar with chloramphenicol after 1 to 7 days incubation at 37°C and 25°C shows creamy white smooth colonies. Microscopically they are gram-positive yeast cells with budding and pseudohyphae **(Figs. 40.15 A and B)**.

Additional characteristic features are chlamydospores production in corneal agar **(Fig. 40.16)** and germ tube formation in human serum at 37°C within two hours.

Other laboratory tests:
1. Precipitation test
2. Agglutination test
3. Indirect fluorescent test.

Clinical picture: It is an acute or chronic, superficial or disseminated mycosis causing thrush (white, creamy patches on the tongue), paronychia (inflammation of subcutaneous tissues at the base of fingernails or toe-nails), vulvovaginitis, bronchocandidiasis

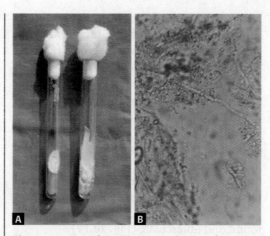

Figs. 40.15A and B: (A) Waxy colonies of *Candida albicans* on SDA medium; (B) Microscopic view of lactophenol cotton blue mount of *Candida albicans*.

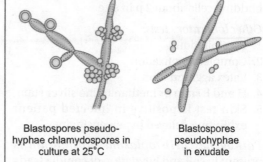

Blastospores pseudo-hyphae chlamydospores in culture at 25°C

Blastospores pseudohyphae in exudate

Fig. 40.16: *Candida albicans.*

(chronic bronchitis), pulmonary candidiasis, endocarditis, meningitis and septicemia.

Treatment: Nystatin and miconazole are useful for candidiasis without the involvement of internal organs. For systemic candidiasis amphotericin B and 5 fluorocytosine are of some value.

Histoplasmosis

Etiology: Histoplasma capsulatum
Specimen:
1. Sputum
2. Scrapings from skin lesions
3. Buffy coat of blood cells
4. Urine
5. Bone marrow
6. Lymph node and skin biopsy.

Direct microscopic examination: KOH preparation, preferably Giemsa stained smear shows round to oval yeast cells (2 to 4 μ) present within macrophages or free in tissue.

Culture and identification: On Sabouraud's dextrose agar with chloramphenicol and cyclohexamide at 25°C for 1 week there is slow growth raised, cottony first and buff brown colored later on. Microscopic examination of this growth shows septate hyphae, delicate and branching with smooth, round or pyriform microconidia which are sessile or short stock. Macroconidia are 7 to 15 μ in size, thick-walled, round and tuberculate **(Fig. 40.17)**.

At 37°C on glucose cysteine blood agar or, after 4 to 6 weeks there grow yeast form, small mucoid, cream colored colonies which on microscopic examination are seen as oval budding cells about 2 μ in size.

Other laboratory tests:
1. Precipitation
2. Complement fixation
3. Latex agglutination
4. H and E stain or methanamine silver stain
5. Skin test is positive in infected patient exhibiting delayed hypersensitivity.

Pathogenesis:Histoplasma capsulatum is present in soil and inhalation of conidia leads to pulmonary infection. Miliary lesions appear throughout the lung parenchyma and hilar lymph nodes become enlarged. With healing the pulmonary lesions become fibrotic and calcified. Sometimes the initial infection may pass unnoticed.

In small number of infected cases the infection becomes progressive and widely disseminated with lesions in practically all tissues and organs. In fact, disseminated form of histoplasmosis often coexists in patients who have tuberculosis, leukemia or Hodgkin's disease.

The tissue lesions are characterized by granulomatosis inflammation with epithelioid cells, giant cells, even caseation necrosis. The characteristic features are swollen, fixed and wandering macrophages containing small, oval yeast cells **(Fig. 40.18)**.

Treatment: Disseminated histoplasmosis can be treated with amphotericin B.

Coccidioidomycosis

Etiology:Coccidioides immitis
Specimen:
1. Sputum
2. Pus
3. CSF
4. Tissue biopsy.

Direct microscopic examination: KOH preparation shows spherules 30 to 60 μ in size with endospores.

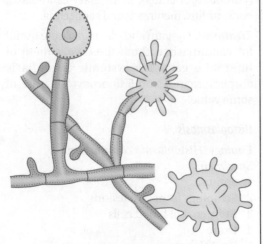

Fig. 40.17: *Histoplasma capsulatum.*

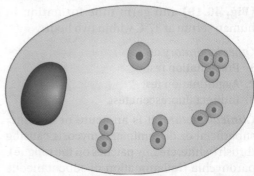

Fig. 40.18: Macrophage containing blastospores of *Histoplasma capsulatum.*

Culture: On Sabouraud's dextrose agar with chloramphenicol and cycloheximide at 25°C for 1 to 3 weeks' incubation there appear white and moist thin cottony colonies. Later on they become matted of buff colored. Microscopically this growth is seen as septate hyphae which break up into endospores.

On blood agar without antibiotics at 37°C for 1 to 3 weeks' incubation there appears yeast-like moist colonies which microscopically is seen as spherules 30 to 60µ in size with thick wall containing endospores (**Fig. 40.19**).

Other laboratory tests:
1. Precipitation test.
2. Complement fixation test.
3. Histological examination of H and E stained section shows spherules 30 to 60 µ in size with endospores.
4. Skin test is positive in infected patients exhibiting delayed type of hypersensitivity.

Pathogenesis: Coccidioides immitis infection is established by inhalation of airborne spores. The infection may remain asymptomatic or mild symptoms like pneumonia may appear. The lesions of lung may heal up by calcification or thin-walled cavity may appear. In blood borne dissemination the lesions may spread to skin, bones and central nervous system.

The inflammatory lesions of acute pneumonitis due to this fungus are histologically like those caused by pyogenic bacteria. However, in chronic pulmonary disease and in disseminated lesions the inflammation is granulomatous characterized by abundant histiocytes, giant cells and caseation necrosis. Small spherules are found within macrophages or giant cells and larger more mature spherules lie freely in tissue spaces.

Treatment: Treatment with amphotericin B is highly encouraging. Failures occur because of prolonged therapy and severe intoxication.

Paracoccidioidomycosis

Etiology: Paracoccidioides brasiliensis
Specimen:
1. Sputum
2. Pus
3. Exudates
4. Skin biopsy.

Direct microscopic examination: KOH preparation shows thick-walled cells 10 to 30 µ with multiple buds.

Culture: On Sabouraud's dextrose agar with cycloheximide and chloramphenicol after 1 to 4 weeks' incubation at 25°C, there grows colonies which are covered with white, velvety hyphae. The underside of the colony is light tan. Microscopic examination of the colony shows septate hyphae, puriform conidia 3 to 4 µ, sessile or with short sterigmata. Occasionally chlamydospores are also seen.

At 37°C the colonies are waxy, wrinkled and cream colored. Microscopically there may be single or multiple thick-walled budding cells.

Other laboratory tests:
1. Precipitation test.
2. Complement fixation.
3. Histological examination reveals large 10 to 30 µ round or oval cells with multiple budding.
4. Skin test is positive (delayed hypersensitivity) in infected patient.

Clinical picture: Coccidioidomycosis is an inapparent, benign, severe or fatal mycosis. There are 3 clinical forms as under:
a. Primary pulmonary form occurs 7 to 28 days after inhalation of a single spore of

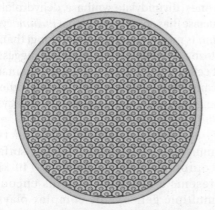

Fig. 40.19: *Coccidioides immitis* (spherule with endospores).

the infectious agent. Symptoms are fever, malaise and cough. Skin test becomes positive. There may be development of rash called erythema nodosum or erythema multiforme.

b. Benign form coccidioidomycosis exhibits precipitin and complement fixation titer positive apart from positive skin test. There is development of lung cavity. Usually this form exists for years and it may go unnoticed, usually causing no problem to the patient.

c. Disseminated form occurs in very few patients. Here disease may involve brain and other organs. Precipitin titer disappears but complement fixation titer continues to rise and there is reversion from skin test positive to skin test negative.

Treatment: Coccidioidomycosis is a difficult disease to manage and carries a grave prognosis. Amphotericin B may be useful.

Blastomycosis

Etiology:Blastomyces dermatitidis.

Specimens:
1. Sputum   2. Pus
3. Exudate   4. Urine
5. Skin biopsy.

Direct microscopic examination: KOH preparation shows broadly attached bud, large (7 to 20 µ), spherical, thick-walled yeast cell **(Fig. 40.20)**.

Culture: On Sabouraud's dextrose agar at 25°C for 1 to 4 weeks' incubation there appears white or brownish cottony growth. Microscopic examination of them shows, septate hyphae with round or pyriform microconidia borne on lateral conidiophores.

At 37°C incubation there appears wrinkled waxy and soft colonies. Microscopically there are round, thick-walled budding cells 8 to 15 µ in diameter.

Other laboratory tests:
1. Precipitation test
2. Complement fixation tests

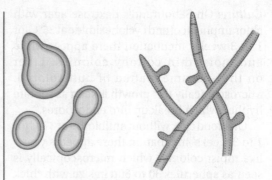

Fig. 40.20: *Blastomyces dermatitidis.*

3. Histological section when studied microscopically shows budding yeast cells which are thick-walled. Each yeast cell carries a single broad based bud.

Pathogenesis: Infection usually begins in the lungs and spreads hematogenously to establish focal destructive lesions in bones, skin, prostate, and other viscera. The gastrointestinal tract is spared.

The lesions are characterized by granulomatous inflammation, microabscesses, and extensive tissue destruction. The yeast cells are visible within the abscesses and granulomata.

Treatment: Amphotericin B or hydroxystibamidine may be used.

Pneumocystis Carinii

Analysis of gene sequences of ribosomal RNA, mitochondrial proteins and major enzymes (thymidylate synthase, dehydrofolate reductase) has demonstrated that *Pneumocystis carinii* is more closely related to fungi than to protozoa. Biochemical studies have suggested that cell wall of *Pneumocystis carinii* contains glucans. Drugs that inhibit glucans synthesis in fungi are highly active against *Pneumocystis carinii* in animals.

Pneumocystis carinii contains two prominent antigen groups. A major surface glycoprotein complex of 95 to 140 kDa represents a family of proteins encoded by multiple genes. This complex plays a central role in the hostparasite relationship in this infection. This antigen facilitates the adherence of *P. carinii* to lung cells, contains protective epitopes and is capable of antigenic variations. The other antigen which migrates as a band of 35 to 55 kDa is most common antigen recognized by host. This may serve as a marker of infection.

OPPORTUNISTIC MYCOTIC INFECTIONS

Aspergillus

Etiology: Aspergillus fumigatus

Specimen:
1. Exudate
2. Sputum
3. Lung biopsy.

Direct microscopic examination: KOH preparation of the specimen shows septate filamentous hyphae.

Culture: On Subouraud's dextrose agar with chloramphenicol after 25°C incubation for 1 to 4 days, there appear gray green colored colonies. Microscopic examination of these colonies shows septate hyphae bearing conidia in chain like fashion on sterigmata of conidiophore **(Figs. 40.21 A and B)**.

Other laboratory tests: Histological examination of H and E stained and methenamine silver stain section shows septate hyphae branching dichotomously.

Aspergillus fumigatus **(Fig. 40.22)** is uniquely positioned for diagnosis by PCR by virtue of the presence of a gene coding for 16 kDa virulent factor. Primers were designed for the 5 and 3 ends of the gene that are virtually specific for the amplification of a 444 bp fragment.

A procedure that uses chitinase and microwave treatment is described for the extraction of genomic DNA of *Aspergillus* species from the sputum and bronchial aspirate of patient with established aspergillosis. A colorimetric method for detection of PCR product is developed based on immunoaffinity reaction. It is established that at least 1 pg of DNA

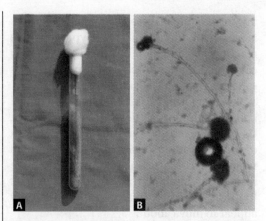

Figs. 40.21 A and B: (A) Growth of *Aspergillus niger* on SDA medium; (B) Microscopic view of lactophenol cotton blue mount of *Aspergillus niger*.

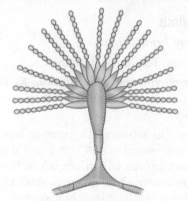

Fig. 40.22: *Aspergillus.*

is extractable from the clinical samples to produce enough quantity of PCR product for detection on agarose gel or by immunoaffinity based color reaction. An absorbance value of 0.9 to 1.5 against 0.2 for negative control at 405 nm for colorimetric PCR is observed. This method is useful for screening a large number of clinical samples from immuno-compromised as well as from suspected cases of aspergillosis. Other methods include agarose gel electrophoresis of PCR products and colorimetric immuno PCR under discussion.

Clinical picture: The disseminated form of aspergillus is granulomatous, necrotizing disease of the lungs which often disseminates hematogenously to various organs. Most often this form of the disease is fatal and diagnosis is usually made at autopsy. Hypersensitive reaction to inhalation of fungal spores may cause asthmatic attack and mucifibrinous sputum containing eosinophils.

Another form of *Aspergillus* is called fungal ball. Here fungus settles in old lung cavity. Usually these lung cavities are the result of old tuberculous lesions. If the organism remains in these cavities it grows into huge mass of mycelium in the form of fungus ball. Radiographically these fungus balls may appear to move about.

Treatment: Amphotericin B may be used. Fungus ball may be removed surgically.

Penicillosis

Etiology: Penicillium

Specimen: Skin lesion scrapings

Direct microscopic examination: KOH preparation shows small, round spores and hyphae.

Culture: On Sabouraud's dextrose agar with chloramphenicol at 25°C for 1 to 4 days the colonies appear which are white first and later on become blue green. Surface of these colonies is usually velvety or powdery.

Microscopic examination of these colonies show brush like arrangement of conidia, sterigmata and conidiophores **(Fig. 40.23)**.

Clinical picture: Penicillium species are implicated in otomycosis and mycotic keratitis. In otomycosis there is inflammation, pruritus, exfoliation of epithelium and often, deafness when ear canal is occluded by a plug of hyphae.

In mycotic keratitis there may be corneal ulcer or hypopyon or both. However, corneal trauma, corneal disease and glaucoma predispose to mycotic keratitis.

There may be pulmonary and cerebral penicillosis.

Treatment: In otomycosis 5% aluminum acetate solution may be used to reduce edema and to remove epithelial debris. Aqueous solution of 0.02 to 0.1% phenyl mercuric

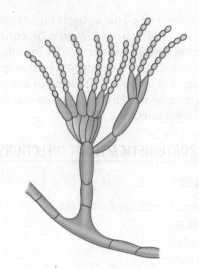

Fig. 40.23: *Penicillium conidia* firm within phialide.

acetate, thymol (1%) in metacresyl acetate and iodochlo rohydroxyquin are more effective drugs.

In mycotic keratitis, topical application of amphotericin B is quite useful.

Zygomycosis

Etiology

1. *Mucor*
2. *Rhizopus.*

Specimen
1. Skin lesion scraping
2. Tissue biopsy.

Direct microscopic examination: KOH preparation may show mycelial fragments and spores.

Culture: On Sabouraud's dextrose agar after 25°C incubation for 1 to 4 days there may be the growth of cottony colonies. For identification whether mucor or rhizopus, microscopic examination of this growth is helpful. *Mucor* colonies, microscopically are seen as non-septate hyphae having branched sporangiophores with sporangium at terminal end whereas in case of rhizopus there are non-septate hyphae and sporangiophores arise in groups exactly above rhizoids **(Fig. 40.24)**.

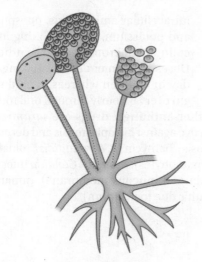

Fig. 40.24: *Rhizopus.*

Histological sections: Microscopic examination shows broad, non-septate, irregular hyphae in thrombosed vessels or sinuses surrounded with leukocytes and giant cells.

Clinical picture: Zygomycosis and phycomycosis (mucormycosis) is a systemic disease which may involve internal organs with predilection for blood vessels. Sometimes phycomycosis may be seen as a chronic infection of subcutaneous tissue.

Treatment: In some cases amphotericin B may be useful.

MISCELLANEOUS MYCOLOGY TOPICS

I. **Mycotoxins:** Some fungi produce myco-toxins (poisonous substance) that are capable of causing acute or chronic intoxication and damage. Severe damage to liver, kidney and bone marrow may be caused as a result of eating of poisonous mushrooms, e.g., *Amantia phalloides.* Ingestion of small quantities of toxin if contaminated food (aflatoxin from *Aspergillus flavus*) may cause chronic damage or neoplasm in animals or man. Also derivatives of fungal products (LSD) may result profound mental derangement.

II. **Antifungal drugs:** Followings are major antifungal drugs:
  1. *Iodides:* It is most commonly used for the treatment of sporotrichosis (cutaneous lymphatic form). Disseminated sporotrichosis is frequently resistant to iodide therapy. It is customary to begin treatment with potassium iodide with a dose of 1 mL of saturated solution three times a day which may be gradually increased to 12 to 15 mL/day. Treatment should be continued for at least 6 weeks.
  2. *Hydroxystilbamidine Isethionate:* It is an aromatic diamidine. Only *B. dermatitides* is susceptible. Contents of vial containing 225 mg should be added to 200 mL of glucose or saline solution and should be administered intravenously in 45 to 70 minutes.
  3. *Amphotericin B:* It is an antibiotic derived from *Streptomyces nodosus.* When suspended in liquid it is unstable at 37°C. Its mode of action is by binding to sterol present in the cell membrane of some fungi. Such binding increases permeability of the cell with leak of essential component like glucose and potassium. Susceptible fungi to amphotericin B are *Blastomyces dermititidis, Histoplasma capsulatum, Cryptococcus neoformans, Candida, Sporthrix schenkili,* etc. *Aspergillus* are most frequently resistant. To the 50 mg vial, 10 mL of sterile water is added and vial is shaken for 3 minutes. This suspension is added to 5% glucose solution in a final concentration no greater than 10 mg/100 mL. The contents are given intravenously over a 2 to 6-hour period.
  4. *Griseofulvin:* It is active against derma-tophytes only. It causes stunting and shrinking of hyphae. Drug is administered orally 10 mg/kg daily. Although symptomatic improvement is noticed after 2 to 3 days of administration, treatment must continue for at least 4 weeks.

5. *Flucytosine:* It is a fluorinated pyrimidine. Fungi like *Cryptococcus neoformans, Candida, Cladosporium* are susceptible to it. It is administered orally 150 mg/kg/day in equally divided 4 doses at 6 hour intervals.

6. *Imidazoles:In vitro* it is effective in yeasts and filamentous fungi including dermatophytes. Little is known about its mode of action. However, its relatively high concentration preferentially damages the fungal cell wall and plasma membrane making them permeable to intracellular amino acids, phosphates and potassium, thus inhibiting intracellular macromolecular synthesis. Doses recommended are 100 mg/kg/day in children whereas in adults 1.5 gm every 6 hourly through oral route.

Other antifungal drugs are *saramycetin* (effective against histoplasmosis and dermatophytosis), hamycin *(B. dermatitidis),* tolnaftate (dermatophytes), nystatin (*Candida* infection of skin and mucous membrane), pimaricin (keratitis due to fusarium), etc.

Parasitology and Medical Entomology

SECTION 7

Protozoa

Protozoa are subdivided into four groups (**Table 41.1**).

RHIZOPODA

Entamoeba Histolytica

Geographical Distribution

Entamoeba histolytica has been found in all populations throughout the world where search has been conducted. It is more prevalent in the tropics and subtropics than the cooler climates. In the Western Hemisphere, *Entamoeba histolytica* has been found from Anchorage, Alaska (60°N) to the strait of Magellan (52°S), and in the Eastern Hemisphere from Finland (60°N) to Natal, South Africa (30°S).

Habitats

Trophozoites of *Entamoeba histolytica* live in the mucous and submucous layers of large intestine.

Morphology

Table 41.2 shows morphological features of *Entamoeba histolytica* and their distinction from macrophages and PMN.

Table 41.1: Classification of the pathogenic protozoa.

Class	Organ of locomotion	Important human pathogens	Graphical prevalence
I. Rhizopoda	Pseudopodia	*Entamoeba histolytica* *Hartmonella and Naegleria*	Worldwide May be worldwide but reported so far in South Australia, USA, New Zealand, Britain and Czechoslovakia
II. Mastigophora	Flagella	1. Flagella of blood and tissues: *Trypanosoma brucei* *Trypanosoma cruzi* *Leishmania donovani*	Africa South Africa Asia, Africa, Southern Europe, South and Central America
		2. Flagellates of the genital and alimentary tract *Trichomonas vaginalis* *Giardia lamblia*	Worldwide Worldwide
III. Sporozoa	None, exhibit a slight amoeboid movement	*Plasmodium falciparum* *P. vivax* *P. malariae* *P. ovale*	Tropical and subtropical areas of Africa, South America, Near East India, Pakistan, Bangladesh, Sri Lanka, Southern China, Malaysia, South Pacific, Islands and North Australia
IV. Ciliata	Cilia	*Balantidium coli*	Worldwide

Table 41.2: Comparison of some host cell in feces confused with *E. histolytica*.

S. No.	Character	Macrophages	PMNs	E. histolytica
1.	Size (μ)	30 to 60	Mean 14	12 to 60
2.	Ratio of nuclear material to cytoplasm	1:4 to 1:6	1 to 1	1:10 to 1:12
3.	Nuclear morphology	Large, may be irregular	2 to 4 segments connected by chromatin strands chromatin	Round, vesicular with a central karyosome and peripheral
4.	Ingested material	PMNs, RBC, tissue debris	—	RBC
5.	Cytoplasm	May contain red staining bodies	Granular	Uniform, finely granular
6.	Trichrome staining characteristics	Green cytoplasm, dark red nucleus	Green cytoplasm, dark red nucleus	Green cytoplasm, dark red nucleus

Three stages are encountered (a) active ameba trophozoite (b) inactive cyst, and (c) intermediate precyst.

Trophozoite

Under the microscope the living parasite on warm stage exhibit remarkable locomotion. Movement results from long finger-like pseudopodial extension of ectoplasm into which the endoplasm flows. It is 15 to 30 μ in size.

Cytoplasm is divisible into a clear translucent ectoplasm and granular endoplasm. Cytoplasm may contain erythrocytes, white blood cells and tissue debris.

Nucleus is 4 μ spherical in shape and placed eccentrically. It has well-defined nuclear membrane, inner line of which is lined with uniform and closely packed fine granules of chromatin. Karyosome is centrally placed.

Precystic Stage

It is colorless, round or oval, smaller than trophozoite but larger than cyst about 10 μ to 20 μ, endoplasm free from RBC, etc. with sluggish pseudopodial activity. Characters of nucleus remain intact.

Cystic stage: Cysts are encountered only in the lumen of intestine under unsuitable conditions. Cyst begins as a uninucleated body but divides by binary fission and develops into binucleated and quadrinucleated structure. The cyst is 6 to 15 μ with clear and hyaline cytoplasm containing oblong bars with rounded ends called chromatoid bars (1 to 4). A distinct glycogen mass is found in the early stages of cyst formation. In quadrinucleate cyst chromidial bars and glycogen mass disappear. It is the mature and infective form.

Life cycle: Cysts of Entamoeba are formed in bowel of man and are passed with stools. Cysts are swallowed with contaminated food and drinks by man. They pass through stomach and reach intestine. Cyst wall is weakened because of alkaline pH and cytoplasmic mass containing 4 nuclei (metacyst) comes out. The nuclei divide by binary fission giving rise to 8 daughter trophozoites. Trophozoites which are actively motile move towards ileocecal region **(Fig. 41.1)**.

Strain differentiation: Strains of *Entamoeba histolytica* can be differentiated from the pathogenic strains by certain physiological differences such as ability to grow at reduced temperatures, genome size, DNA base ratio contents and DNA homology. Strain differentiation can also be done on the basis of phenotypic isoenzyme patterns called zymodemes. These zymodemes are identified using phenotypic isoenzymes, e.g., glucose phosphoisomerase (GPI),

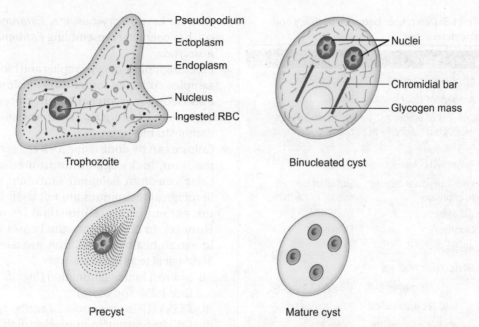

Fig. 41.1: Life-cycle of *Entamoeba histolytica*.

phosphoglucomutase (PGM), malate NADP oxidoreductase (ME), hexokinase (HK), etc. On the basis of different isoenzyme patterns *Entamoeba histolytica* can be divided into 22 zymodemes. Out of these 22 zymodemes only 7 (II, VI, VII, IX, XII, XIII and XIV) are potentially pathogenic.

Pathogenesis

❖ Invasiveness depends with particular zymodemes
❖ Invasiveness also correlates with phagocytic process, collagenase, immunologic cytotoxic proteins, host's inflammatory response and capacity to induce histolysis
❖ Bacteria may enhance pathogenicity.

Pathology

❖ Bacteria may enhance pathogenicity
❖ Man is the reservoir of infection. Infections occur by 4 nucleated cysts
❖ *Entamoeba histolytica* produces dysentery with frequent passing of stools mixed with mucus and blood

❖ Intestinal lesions are acute amebic dysentery and chronic intestinal amebiasis
❖ Extraintestinal lesions (metastatic) include: liver (amebic hepatitis and amebic liver abscess), lungs (primary small abscess or multiple abscess in one or both lungs or secondary single abscess in lower lobe of right lung which is contacted from amebic liver abscess), brain (a small cerebral abscess), spleen (splenic abscess), skin granulomatous lesion (ameboma) near visceral lesion, e.g., liver.
  ▪ Amebic vaginitis
  ▪ Amebic ulcer of penis.

The differences between bacillary and amebic dysentery are given in **Table 41.3**.

Characters of Amebic Intestinal Ulcers

Size varies from pinhead to one inch. Other features of lesions include shape which is round or oval with narrow neck and broad base (flask-like). Margins are ragged or undermined. Superficial ulcers do not extend beyond muscularis mucosa but deep ulcer may extend to submucous coat. Superficial ulcer

Table 41.3: Differences between bacillary and amebic dysentery.

Bacillary	Amebic
• Frequency 10 per day	6 to 8 per day
• Amount of stool small	More
• Consists of blood, mucus but hardly fecal matter	Feces mixed with blood and mucus
• Bright red colored	Dark red
• Viscid, mucus adherent to container	Liquid or formed mucus not adherent to container
• Odorless	Offensive
• Alkaline	Acidic
• Microscopic findings	
i. Pus cells numerous	Less in number
ii. RBC lies discretely	RBC in clumps
iii. Macrophages with ingested RBC	Absent
iv. Charcot Leydon crystals absent	Present
v. *Entamoeba histolytica* absent	Present
vi. Bacteria scanty	Numerous

heals without any scar but deep ulcer healing invites scar formation. If ulcer is studied microscopically, it consists of central area of necrosis (no ameba seen) but towards periphery, trophozoites of *Entamoeba histolytica* are seen in large numbers. The ulcers might be distributed along the whole length of intestine more at cecum, hepatic flexure and rectum.

Chronic ulcers are small, superficial, causing scarring, thinning, dilatation, succulation of intestinal wall, extensive adhesion with neighboring areas and formation of tumor-like mass.

Laboratory Diagnosis

❖ Macroscopic examination of stool (dark red stool mixed with blood and mucus)
❖ Microscopic examination of stool for demons-tration of trophozoite or cyst of *Entamoeba histolytica*, cellular exudate, Charcot Leydon crystals, etc. *Entamoeba coli* has characters resembling *Entamoeba histolytica*

❖ Proctosigmoidoscopy, scraping and biopsy samples collected under direct vision by endoscopy may reveal trophozoites of *Entamoeba histolytica*, if otherwise not demonstrable
❖ Culture can be done using lock egg serum medium, locks egg albumin medium, Craig's medium, Balamuth's medium, etc
❖ Serological techniques are not useful for the patient of acute intestinal lesions. However, in chronic intestinal cases and in extraintestinal cases, they are useful. Serological tests include:
  i. Indirect hemagglutination (Significant titer 1:256 and more)
  ii. ELISA (Using monoclonal antibody)
  iii. Counter current immunoelectrophoresis
  iv. Latex agglutination
  v. Gel diffusion precipitation
  vi. Indirect immunofluorescence.
❖ DNA probes make the diagnosis rapid and specific.

SEROLOGICAL TESTS IN INVASIVE AMEBIASIS

1. Latex agglutination slide test to detect antibodies to *Entamoeba hislolytica*.
2. Cellulose acetate precipitin test is simple specified and inexpensive. It becomes positive early during early invasive amebiasis. It becomes negative in 3 months after successful treatment.

The principle is based on the fact that specified antibodies and soluble antigen diffuse on cellulose acetate paper towards each other. It forms a line of precipitation where they meet.

Treatment

Metronidazole, chloroquine, tinidazole, diloxanide furoate, emetine and secnidazole are effective drugs.

Table 41.4: Differences between Entamoeba histolytica and *Entamoeba coli.*

Entamoeba histolytica	Entamoeba coli
Cyst	
• 5 to 20 μ	10 to 40 μ
• Nuclei 4 or less	Up to 8
• Chromatoidal body cigar like	Thread like
• Karyosome smaller and central	Large and eccentric
Trophozoite	
• 10 to 60 μ in size	10 to 50 μ
• Single pseudopodium	Multiple
• Cytoplasm finely granular	Coarsely granular
• Cytoplasm encloses RBC	Cytoplasm encloses bacteria debris as inclusion bodies
• Actively motile	Sluggishly motile
• Nucleus invisible	Visible

Nonpathogenic Amebae

Entamoeba Coli (Table 41.4)

❖ It habitates in the lumen of large gut but does not invade tissues
❖ Trophozoite is 10 to 40 μ, blunt granular slow pseudopodia
❖ Cyst is 10 to 30 μ thread-like pointed chromo-toid bodies (1 to 8)
❖ It is commensal of large intestine.

Entamoeba Gingivalis

❖ It is found only in trophozoitic form and cystic forms are absent
❖ Trophozoite is 5 to 35 μ, having hyaline, blunt but rapid pseudopodia and actively motile
❖ Present in pyorrhea alveolaris and may cause pyorrhea.

Endolimax Nana

❖ Trophozoite is 6 to 15 μ, pseudopodia blunt, hyaline, slow, motility is sluggish

❖ Cyst is 5 to 14 μ, glycogen mass absent, chromoidal bodies are spherical and nuclei 1 to 4
❖ Present as commensal in human intestine.

Iodamoeba Butschlii

❖ Trophozoite is 6 to 20 μ, pseudopodia blunt, hyaline and slow showing sluggish motility
❖ Cyst is 5 to 18 μ with large mass of glycogen (dark brown) and nucleus is one
❖ It is found in the lumen of colon
❖ It is nonpathogenic.

▮ FREE LIVING SOIL AMEBA

Primary Amebic Meningoencephalitis (PAM)

Etiologic Agent

Naegleria fowleri: It occurs in trophozoitic form and cystic form **(Fig. 41.2)**. Trophozoite may be in ameboid form (10 to 30 μ exhibiting eruptive locomotion) or flagellated form (pear-shaped with two flagella at anterior end and is non-replicating). Both forms are uninucleated with large karyosome.

Cystic form measures 7 to 10 μ having smooth double cyst wall. Cysts are not formed within tissue.

Table 41.5 lists the differences between free living ameba and *Entamoeba histolytica.*

Granulomatous Amebic Encephalitis

Etiologic Agent

Acanthamoeba culbertsoni: Trophozoites are larger than Naegleria organisms (15 to 40 μ in

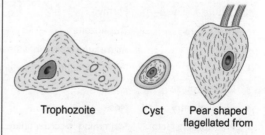

Trophozoite   Cyst   Pear shaped flagellated from

Fig. 41.2: *Naegleria fowleri.*

Table 41.5: Differentiation between free living Amebae and *Entamoeba histolytica*.

Free living ameba	Entamoeba histolytica
• Nucleolus large and distinct and indistinct	Nucleolus small
• Contractile vacuoles present	Absent
• One nucleus in cyst	1 to 4 nuclei
• Glycogen and chromatoid bodies in the cyst are absent	Present
• Mitochondria present	Absent
• Cell wall has pores	Pores absent in cell wall

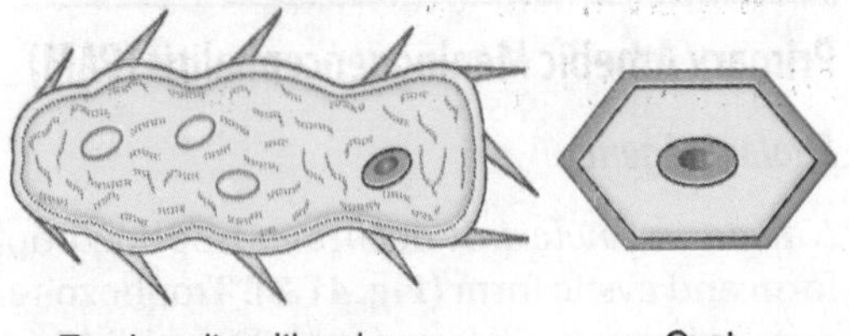

Trophozoite with spinows acanthopodia acanthamoeba   Cyst

Fig. 41.3: Acanthamoeba.

size, produce fine hyaline projection called acanthopodia without any flagella). Cystic form is 10 to 25 μ with double wall. The outer wall is wrinkled one (ectocyst) and polygonal or round inner wall (endocyst). Nucleus is single, large, dense with centrally located nucleolus (**Fig. 41.3**). It differs from Naegleria in not having flagellated form and in forming cyst in tissue (**Table 41.6**).

Incubation period is 1 to 7 days in case of Naegleria and several weeks to several months in case of acanthamoeba. Swimming in lakes, ponds and swimming pool causes infection in Naegleria. In Acanthamoeba inhalation, ingestion through skin (traumatic) and eyes are the modes of infection.

Life cycle: In case of *Naegleria amebae* invade the nasal mucosa, pass through olfactory plate into the meninges and start an acute purulent meningitis.

In Acanthamoeba, it reaches brain by way of bloodstream from lower respiratory tract and ulcers of skin and mucosa.

Clinical Picture

Naegleria disease is acute in onset resulting in rapid worst condition of the patient. To start with there is upper respiratory tract infection, low fever, and headache. Within 1 to 2 days meningitis develops with symptoms of frontal

Table 41.6: Differentiation between *Naegleria* and *Acanthamoeba*.

	Naegleria	Acanthamoeba
• Trophozoite	10 to 30 μ with single pseudopodium	15 to 40 μ with thorn-like pseudopodia
• Cyst	7 to 10 μ with smooth surface	10 to 25 μ with wrinkled surface
• Flagellate form	Present	Absent
• Mitosis and nuclear membrane persists	Nucleolus divides	Nuclear membrane dissolves
• Culture	Positive	Positive
• Tissue form	Trophozoite	Cyst and trophozoite
• Lesion	Acute suppurative inflammation	Granulomatous inflammation
• Disease	Primary amebic meningoencephalitis	Granulomatous amebic encephalitis
• Clinical course	Acute	Subacute or chronic
• Portal of entry	Nose	Upper respiratory tract
• Predisposing factor	Swimming in contaminated water	Immune incompetence
• Leukocytes in CSF	Predominantly neutrophils	Predominantly lymphocytes

headache, high fever, nausea, vomiting and nuchal rigidity. Finally, there is cerebral edema and patient becomes comatosed and dies within few hours. It causes primary amebic meningoencephalitis (PAM).

In Acanthamoeba course of infection is subacute or chronic. There is focal granulomatous lesion of the brain called granulomatous amebic encephalitis (GAE).

Laboratory Diagnosis

It is established by demonstration of amebae, culture on nutrient agar plate with a suspension of *Escherichia coli*, *Klebsiella*, etc. serology (immunofluorescent test and immunoperoxidase in Acanthamoeba only).

Treatment

Amphotericin B may be used for *Naegleria*. Ketoconazole with topical miconazole is useful for *Acanthamoeba keratitis*.

Differences between Naegleria and Acantha-moeba is depicted in **Table 41.6**.

◼ MASTIGOPHORA

Giardia lamblia

Geographical Distribution

It occurs all over the world. It is prevalent in 2 to 25% population.

Habitat

Duodenum and upper part of intestine.

Morphology

It is found in the following two forms (**Fig. 41.4**):

Trophozoite: It resembles longitudinally-cut pears. It is 10 to 20 μ in length and 6-15 μ in width and 1 to 3 μ in thickness. The dorsal surface is convex and ventral surface is concave. There is an oval shaped adhesive area in the anterior ventral surface. The dorsal surface area is meant for diffusion of nutrients.

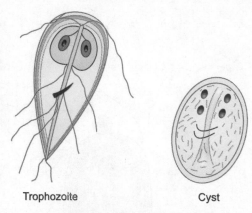

Trophozoite   Cyst

Fig. 41.4: *Giardia lamblia.*

The anterior end is rounded and posterior end is pointed. It is bilateral symmetrical. There are a pair of axostyles, two nuclei and 4 pairs of flagellae. It multiplies by binary fission.

Cyst: Trophozoites are transformed into cysts under unfavorable conditions. The cyst is:

❖ Oval
❖ 8 to 14 μ × 6 to 10 μ.
❖ Contains 4 nuclei usually lying at one end or lie in pairs at opposite poles.
❖ Ramnant flagellae and margins of sucking disk lie inside cytoplasm.
❖ They are passed in stools.

Life cycle: Cyst is the infective form. Cysts are ingested through water and edibles. Acidic pH of stomach initiates excystation which is completed in duodenum thus releasing trophozoites (2 trophozoites from each cyst). The trophozoites establish themselves in the intestinal villi and start multiplying by binary fission. It can also localize itself in biliary tract.

Symptomatology

The role played by this parasite in pathogenesis is not fully understood. Acute manifestations of giardiasis are nausea, anorexia, explosive watery stools, steatorrhea, malabsorption, severe flatulence with abdominal distention and mid epigastric cramps. The foul smelling stool, flatus, marked abdominal distention along with the absence of pus and the blood

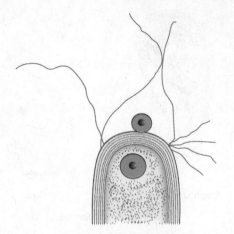

Fig. 41.5: *Giardia lamblia* trophozoite perched on top of an epithelial cell.

are more suggestive of giardiasis. The most common chronic complaints are periodic bouts of soft, mushy, foul smelling stools, flatulence and abdominal distention. Biliary disease is simulated in adults, whereas children show predominantly a diarrheal syndrome often steatorrheal in nature.

Pathology

Mucosal suction biopsies from duodenum and adjacent to duodenum have shown invasion of the mucosa but there are no signs of host cell injury. Electron microscope studies suggest that the organism may be attacking the fuzzy coat of the microvilli **(Fig. 41.5)**. Trophozoites have been demonstrated inside host cells by some investigators. Autopsy findings, in some instances, have shown extensive ulceration and sloughing of mucosa in the presence of heavy infection. Passage of *Giardia lamblia* trophozoites up to the bile duct to the gallbladder may occur with signs and symptoms of biliary tract disease.

Secondary vitamin A deficiency has been suggested by the lower carotene levels in children infected with giardia.

Two predisposing factors to symptomatology appear to be achlorhydria and hypogammaglobulinemia. Giardiasis appears to cause general disaccharidase deficiency, resulting in lactose intolerance which is usually restored after chemotherapy. Immunoglobulin deficiency has also suggested that lack of secretory IgA in patients may lead to colonization of bacteria in the jejunum and increased susceptibility to giardia. By deconjugating bile acids the bacteria may cause steatorrhea, but opportunist *Giardia lamblia* may aggravate the condition.

Laboratory Diagnosis

❖ Demonstration of cysts in the stool micro scopically
❖ Demonstration of trophozoites in duodenal aspirate
❖ Intestinal biopsy
❖ Immunological techniques like ELISA, indirect immunofluorescence, counter-current immuno-electrophoresis
❖ *Giardia lamblia* specific antigen can be detected using enzyme immunoassay (EIA) technique performed on microplate or micromembrane. It gives result in 10 minutes.

Treatment

Metronidazole, quinacrine, furazolidone and tinidazole may be effective.

Prevention

❖ Safe water supply (boiled treatment with hypochlorite or iodine)
❖ By checking fecal contamination
❖ Treating properly giardiasis patients.

◼ TRICHOMONAS VAGINALIS

Geographical Distribution

It is encountered in all climates and all social groups.

Habitat

❖ In female, it is found mainly in vagina and in male it is in urethra.

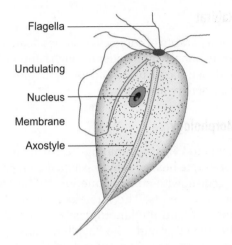

Fig. 41.6: *Trichomonas vaginalis.*

Morphology

It is found only in trophozoitic form which bears following characters **(Fig. 41.6)**:

❖ Pear-shaped measuring 10 to 30 μ × 5 to 10 μ
❖ It has short undulating membrane which comes up to the middle of the body
❖ Possesses 4 anterior flagellae, a prominent axostyle which bifurcates the body into two and projects posteriorly
❖ There is a costa, parabasal body, rounded nucleus (anteriorly)
❖ Chromatin granules are present all over, more densely near costa and axostyle
❖ Flagellae give characteristic webbing or rotatory motility
❖ It multiplies by binary fission in longitudinal axis.

Mode of Transmission

It is primarily a venereal disease in which transmission can also be from person-to-person contact. However, newborns may get infected during birth. Fomities also form another way of transmission of infection.

Incubation Time

It varies from 4 to 30 days.

Pathogenesis and Pathology

Within a few days following the introduction of viable *Trichomonas vaginalis* into the vagina, the proliferating colonies of this flagellate cause degeneration and desquamation of the vaginal epithelium. It is followed by leukocytic inflammation of the tissue layer. Very large numbers of trichomonads and leukocytes are now present in the vaginal secretion, which is liquid, greenish or yellow, and covers the mucosa down to the urethral orifice, vestibular glands and clitoris. As the acute condition changes to the chronic stage the secretion loses its purulent appearance due to decrease in number of trichomonads and leukocytes, increase in epithelial cells and establishment of a mixed bacterial flora.

Trichomonas vaginalis in male genitalia may be symptomless or may be responsible for an irritating, persistent or recurring urethritis.

Clinical Picture

The vaginal secretion is extremely irritating, almost unbearable and is constantly flowing. These symptoms may continue from a few days to many months. After each menstruation there is a tendency for acute stage to recur. Eventually, the chronic condition transforms into latent one and secretions become normal with no manifestation although trichomonas are still present. Difference in the intensity of symptoms may be due to differences in virulence of strains of this organism.

In male patients it may be symptomless or may cause urethritis and prostatitis.

Laboratory Diagnosis

1. In female patient, *Trichomonas vaginalis* may be demonstrated in sedimented urine, vaginal secretion or from vaginal scraping.

   In male patient *Trichomonas vaginalis* may be found in the centrifuged urine and prostatic secretions following massage of the prostatic gland.

However, care should be taken to prevent contamination of the specimen with feces, since *Trichomonas hominis* may be seen and thus misdiagnosed as *Trichomonas vaginalis*. The smear is stained using Giemsa, PAS, Papani-colaou, Leishman, Diff Quick and acridine orange.

2. *Culture:* It is quite sensitive technique. Media used for culture include, CPLM (cysteine, peptone, liver maltose), Bushley's, Feinberg, Whittington, etc.
3. Indirect hemagglutination test (IHA) employing glycoprotein obtained from *Trichomonas vaginalis* as an antigen. It is considered to be highly specific.

Treatment

1. Administration of metronidazole 250 mg thrice daily orally for five days.
2. Suppositories of diiodohydroxyquin are also useful.
3. Douching with lactic acid and vinegar to promote acid pH is also advocated.

TRICHOMONAS TENAX

❖ Harmless commensal of oral cavity, perio-dontal area, carious cavities of tooth, tonsillary crypts, etc.
❖ Measures 5 to 10 µ, i.e., smaller in size as compared to *Trichomonas vaginalis*
❖ Transmission is through fomites, salivary droplets and kissing.

TRICHOMONAS HOMINIS

❖ Measures 8 to 12 µ
❖ Carries 5 flagellae, undulating membrane going over the full length of protozoal body.
❖ It is a common commensal of cecum.

TRYPANOSOMA BRUCEI

Geographical Distribution

Western and central parts of Africa.

Habitat

It is a parasite of connective tissues. It attacks the regional lymph nodes through lymphatics and then goes to blood and finally may involve central nervous system.

Morphology

It occurs in trypomastigote form in the vertebrate host as spindle-shaped elongated organism with pointed anterior and blunted posterior ends. The nucleus is central in position and the kinetoplast is situated at the posterior end. The flagellum starts just adjacent to the kinetoplast, curves around the body to form an undulating membrane and continues beyond the anterior end as free flagellum. The trypomastigotes of *T. brucei* are highly pleomorphic, varying in shape and size in different stages. The size may vary from $10\,\mu \times 3\,\mu$ to $20\,\mu \times 3\,\mu$. Many antigenic variants of the organism occur.

Life Cycle

The definitive hosts are man, domestic animals and wild game. The intermediate hosts are several species of Tsetse fly (Glossina), e.g., *Glossina palpalis*. The infective metacyclic form of the organism is introduced into man by the bite of the insect (tsetse fly). After multiplication at the site of inoculation, the parasite attacks the blood of the definite host. The trypomastigote forms are picked up by the tsetse fly during its blood meal from the infective definitive host to continue cycle.

Clinical Picture

A typical trypanosomal chancre appears at the site of insect bite. There is an enlargement of lymph node and involvement of central nervous system. There may be fever, headache, loss of sleep at night. Later there is meningoencephalitis manifested as sleeping sickness. If not treated, the disease is fatal one.

Laboratory Diagnosis

It comprises:
1. *Demonstration of trypanosomes form:*
    i. Peripheral blood
    ii. Bone marrow
    iii. Lymph node aspirate
    iv. Cerebrospinal fluid
       Demonstration of trypanomastigote may be done as under:
       a. Unstained preparation by direct microscopy.
       b. Leishman's stained smears.
       c. Culture on NNN medium.
       d. Animal inoculation (white rat, white mice, guinea pig).
2. *Serological diagnosis:*
    i. Indirect immunofluorescence (IIF).
    ii. Indirect hemagglutination (IHA).
    iii. ELISA.
    iv. Complement fixation test (CFT).
    v. Card agglutination trypanosomiasis test (CATT).

Treatment

Suramin and pentamidine are the drugs of choice. Nitrofurazone, arsenicals and malaresopal are also useful.

TRYPANOSOMA CRUZI

Geographical Distribution

Central and South Africa.

Habitat

A parasite of the muscular and nervous tissues and also of reticuloendothelial system.

Morphology

It is same as *Trypanosoma brucei* except that it is C or U shaped in stained films of blood measuring 3 μ × 3 μ. It does not multiply in peripheral blood. Amastigote forms are seen in cells of striated muscle (heart and skeletal muscle) neurological and reticuloendothelial cells as round or oval bodies 2 to 4 μ with nucleus and kinetoplast. Multiplication occurs only at this stage.

Culture: NNN medium

Life cycle: It is similar to that of *T. brucei* except that it is transmitted by the reduviid bug. Within bug the trypomastigote forms taken up during the bite, are transformed to epimastigote form and finally trypomastigote forms are excreted into the feces of insect. Man is infected by fecal matter rubbed into the site of the insect bite or by infection of conjunctiva or other exposed membranous surface with finger.

Clinical Picture

After 7 to 14 days of incubation period patient suffers from acute or chronic symptoms of Chaga's disease. It is characterized by fever, conjunctival congestion, edema of one side of face, enlargement of spleen and lymph nodes, anemia and lymphocytosis. These manifestations last for 30 days and often end fatally because of myocardial failure and meningoencephalitis.

The chronic form is found in adults and characterized by cardiac arrhythmia and neurological problems like psychic change and spastic paralysis. The disease lasts for 10 to 12 years. Degeneration of the intramural autonomic nervous system may cause megaesophagus or megacolon. Cardiomyopathy is the other complication.

Laboratory Diagnosis

❖ Direct microscopic examination of peripheral blood smear (Leishman's stained) shows trypomastigote form
❖ Inoculation in animals (Guinea pig)
❖ Xenodiagnosis by allowing laboratory bug to feed on patient blood and examining its intestinal contents after 2 weeks
❖ Biopsy of lymph node or muscle
❖ Serological tests like:
    a. Complement fixation test
    b. Immunofluorescence test
    c. ELISA

d. Intradermal test (delayed hypersensitivity) using *T. cruzi* antigen.

Treatment: Nitrofurazone is effective.

LEISHMANIA DONOVANI

Geographical Distribution

Visceral leishmaniasis is widely distributed but local endemicity is usually rather sharply delimited. It is endemic in many places in America, Africa, China, South Europe, Europe and India. In India, it is common in Assam, Bengal, Bihar, Odisha, Tamil Nadu and eastern parts of Uttar Pradesh up to Lucknow.

Habitat

The natural habitat of *Leishmania donovani* in man is reticuloendothelial system especially spleen, liver, bone marrow, intestinal mucosa. It may be found in endothelial cells of kidneys, suprarenal capsules, lungs, meninges, cerebrospinal fluid and also in the macrophages of intestinal wall.

Morphology

Leishmania donovani exists in two forms: (a) amastigote form also called a flagellar form and (b) Promastigote form also called flagellar form or leptomonad form **(Fig. 41.7)**.

Amastigote Form

In this form, this parasite is found in the cells of reticuloendothelial system of vertebrate hosts like man, dog, hamster, etc.

Promastigote Form

They are found in sandfly and in cultures.
a. Shape: Pear-shaped bodies (early stage) to long slender spindle-shaped bodies.
b. Size: 5 to 10 μ × 2 to 3 μ (early stage). 15 to 20 μ × 1 to 2 μ (fully developed).
c. Nucleus: Centrally placed.
d. Kinetoplast: It lies transversely near the anterior end and consists of parabasal body and blepharoplast.
e. Eosinophilic vacuole: It is a light staining area lying in front of kinetoplast over which axoneme runs.
f. Flagellum: It projects from the front and may be of the same length as the body of parasite. Undulating membrane is absent.

Culture

In vitro it can be cultured in NNN (Novy, MacNeal and Nicolle), bacto-agar biphasic medium, Schneider's medium with 20% calf serum (proved to be excellent), etc. Apart from this tissue, culture media and insect culture are also found useful.

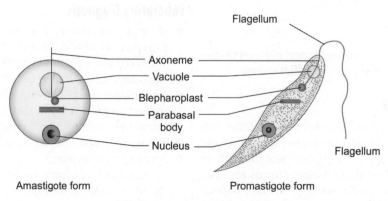

Amastigote form   Promastigote form

Fig. 41.7: *Leishmania donovani.*

The incubation in NNN medium is undertaken in water of condensation and incubation is done at 22°C to 24°C. To prevent contaminants, antibiotics and antifungal drugs may be added to above medium.

The salient features of amastigote form are as below:

a. Shape: Rounded or ovoidal.
b. Size: 2 to 4 μ along the longitudinal axis and living intracellularly in monocytes, polymorphonuclear leukocytes or endothelial cells.
c. Cell membrane: It is very delicate.
d. Nucleus: Lying within the cytoplasm is a relatively large nucleus measuring about 1 μ in diameter and it is oval or round lying in the middle or along the side of cell wall.
e. Kinetoplast: It lies tangentially at right angles to the nucleus. It consists of:
   i. Parabasal body which is a rod-like structure.
   ii. Blepharoplast is a dot-like structure lying near parabasal body.
f. Axoneme: It is a delicate filament which arises from blepharoplast and extends to the margin of the body.
g. Vacuole: It is a clear, unstained space lying along side the axoneme.

Animal Models

Hamster is the most commonly used animal in routine.

Mode of Transmission

❖ Natural transmission by the bite of sandfly (Phlebotomus)
❖ Mother to fetus (vertical transmission)
❖ Blood transfusion
❖ Accidental inoculation of culture in the laboratory.

Life Cycle

The female sandfly (Phlebotomus) after sucking leishmania along with blood of the patient, invariably require fruit juice feed before it becomes infective. Phlebotomus is small hairy fly (1.5 to 3.5 mm). Its usual biting time is at dusk or night.

Leishmania donovani undergoes development inside the body of female sandfly. The promasti-gote forms after multiplication ascend to pharynx and reach the proboscis. It takes 9 days to complete the cycle in sandfly. Ultimately, the buccal cavity of sandfly is blocked by promastigote form. For taking second meal the sandfly has to release the promastigote form from its mouth into the bite wound caused by its proboscis.

The promastigotes thus enter the circulation are mainly destroyed by vertebrate host (man). Still some promastigotes take shelter inside cells of reticuloendothelial system where promastigote form is transformed into amastigote one. They undergo multiplication there at a slow rate. When the infected cells of reticuloendothelial system rupture, the free amastigote forms attack other cells. Sometimes they may be phagocytosed.

■ PATHOLOGY AND CLINICAL PICTURE

Spleen

Macroscopic Picture

❖ Enlarged grossly
❖ Capsule thickened
❖ Soft in consistency
❖ Cut surface shows congestion.

Microscopic Picture

❖ Vascular space engorged with blood and widely dilated
❖ Reticular cells of Billroth cords are increased and packed with amastigote form of parasite (*Leishmania donovani* bodies, i.e., L.D. bodies)
❖ Trabeculae are thin and atrophied
❖ Malpighian corpuscles disappear
❖ No fibrosis occurs.

Liver

Macroscopic Picture
- Enlarged
- Congested
- Cut surface shows nutmeg appearance.

Microscopic Picture
- Kupffer cell hyperplasia and loaded with LD bodies.
- Engorgement with blood of sinusoidal capillaries. They are dilated too.

Bone Marrow

- Macrophages (loaded with LD bodies) and plasma cells abundantly replace hemato genous tissue.

Miscellaneous

- Cloudy swelling of kidney
- Degenerative myocarditis
- Anemia
- Intestine may be present with ulcer because of secondary infection
- Lymph nodes are not involved in Indian infection.

The clinical picture is as under (Kala-azar):
- Irregular fever
- Hepatosplenomegaly
- Marked emaciation and anemia
- Loss of weight
- Dry skin and brittle hair
- Pigmentation of the skin
- Perverted appetite
- Epistaxis, cancrum oris, lung infection, edema, etc. are some of the complications. The incubation period is 3 to 6 months.

AIDS and Visceral Leishmaniasis

- Sera of visceral leishmaniasis patients co-infected with HIV may be non-reactive in serodiagnostic tests.
- Visceral leishmaniasis rapidly accelerates the onset of AIDS and shortens the life span of HIV infected patients.

- HIV spurs the spread of visceral leishmaniasis. AIDS increases the risk of 100 to 1000 times in endemic regions.
- Both visceral leishmaniasis and HIV produce cumulative deficiency of immune responses thus increasing disease severity complications and net consequences.

Laboratory Diagnosis

1. Non-specific tests
   a. TLC indicates leukopenia.
   b. DLC shows neutropenia with relative lymphocytosis and monocytosis.
   c. WBC: RBC ratio 1:2000 (Normal: 1:750).
   d. Reverse albumin globulin ratio detected by following tests.
      i. Naplier Aldehyde test where 1 mL of patient's serum is mixed with 1 drop of formalin (40%) and incubated at room temperature. Gellification means test is positive.
      ii. In 2 mL of patient serum, few drops of 4% stibamine solution is added. Positive test means appearance of profuse flocculant precipitate. However, this test is less sensitive as compared to aldehyde test.
      iii. Electrophoresis.
2. Demonstration of LD bodies (amastigote) from specimens (Blood, spleen, bone marrow, liver, etc).
   a. Biopsy or aspirate from these specimens is smeared on clean glass slide fixed with methyl alcohol and stained with Giemsa stain. LD bodies are demonstrated. LD bodies should be differentiated from *Histoplasma capsulatum, Toxoplasma gondii*. Konetoplast is characteristically present in LD bodies which is absent in *Histoplasma capsulatum* and *Toxoplasma gondii*.
   b. Culture may be done on following media.
      i. Grace, insect medium.
      ii. Schneider's drosophila medium.
      iii. Brain-Heart infusion agar medium.
      iv. Tobie's medium.

v. NNN (Novy, MacNeal, Nicolle) is the popular medium used all over. Basically, it is rabbit blood agar slope to which antibiotics are added to check contamination. The specimen is inoculated in the water of condensation and incubated at 24°C for 7 days. Growth in the form of PROMASTIGOTE ONLY is demonstrated. The specimen is declared negative only after 5 to 6 weeks of incubation.

3. Animal inoculation is performed by injecting intraperitoneally the specimen in either hamster or mice. The inoculated animals are kept at 26°C. Amastigote form of parasite is recovered from injected animal.

4. Leishmanin skin test is also called Montenegro test. It is based on the principle of delayed hypersensitivity. About 0.1 mL of antigen suspension (10%) is injected intradermally on dorsoventral part of forearm. Induration of 5 mm or more after 48 to 72 hours means test is positive. Skin test is negative in Indian Kala-azar.

5. Immunological tests include tests to detect antigen (e.g., ELISA and Indirect fluorescence test) and tests to detect antibodies (e.g., complement fixation test—CFT) using Witebsky, Klingenstein and Kuhn antigen also called WKK antigen (obtained from human tubercle bacille) and CFT using Kedrowsky's acid fast bacilli. Other tests used to demonstrate antibodies are using antigen procured from culture are:
   i. CFT
   ii. Counter-current immunoelectrophoresis
   iii. Indirect immunofluorescence (1:32)
   iv. ELISA
   v. Indirect hemagglutination.

6. Some newer test are:
   i. DOT ELISA
   ii. IIF using monoclonal antibodies
   iii. Nodular lesions may appear on depigmented macules or erythematous patches. Characteristic feature of the nodule is that they never ulcerate.

Direct Agglutination Test (DAT)

❖ It is a rapid and reliable screening test for visceral leishmaniasis. The antigen used is a suspension of trypsin treated amastigotes. A titer of 3200 or more indicates positive result.

❖ A rapid latex agglutination test detects leishmania antigen in urine of patients suffering from visceral leishmaniasis.

Treatment

❖ Pentavalent antimonial drugs, e.g., meglumine antimonate, sodium stiboglucomate.

❖ Other drugs like pentamidine, amphotericin B and allopurinol are used as an alternative to pentavalent antimonial drugs.

Preventive Measures

❖ Treatment should be continued with adequate dose for recommended duration and control over the cases of leishmaniasis.

❖ Use of insecticidal spray like DDT.

❖ Use of mosquito net, mesh doors and repellents.

   Preliminary work in Brasil suggests vacci-nation with multiple recombinant leishmania antigen may be useful.

❖ A killed promastigote plus BCG vaccine preparation is being investigated as prevention measure.

POST KALA-AZAR DERMAL LEISHMANIASIS (DERMAL LEISHMANIASIS)

Geographical Distribution

Mainly, it is seen in Indian regions like Bihar, West Bengal, etc.

Pathogenesis and Clinical Picture

It occurs in patients residing in endemic areas who take drugs for a short while or drugs not in recommended doses. It usually occurs in 2 to 8% cases of visceral leishmaniasis about 2 years after recovery from visceral lesions.

It is manifested as:

i. Depigmented macules distributed over trunk and extremities.

ii. Erythematous patches on face resembling distribution like butterfly.

Laboratory Diagnosis

Biopsy from lesions shows amastigote form in a stained smear/section. The biopsy material may be cultured on NNN medium or inoculated into animals for establishing diagnosis.

Treatment

Such patients require treatment with pentavalent antimonial drugs in double doses and this treatment should be continued for long time.

■ LEISHMANIA TROPICA

Along Mediterranean Sea coast.

Geographical Distribution

Central and Western India. The infection does not coexist with kala-azar.

Habitat

Amastigote in reticuloendothelial cells of skin (clasmatocyte). Promastigote form in sandfly, i.e., *Phlebotomus sergenti* in India.

Morphology

Resembles *Leishmania donovani*.

Culture: NNN medium.

Clinical Features

Incubation period is 6 months. It causes disease called oriental sore, Delhi boil, Baghdad boil, etc. Lesions are cutaneous (exposed parts). Lesion starts as a granulomatous nodule surrounded by red margin. The lesion ulcerates in the center. Later satellite lesions appears around the ulcer.

Pathology

Deposition of promastigotes as a result of bite of infected sandfly on the surface of skin. Promastigote enters through punctured wound and transform into amastigote form inside histiocytes and endothelial cells. Inflammatory granulomatous reaction occurs with infiltration of lymphocytes and plasma cells. As a result of disturbance of blood supply, necrosis and then ulcer formation occurs.

Laboratory Diagnosis

Smear from specimen collected by puncturing the edge of lesion is prepared and stained with leishman stain to demonstrate amastigote form. Material may also be cultured on NNN medium to demonstrate promastigote form.

Treatment: Same as in kala-azar.

■ LEISHMANIA BRAZILIENSIS

Geographical Distribution

Central and South America.

Habitat

Amastigote form occurs in the macrophages of skin and mucous membrane of the nose and buccal cavity.

Morphology

Resemble *Leishmania donovani*.

Life Cycle

Same as *Leishmania donovani* but the vector is forest sandfly (Lutzomyia).

Reservoir: Small forest rodent.

Culture: NNN medium.

Clinical Features

A specific ulcerative granuloma of the skin occurs after incubation period (few days). Later the lesion involves mucosa of mouth, nose, pharynx and larynx. The lesions may appear as papules, nodules or ulcers.

Pathology

The initial lesion has tendency to enlarge radially forming an ulcer with clearcut margin and oozing surface. Amastigotes are there in large numbers towards the periphery of lesion.

Laboratory Diagnosis

Direct smear, culture and animal inoculation and serological techniques (IFA, ELISA and Leishmanin skin test) are of immense value in establishing the diagnosis.

Treatment: Antimonial preparation.

■ SPOROZOA

Malarial Parasite

Geographical Distribution

It occurs in all countries in the tropics and subtropics (40°S to 60°N). *Plasmodium ovale* is not reported in India whereas *Plasmodium vivax, Plasmodium falciparum* and *Plasmodium malariae* exist in India.

Habitat

It is found in parenchymal cells of liver, erythrocytes and other organs.

Life cycle: All species complete life cycle in man and female anopheles mosquito.

Life Cycle in Man (Schizogony)

Female anopheles mosquito bite to man results in the injection of sporozoites which circulate in blood (about 1 hour) when some sporozoites attack liver cells and start pre-erythrocytic cycle. In 6-15 days' time release of thousands of merozoites occurs after completion of pre-erythrocytic cycle. Some of these merozoites are phagocytosed whereas others start erythrocytic schizogony.

In *Plasmodium vivax* and *Plasmodium ovale* hepatic form known as hypnozoites persist and remain active in hepatocytes for considerable time before they grow and undergo pre-erythrocytic schizogony with liberation of merozoites in bloodstream causing lapse of the infection.

During erythrocytic schizogony **(Table 41.7)** parasite assumes a form of ring and then of trophozoite. In trophozoitic form malarial

Table 41.7: Morphological features in different species.

	P. falciparum	P. vivax	P. malariae	P. ovale
RBC				
Size	Normal	Enlarged	Normal	Enlarged
Shape	Round and crenated	Round	Round	Oval or round
Color	Normal	Pale	Normal	Normal
Stippling	Maurer's dots (large red)	Schuffner's dots (small red)	Ziemann's dots	James dots (many small red)
Pigment	Black or dark brown	• Fine golden brown in cytoplasm	Black or brown large	Black or brown
Parasite	Small, dark multiple infection of one RBC	• Large	Tendency to form band across the RBC otherwise of moderate size	Regular shape

Contd...

Contd...

	P. falciparum	P. vivax	P. malariae	P. ovale
Stages in PBF	Only rings and Gametocytes	Trophozoites Schizonts Gametocytes	Trophozoites Schizonts Gametocytes	Trophozoites Schizonts Gametocytes
Ring stage	Small, 1.5 µ, double chromatin multiple rings and vacuole formation	Large 2.5 µ single Thicker chromatin	Characters of *P. vivax*	Characters of *P. vivax*
Trophozoites	Compact, small, no vacuole seen	Large irregular ameboid, vacuole prominent Thick chromatin	Band formation	Compact chromatin is large irregular clumps
Schizont	• Small • Compact • Not seen in PBF	Large, filling RBC Yellow brown pigment	Fills RBC Segmented, Daisy head pigment (dark brown)	Fill 3/4th RBC Segmented Dark yellow brown pigment
Micro-gametocyte	• Larger than RBC • Kidney shaped • Cytoplasm blue • Fine granules scattered • In smear many in number	• Fills enlarged RBC • Round • Cytoplasm pale blue Many brown granules	• Smaller than RBC • Round • Cytoplasm pale blue • Pigment and chromatin like *P. vivax*	• Of the size of RBC • Round • Cytoplasm pale blue • Pigment and chro-matin as in *P. vivax*
Macro-gametocyte	• Crescent • Deep blue • Cytoplasm • Ends sharply rounded • In abundant in PBF	• Round • Fills enlarged • RBC • Pigment as small masses • Many in PBF	• Round • Smaller than RBC • Cytoplasm dark blue • Scanty in PBF	• Round • Of RBC size • Cytoplasm dark blue • Rarely in PBF
Number of merozoites in a schizont	20–24	16	8	8
Erythrocytes infected	Any age	Young	Old	Young
Maximum parasitemia	1,000,000/µl	25,000/µl	10,000/µl	25,000/µl
Relapse	No	Yes	No	Yes
Drug resistance	Yes	No	No	No
CNS involvement	++++	+	+	±
Nephrotic syndrome	+	+	++++	+
Anemia	++++	++	++	–

pigments start appearing. Trophozoites are transformed to schizont with division of chromatin surrounded by pieces of cytoplasms. On attaining maturity schizont ruptures with the liberation of merozoites. They, in turn, invade fresh erythrocytes.

After undergoing erythrocytic schizogony some macrozoites are transformed into gametocytes. Gametogony occurs in the erythrocytes of capillaries of internal organs. Mature gametocytes seek entry to peripheral blood from where they are carried to vector (mosquito) when it bites the patient.

Life Cycle in Mosquito (Sporogony)

The female anopheles mosquito during blood meals from malarial patient sucks blood containing plasmodia in various forms and stages. The presence of male and female mature gametocytes should be there for continuing sexual cycle (sporogony) in the mosquito. At least 12 gametocytes per cu mm of blood and macrogametocytes must be in excess. The other forms of plasmodia, i.e., asexual forms are destroyed in the stomach of mosquito.

First of all gametocytes become rounded and exflagellation occurs with the formation of 4 to 8 filamentous structure (microgametocyte). These filaments are detached and form microgametes. One of these microgametes penetrates the macrogamete. This follows the transformation of fertilized macrogamete into zygote. It happens from 20 minutes to 2 hours after ingestion of blood by mosquito.

Zygote becomes very active and now called ookinete which penetrates the muscle wall of stomach and comes to lie below the outer limiting membrane of stomach wall in the form of oocyst (6 to 12 μ). Oocyst further increases in size to 60 μ in diameter, containing many sickle-shaped structures called sporozoites. Oocyst containing sporozoites is called sporocyst.

Sporocyst ruptures with the liberation of sporozoites in body cavity of mosquito. Sporozoites are disseminated in all parts of body except ovaries. Sporozoite has special affinity for salivary glands. They pass through the glands and reach the lumen of salivary duct with maximum concentration of sporozoites. The mosquito is now infective.

Pathogenesis of Plasmodium

1. The plasmodia that invade the red blood cells grow and segment at the expense of these host cells, which rupture when schizogony is complete. The debris of ruptured cells, the released merozoites, and their metabolic products, stimulate chemoreceptor of the temperature regulating mechanism of the host to conserve heat. As the number of the invaded red cells increases and the asexual cycle of parasite becomes more synchronized, the quantity of pyrogen released at one line becomes sufficient to produce the characteristic chills and fever of a malaria attack.

2. The species of plasmodia differ greatly in their ability to multiply in the blood Plasmodium vivax prefers to invade the youngest erythrocyte, whereas Plasmodium malariae prefers the older red cells. Hence these species parasitize around 2% of host red blood cells. Plasmodium falciparum, on the other hand, invade erythrocytes of all ages and, thus, is capable of parasitizing a very high percentage of erythrocytes.

3. Due to the varying number of merozoites produced in schizogony by the species of plasmodium, Plasmodium falciparum multiplies more rapidly than Plasmodium vivax which, in turn, multiplies more rapidly than Plasmodium malariae and Plasmodium ovale. The parasitemia of Plasmodium falciparum also tends to be higher because more than one parasite frequently develop in a single erythrocyte.

4. With each schizogony, the parasitized cells are destroyed, but there also in considerable destruction of unparasitized cells due to lysis and phagocytosis, phagocytosis especially occurs in the spleen and liver. In falciparum malaria with a very high parasitemia, hemolytic jaundice may be evident and anemia may be severe.

5. Malignant character of falciparum malaria is not so much related to its rapid multiplication and invasiveness as to the

manner in which it causes lesions in the human host. Characteristic lesions are due to blockade of small vessels by sticky parasitized erythrocytes. The blockade causes stasis, then local anoxia, then increased vascular permeability, which allows plasma and unparasitized cells to leak into the perivascular space. This incidently results in additional loss of erythrocytes.

6. These factors combine to cause a decrease in circulating erythrocytes in the circulating blood volume, local tissue anoxia and edema.

Clinical Picture

❖ Fever peaks (exhibits cold, hot and sweating stages)
❖ Anemia
❖ Splenomegaly and hepatomegaly.

Complications of *P. falciparum*

❖ Cerebral malaria occurs when nonimmune person remains untreated for 7 to 10 days after plasmodial infection. It is associated with fever, confusion, convulsion, coma and death.
❖ Black water fever is characterized by sudden massive hemolysis followed by fever and hemoglobinuria. It is always associated with consumption of small doses of quinine. There is intravascular hemolysis with the mani-festations like methemalbuminemia, hyper-bilirubinemia, hemoglobinuria. Kidneys and liver are particularly involved. RBC and hemoglobin fall considerably. Sequelae of black water fever includes uremia, renal failure, circulatory failure, liver failure, anemia and pigment calculi. Renal failure is the cause of death.
❖ Pernicious malaria results from anoxia due to obstruction of capillaries in various organs followed by necrosis of tissues. It occurs in recently infected persons (*P. falciparum*) without immunity to plasmodium.

It may involve:
  i. Nervous system (cerebral malaria) cerebrospinal involvement and peripheral nerves plus cord nerves rarely
 ii. Gastrointestinal having gastric, choleric and dysenteric forms
iii. May involve cardiovascular, respiratory and genitourinary system. Hence, pernicious malaria may be of following types:
   a. Septicemic form may eventually cause cardiac failure and death.
   b. Acute hemolytic form may cause anemia.
   c. Hemorrhagic form may manifest like purpura.
   d. Pneumonic form may result in pulmonary edema.
   e. Nephrotic form with nephritis, nephrosis, etc.

Transmission Modes

❖ Mosquito bite **(Table 41.8)**
❖ Transfusion malaria
❖ Congenital malaria
❖ Use of contaminated syringe as in drug addicts.

Immunity

❖ Glucose 6-phosphate dehydrogenase deficients are protected from malaria as

Table 41.8: Differences between sporozoite induced and trophozoite induced malaria.

Sporozoite induced	Trophozoite induced	
Transmission	Mosquito bite	Blood, e.g., blood transfusion
Pre-erythrocytic schizogony	+	
Incubation time	Prolonged	Short
Relapses	May occur	Absent
Severity	Less	More severe
Radical drug	Indicated	Not required

this enzyme is necessary for respiration of plasmodium.

❖ Absence of Duffy blood group protects against *Plasmodium vivax* as this blood group antigen seems to be receptor for *Plasmodium vivax*.

❖ *Plasmodium falciparum* does not multiply in sickle red cells as they contain abnormal hemoglobin S.

❖ Severe malnutrition and iron deficiency appear to offer some protection against malaria.

❖ Infants are immune to malaria because of presence of fetal hemoglobin (Hb-F), diet deficient in amino benzoic acid and passive antibodies, i.e., maternal antibodies.

❖ Premunition is a state of resistance in an infected person which harbors parasites but remains asymptomatic. This immunity disappears soon after eradication of plasmodial infection. Hence low levels of parasitemia must be there to maintain immunity.

Pathology: Changes in various organs are mentioned as under:

Liver

Macroscopic (Gross)

❖ Liver enlarged
❖ Color differs from dark red to slate gray.

Microscopic

❖ Dilatation of capillaries and sinusoids
❖ Hypertrophy and hyperplasia of Kupffer's cells lining sinusoids.

Spleen

Macroscopic

❖ Enlarged
❖ Congested
❖ Dark red
❖ Soft
❖ Capsule tense.

Microscopic

❖ Hyperemia
❖ Hyperplasia of reticuloendothelial and lymphoid elements
❖ Macrophages loaded with red cells and parasitic debris plus pigments.

Kidney

Macroscopic

❖ Congested.

Microscopic

❖ Degenerative changes in the epithelium of tubules
❖ Acute tubular necrosis
❖ Immune complex deposition especially in *Plasmodium malariae*.

Bone Marrow

Macroscopic

❖ Dark red.

Microscopic

❖ Hyperplasia of reticuloendothelial cells containing pigments
❖ Parasitized erythrocytes.

Brain

Macroscopic

❖ Congested and edematous
❖ Petechial common in white matter.

Microscopic

❖ Capillaries congested and loaded with parasitized erythrocytes
❖ Ring hemorrhages
❖ Necrosis.

Heart

❖ Petechial hemorrhage in epicardium
❖ Congested capillaries engorged with parasitized erythrocytes
❖ Degenerative changes in heart muscles.

Lungs

❖ Congested
❖ Capillaries contain parasitized erythrocytes
❖ Pulmonary edema may be there.

Gastrointestinal Tract

❖ Edematous
❖ Congested
❖ Petechial hemorrhage, but necrosis and ulceration only in *Plasmodium falciparum.*

Laboratory Diagnosis

❖ Peripheral blood film for parasites (thick and thin smear) is studied microscopically after staining often with Leishman technique. Morphological features are noted and plasmodium is identified in thin film.
❖ Serological techniques like IHA, ELISA, etc. These tests are of very limited importance in establishing diagnosis. However, it does carry epidemiological importance.

Newer diagnostic techniques are:
   i. Use of fluorescent dyes
  ii. Radioimmunoassay
 iii. Agar gel diffusion
  iv. Dot-blot assay
   v. Use of automated equipment
  vi. Visualization of parasite by quick buffy coat method
 vii. ELISA using polyclonal or monoclonal antibodies
viii. DNA probe
  ix. RNA probe
   x. PCR
  xi. Immunochromatographic test kit which is a credit card size manual kit based on capture of a circulating *Plasmodium falciparum* histidine rich protein-2 (Pf HRP-2) in whole blood
 xii. A rapid immunodiagnostic: Strep test for detection of *Plasmodium falciparum* specific parasite lactate dehydrogenase (PLDH) may be used.

Treatment

❖ Quinine
❖ Chloroquin
❖ Primaquin
❖ Pyrimethamine + sulfadoxine.

Prevention and Control

❖ Mosquito repellants and bed nets
❖ Spray of chemicals
❖ Biological control measures like use of special fishes (Gambiens) in water, destruction of reproductive system using radiations, etc.
❖ Proper treatment of malarial patients
❖ Use of malarial vaccine which are under trial, e.g., sporozoites vaccines, vaccine with exo-erythrocytic merozoites, merozoites of erythrocytic stage vaccine, vaccine prepared from purified gametocytes and SPF-66.

Now PCR and genetic engineering techniques have brought new hopes in the preparation of ideal vaccine against malarial infection.

TOXOPLASMA GONDII

Geographical Distribution

It is worldwide in distribution.

Habitat

Endothelial cells, leukocytes, body fluid and tissue cells.

Morphology

It occurs in following three forms:

Trophozoites (Fig. 41.8)

❖ Oval-shaped or crescent-shaped with one end pointed and the other rounded
❖ Measure 7 × 7 μ
❖ Lack flagella, cilia and pseudopodia
❖ Staining by Giemsa's or Wright's technique.
❖ Nucleus lies near blunt end
❖ Multiplication by endogeny which means internal budding
❖ Rapid proliferation of trophozoites in acute infection (invade mammalian cells) is called tachyzoites **(Fig. 41.9)**
❖ Trophozoites may be found extracellular too
❖ Exhibit asexual multiplication, i.e., schizogony.

Tissue Cysts

❖ Measure 10 to 200 μ
❖ Contain thousands of organisms

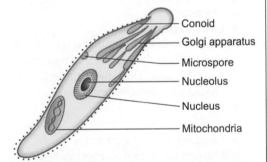

Fig. 41.8: Trophozoite of *Toxoplasma gondii*.

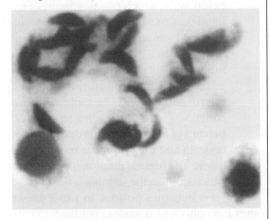

Fig. 41.9: *Toxoplasma gondii*.

❖ Demonstration by periodic acid Schiff stain
❖ Slowly multiplying parasites within cyst are named bradyzoites.
❖ Act as a source of infection and thus responsible for transmission of infection.
❖ Tissue cysts are formed during the chronic stage of infection.
❖ May involve any organ of the body predominantly skeletal muscles, heart muscles and brain.
❖ Exhibit asexual multiplication, i.e., schizogony.

Oocysts

❖ Spherical or oval 10 to 12 μ
❖ Contain sporoblast
❖ Freshly passed oocysts are not infective
❖ They attain infectiveness only after development in soil or water. Infective form contains 8 sporozoites
❖ Oocysts are formed as a result of sexual reproduction, i.e., gametogony or sporogony
❖ Oocysts develop only in the definitive host, i.e., cat and members of felidae family.

Life Cycle

Life cycle is completed as under:

Enteric Cycle in Cat

Ingested oocyst releases sporozoites. These sporozoites penetrate the epithelial cells of the intestine. They become rounded and grow within host cells. Thereafter, asexual division occurs resulting in the formation of merozoites. Some merozoites manage to seek entry in extraintestinal tissues and thus tissue cysts formation occurs in other organs of body. Other merozoites are changed into sexual forms and thus start sexual reproduction named gametogony. A motile microgamete fertilizes a macrogamete which results in the formation of oocyst which undergo development through various stages before it becomes infective.

Exoenteric Cycle in Man

Ingestion of oocyst contaminated improperly cooked meat results in infection. Alternatively, oocyst from cat may be ingested. Only asexual form of reproduction occurs in man with the formation of merozoites only. Merozoites enter lymphatics and blood. They develop into tissue cysts in different organs of the body. Human-to-human infection is possible through placenta giving rise to congenital toxoplasmosis. It is worthwhile to point out that oocysts are not formed in the intestine of man.

Mode of Transmission

It is by ingestion of oocyst or tissue cyst containing edibles, through placenta to the fetus, occupational (laboratory or slaughter house workers), etc.

Pathogenesis

Many organs are involved once parasites gain access to bloodstream. Initial invasion of cell occurs followed by their multiplication and finally disruption of cell. It results in focal area of necrosis with lymphocytes, and monocytes around it. By and large the infection is asymptomatic and its reason may be effective protection immunity (extracellular antibody and intracellular T cell factors).

Clinical Picture

❖ Congenital toxoplasmosis with manifestation in newborn like chorioretinitis, blindness, epilepsy, mental retardation. It may give rise to abortion or stillbirth. Other less important lesions are of eyes, liver and spleen.
❖ Infection of mother during pregnancy.
❖ Ocular toxoplasmosis with lesions like chorioretinitis.
❖ Widespread infection in immuno-compromised persons, e.g., AIDS, organ transplantation recipients, malignancies, etc. Other lesions are encephalitis, meningitis, chorioretinitis, myositis, etc.

❖ However, acquired toxoplasmosis has presentation like lymphadenitis, maculo-papular rash, myocarditis, etc.

Laboratory Diagnosis

1. **Isolation of *Toxoplasma gondii*:** It is possible by injecting body fluid or infected tissue into peritoneal cavity of mice or tissue culture. Mice should be examined for demonstration of *T. gondii* in the peritoneal fluid, 6 to 10 days after injection of material.
2. **Demonstration of trophozoites or cysts:** Their demonstration in placenta or tissues of the newborn confirms the diagnosis of congenital toxoplasmosis. They may also be demonstrated in brain biopsy, bone marrow biopsy, CSF, amniotic fluid, etc. thus diagnosing the infection as an acute one.
3. **Lymph node biopsy** shows reactive follicular hyperplasia and irregular clusters of epithelioid histiocytes.
4. **Serological tests:**
   ▪ Latex agglutination.
   ▪ Toxoreagent agglutination test is simple, rapid test exhibiting over 94% agreement with dye test. Here latex particles are coated with soluble antigen.
   ▪ IHA
   ▪ ELISA
   ▪ Complement fixation test
   ▪ Indirect immunofluorescence test
   ▪ Methylene blue dye test of Sabin and Feldman in which equal amount of diluted patient serum, *Toxoplasma gondii*, normal human serum are mixed and incubated at 37°C for one hour. To each tube, 1 drop of methylene blue (pH 11) is added and a drop of mixture is examined microscopically. If the patient serum contains specific antibodies, less than 50 percent of free toxoplasma does not take up stain and the cytoplasm remains colorless. The highest dilution of test serum which inhibits the staining is the titer.

The test becomes positive in 1 to 2 weeks after infection and remains positive for years altogether.

Presence of specific IgM/IgA antibodies in serum, a high dye titer value (>300 IU/ml) are the tests indicative of recent toxoplasma infection. However, all these tests are unreliable because sometimes IgA antibodies persist for months while IgM may persist for years following primary infection. Sabin and Feldman dye test titers also remain very high for several months. Avidity ELISA test is found to be a useful complementary test to differentiate recent infection from chronic infection.

Treatment

❖ Pyrimethamine and sulfadiazine combination is quite useful.
❖ Spiramycin as such or in combination with sulfadiazone may be tried.

▓ ISOSPORA BELLI

It is the protozoa of intestine of man. It is frequently found in Asia, Africa and South America.

Morphology

❖ It is oval in shape
❖ Measures 20 to 30 × 10 to 20 micron
❖ Oocyst develops to 2 sporoblasts which transform to sporocysts
❖ Each sporocyst measures 9 to 15 × 8 to 14 micron and contains 4 crescent-shaped sporozoites

❖ Oocyst is surrounded by thin, smooth and two layered cyst wall.

Life Cycle (Fig. 41.10)

❖ Ingestion of contaminated food or water is the source of infection in man
❖ Eight sporozoites are released from each oocyst in the upper part of small intestine where they invade epithelial cells
❖ In the cytoplasm asexually multiplication of parasite occurs to produce trophozoites
❖ Some trophozoites undergo sexual reproduction (gametogony) and produce oocysts.
❖ Sporulation of oocyst occurs in 5 days both within the host and external environment.
❖ Sporulated and unsporulated oocysts are passed through stools.

Pathogenicity

❖ May cause mild and self-limiting diarrhea.
❖ In AIDS cases, it may be associated with more severe infection.
❖ Patient may present with:
  ▪ Fever
  ▪ Headache
  ▪ Malaise
  ▪ Cholecystitis
  ▪ Persistent diarrhea
  ▪ Weight loss
  ▪ Steatorrhea
  ▪ Death.

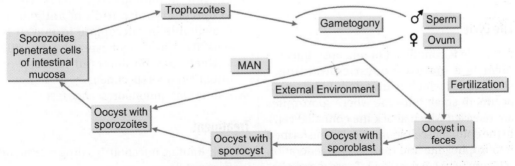

Fig. 41.10: Life cycle of *Isospora belli.*

Laboratory Diagnosis

❖ Demonstration of characteristic oocysts in stool examination in unstained and iodine stained direct smear preparation as well as by zinc sulfate and formalin ether concentration methods.
❖ Intestinal biopsy to demonstrate oocysts.
❖ Trophozoites may be demonstrated in tracheobronchial, mediastinal and mesenteric lymph nodes, gallbladder, liver and spleen of especially AIDS patients.

Treatment

Cotrimoxazole is the drug of choice in case antimicrobial treatment is indicated.

CRYPTOSPORIDIUM PARVUM

Geographical Distribution

It is cosmopolitan reported from USA, Russia, Australia, Denmark, Brazil, UK, Bangladesh, etc.

Morphology

Oocyst is demonstrable in stool and it bears following characters:
❖ It is 4 to 5 µ in diameter
❖ Contains 1 to 6 large dark granules and many small granules
❖ Mature oocyst (postsporulation) in which 2 to 4 sausage-shaped sporozoites are seen
❖ Oocyst exists in 2 forms:
    i. Thin wall oocyst
    ii. Thick wall oocyst.

Life Cycle

Life cycle is completed in one host. Infected form is a mature oocyst containing 4 sporozoites which is ingested. Excystation occurs in small intestine where sporozoites are released which attack the epithelial cells. In the epithelial cell sporozoite is transformed into trophozoite and then to first generation schizont (eight merozoites). These merozoites attack other epithelial cells and form second generation schizont (4 merozoites). These merozoites may attack other epithelial cells and later on develop into microgametocytes or macrogametocytes. A microgametocyte may give rise to 12 to 16 microgametes. On the contrary one microgametocyte gives rise to only one microgamete. A zygote is formed as a result of fertilization which develops into oocyst. Thus life cycle is completed.

Pathogenesis and Clinical Picture

This protozoa can be seen on brush borders of intestinal epithelial cells and in the crypts of Liberkuhn. The lesions may be located in small intestine and also in colon, cecum or rectum.

Cryptosporodiasis clinically resembles giardiasis. It appears as short-term cholera-like diarrheal disease. Diarrheal stools are foul smelling. It has high incidence in AIDS patients.

Laboratory Diagnosis

❖ Microscopic examination of stool for the demonstration of oocyst.
❖ Concentration method of stool examination is sugar floatation or Sheather's method.
❖ Cryptosporidium takes red stain when stained with modified acid fast method.
❖ Intestinal biopsy for microgametes and macrogametes. We can also demonstrate schizont.
❖ ELISA.
❖ Enzyme immunoassay (EIA) is useful to detect cryptosporidium antigen. It is available in microplate format. It is sensitive, specific but expensive. Specific antigen may be detected in fresh or preserved stool specimens.
❖ Indirect immunofluorescence test.

Treatment

It is self-limiting infection. No drug treatment is effective till now.

BABESIA

Geographical Distribution

Northeast USA, France, Ireland, Mexico, Russia and Scotland.

Habitat

Erythrocytes.

Morphology

Babesia are small plasmodiae-like protozoan which are pear-shaped. Human infections are reported by *Babesia bovis*, *Babesia divergens* and *Babesia microti* species.

Transmission of Infection

It is by ticks of genera Ixodes and Dermacentor. Like malaria it may be transmitted by blood transfusion too.

Incubation Period

1 to 2 weeks.

Life cycle: Like malaria, sexual cycle occurs in mammals whereas asexual cycle occurs in ticks. Ring-shaped and ameboid-shaped parasites appear in peripheral blood film. The parasite multiplies by binary fission or budding, dividing up to 4 buds at a time. A cluster of 4 small merozoites (tetrad) is a primary diagnostic finding of babesiosis.

Pathogenesis and Clinical Features

There is invasion and destruction of erythrocytes. Manifestations include splenomegaly, swelling, cellular degeneration and necrosis of hepatic sinusoids.

Laboratory Diagnosis

* Peripheral blood smear examination after staining with Giemsa or Wright stain
* Animal inoculation in which blood of patient is inoculated in hamster or gerbil. It is sensitive technique for recovery of babesia

* Serological techniques like indirect immunofluorescent antibody, complement fixation, ELISA, IHA and rapid agglutination are useful.

Treatment

Pentamidine.

PARASITES ASSOCIATED WITH AIDS

1. *Cryptosporidium*
2. *Isospora belli*
3. *Cryptospora*
4. *Microsporidia*
5. *Pneumocystis carinii*
6. *Blastocystis hominis*
7. *Leishmania species*
8. *Toxoplasma gondii*
9. *Acanthameba species*
10. *Trypanosoma cruzi*

CILIATA BALANTIDIUM COLI

Geographical Distribution

Worldwide.

Habitat

Largest protozoal parasite inhabiting large intestine of man. Also found in pigs and monkeys.

Morphology

Trophozoites (**Fig. 41.11**):
* Oval
* 50 to 200 μ × 40 to 70 μ.

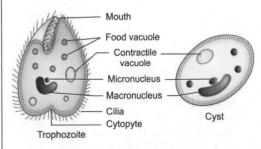

Fig. 41.11: *Balantidium coli.*

❖ Surface is pointed with delicate cilia.
❖ Anterior endpointed and has cytostome.
❖ Posterior end is round.
❖ Cytoplasm contains kidney-shaped large macronucleus and small micronucleus.

Cyst (Fig. 41.11)

❖ Oval
❖ Thick outer wall
❖ Cilia absent
❖ Protozoa is enclosed in double layered wall.

Life cycle: No intermediate host is required. The cysts are passed in stool. Infection occurs by ingestion of cyst with contaminated food or drinks. In the wall of intestine excystation occurs and trophozoites develop which live and subsequently multiply by binary fission on the mucosa of large intestine.

Pathology

Rarely, there is mucosal damage caused by trophozoites. Because of enzyme hyaluronidase produced by parasite may cause mucosal damage resulting in small superficial ulcer which may penetrate up to submucosa. Thus there is diarrhea and later frank dysentery develops. Abdominal colic, nausea and vomiting may occur.

Laboratory Diagnosis

The trophozoites and cysts may be demonstrated in the stool of patient.

Prophylaxis

❖ Improvement of personal hygiene
❖ Prevention of food contamination with stools of man as well as pigs or monkeys.

Helminths

NEMATODES

Trichinella Spiralis

Geographical Distribution

Common in Europe and USA.

Habitat

It is a parasite buried in duodenum or jejunal mucosa, fertilization of female occurs which discharges ova in circulating blood which encyst in striated muscle of man, pig or rat.

Morphology

Adult worm (male) measures 1.4 to 1.6 mm (smallest nematode) and female is 3 to 4 mm long. Larvae measure $100 \times 6 \mu$. They remain encysted in striated muscle of host and keep growing till maximum size is attained in 35 days. Lifespan of male worm is 1 week and female dies in 16 weeks. Most of larvae die within 6 months while others survive for 10 to 30 years.

Life cycle: It is passed in one host (man, pig, etc.). Male and female worms lie in the folds of intestinal villi. Fertilized female bores its way into intestinal wall. Larvae discharged into blood stream are localized in the striated muscle where encystation of larvae occurs. Infection of a new host is by ingestion of raw flesh containing encysted larvae.

Pathogenicity and Clinical Picture

Mode of infection is by ingesting infected pig's flesh. During intestinal invasion gastrointestinal symptoms appear. During invasion of muscle patient complains of remittent fever, urticarial rash, respiratory, myocardial and neurological symptoms. Stage of encystation occurs in striated muscle.

Laboratory Diagnosis

❖ Stool examination for adult worm or larvae demonstration
❖ Blood examination to detect eosinophilia
❖ Muscle biopsy
❖ X-ray examination to detect calcified cyst
❖ Serological tests like complement fixation test, latex agglutination test, etc.

Treatment

Thiabendazole is quite effective.

Trichuris Trichiura (Whipworm)

Geographical Distribution

Worldwide.

Habitat

Adult worm lives in large intestine of man.

Morphology

Adult worm in large, small, whip-shaped parasite having thin anterior end. Female worms measure 3 to 5 cm while male is slightly smaller. Cephalic end of parasite has a stylet which helps in the penetration into intestinal mucosa. The worm is oviparous.

Eggs are barrel-shaped, 25 × 50 µ containing mucous plug at both the ends. The outer shell is bile pigmented which encloses unsegmented embryo.

Life cycle: No intermediate host is required. Eggs are passed in stools of infected patient. A rhabditiform larva develops from egg and infection to healthy person occurs by ingestion of embryonated eggs in food and water. The egg shell is dissolved in the stomach and larvae liberated pass down the cecum which grow into adult worms and embed their anterior parts in the intestinal mucosa. They grow in adult form. The life-cycle is completed in one host, i.e., man.

Pathogenicity and Clinical Picture

In severe infection, abdominal pain, anorexia, vomiting, flatulence and in chronic cases anemia may develop.

Laboratory Diagnosis

It is established by detecting characteristic eggs in stool. Sometimes adult worm may be detected in stools but rarely.

Treatment

Thiabendazole, mebendazole are effective drugs.

Ascaris lumbricoides (Roundworm)

Geographical Distribution

It is cosmopolitan.

Habitat

Adult worm lives in the lumen of the small intestine (jejunum) of man.

Morphology

Adult Worm:
❖ Elongated cylindrical measuring 15 to 50 cm × 2 to 6 mm

❖ Oral cavity has 2 lateral lips and one median lip
❖ Body cavity contains toxin (ascaron) in which digestive and reproductive organs float. Ascaron is allergic.
❖ Posterior end of male is curved ventrally.
❖ Male worm is smaller than female worm.

Egg Fertilized:
❖ 45 to 75 µ × 35 to 50 µ
❖ The shell has innermost very thin vitelline membrane, a thick glycogenous middle layer and coarsely laminate outermost layer
❖ Embryo is unsegmented and made up of coarse lecithin granules
❖ Floats in saturated salt solution.

Unfertilized:
❖ Larger in size 88 to 94 µ × 45 µ
❖ The shell is relatively thin
❖ The innermost layer vitelline is absent
❖ Embryo contains disorganized mass containing refractile granules
❖ It does not develop into larvae
❖ It does not float in saturated salt solution.

Life Cycle:
❖ The female adult worm liberates fertilized eggs in small intestine which are passed with stools. The freshly passed fertilized eggs contain unsegmented ovum. At this stage they are not infective to man
❖ Rhabditiform larvae develop inside in 9 to 15 days in moist soil (22° to 33°C). A moulting occurs within the egg and then the egg becomes infective
❖ Infective eggs are swallowed with raw food material which pass through stomach into small intestine
❖ Outer shell of egg is dissolved and larva comes out in the intestinal lumen measuring 250 µ × 14 µ
❖ The larvae penetrate the mucosa and reach portal circulation thereafter to liver (live for 3 to 4 days), heart and finally to the lung alveoli.
❖ Larvae grow up to 2 mm and moult twice (5th and 6th days)

❖ The larvae from alveoli migrate to bronchioles, trachea and are swallowed back in the stomach. During this period two more moulting occur (in 25th to 29th days). In the intestine larvae develop into adult worm.

Pathogenicity and Clinical Picture

The larvae in lung alveoli cause migrating pneumonitis (allergic reaction) and this allergic reaction may be due to ascaron.

Adult worm may cause malnutrition, vague abdominal pain, colic pain, poor digestion, diarrhea, etc.
❖ Perforation of bowel, appendicitis, diverti-culitis may occur.

Laboratory Diagnosis

❖ Detection of adult worms in stool
❖ Microscopic detection of eggs in feces or bile obtained by duodenal intubation
❖ Eosinophilia
❖ Dermal reaction (allergic), scratch test with powdered ascaris antigen.

Treatment

Piperazine, decaris, albendazole, mebendazole are effective.

Ancylostoma Duodenale (Hookworm)

Geographical Distribution

It is widely found in tropical and subtropical countries.

Habitat

The adult worm resides in small intestine of man particularly in jejunum.

Morphology

Adult Worm:
❖ It is small, pinkish, fusiform in shape
❖ The anterior end is curved

❖ Female worm is 13 mm × 0.6 mm with pointed posterior end
❖ Male worm is smaller 11 mm × 0.4 mm having copulatory bursa with tripartite dorsal rays and a pair of long copulatory spicules
❖ The oral cavity has single pair of dorsal teeth and 2 pairs of ventral teeth which help the worm to get attached to the mucosa.

Egg:
❖ Oval, measuring 75 μ × 40 μ
❖ It has thin outer shell enclosing a segmented ovum with 4 segments
❖ There is a clear space between egg shell and segmented ovum
❖ It floats in saturated saline
❖ It is non-bile stained.

Life Cycle:
The adult worm lives in small intestine of man attached to the mucosa. After fertilization female lays eggs which are passed out with stool. The larvae develop from eggs outside the body of host. Freshly passed egg contains segmented embryo and in 24 hours free living rhabditiform larva is liberated. After 7 to 8 days rhabditiform larva moults twice (once on 3rd day and second on 5th day) and transforms into filariform larva which is infective. On coming in contact with skin of foot, it penetrates into hair of follicle or bores through intact skin to reach right side of heart (through lymphatics and venous blood). Thereafter larvae reach lung and after piercing capillary wall reach alveolar space. Third moulting occurs at this stage. From alveolar space larvae reach bronchioles, trachea, larynx and are swallowed back to stomach. On reaching duodenum and jejunum another moulting occurs. Here, in 5 to 7 weeks, larvae grow to mature adult form which are sexually mature.

Pathogenicity and Clinical Picture

Ancylostomiasis or hookworm disease is characterized by anemia. At the site of filariform larvae penetration, dermatitis may occur. The larvae then migrate to subcutaneous vessels and cause creeping eruption. When larvae reach lung multiple hemorrhage and transient bronchopneumonia occur. Adult worms cause irritation and petechial hemorrhage in the intestinal mucosa.

Laboratory Diagnosis

❖ Stool examination for adult worm (naked eye)
❖ Microscopic examination of stool for ova
❖ Study of duodenal contents for adult worm and ova.

Indirect Evidences:

❖ Blood examination for anemia and eosino philia
❖ Stool examination for occult blood and Charcot-Leydon crystals.

Treatment

❖ Thiabendazole, mebendazole, etc.
❖ Anemia is treated with iron, folic acid and vitamin B_{12}.

Necator Americanus (Table 42.1)

Geographical Distribution

It is the most common species in Sri Lanka and India (except Punjab and UP). It was first discovered in America. It occurs in tropics and South Africa, Far-east and Australia.

Strongyloides Stercoralis

Geographical Distribution

It is worldwide in distribution, more predominant in Brazil, Far-east and Africa.

Habitat

The female adult worm lives in the mucous membrane of small intestine.

Morphology

Females are 2.5 mm × 40 to 50 µ (hardly visible to naked eye). Males are shorter and broader than female.

Eggs measure 30 µ × 5.5 µ, thin shelled, transparent and oval, containing larvae ready to hatch. Rhabditiform larvae come out of eggs into the lumen of intestine from where they are passed with stool. Hence larvae are detected in man's stools.

Larvae are of two types—rhabditiform and filariform larvae.

Life Cycle

No intermediate host is required. Life cycle is completed in one host only. Man is the optimum host.

Table 42.1: Differences between Ancylostoma duodenale and Necator americanus.

Ancylostoma duodenale	Necator americanus
• Adult worm larger and thicker	Smaller and more slender
• Anterior end bends in the same direction as body curvature	Bends in opposite direction to body
• A spine is present at posterior end of female	Absent
• Buccal capsule has 6 teeth	4 chitinous plates
• Vulval opening behind the middle of the body	It is in front of the middle of the body
• More pathogenic because of	Less pathogenic
– large size	
– armed with teeth	
– more migratory leaving more bleeding points	

Pathogenesis and Clinical Picture

The skin lesions include urticarial rash at the site of entry and a linear, erythematous urticarial wheal around anus caused by migrating filariform larvae. Pulmonary lesions include hemorrhages in the lung alveoli and bronchopneumonia.

Laboratory Diagnosis

❖ Detection of rhabditiform larvae in freshly passed stools
❖ Eosinophilia
❖ Microscopic examination of duodenal biopsy for larvae
❖ Sputum examination for larvae
❖ Complement fixation test using filarial larvae as an antigen.

Treatment

❖ Thiabendazole.

Enterobius Vermicularis (Threadworm)

Geographical Distribution

It is cosmopolitan.

Habitat

Adult worm (female resides in cecum and appendix of man).

Morphology

The male adult worm is 5 mm × 0.5 mm in diameter while female measures 8 to 12 mm × 0.3 to 0.5 mm. The posterior end of female is sharp and pointed while it is curved in males. Male dies after fertilization while gravid female dies after oviposition within 2 to 3 weeks.

Eggs are colorless, planoconvex, 50 to 60 μ × 30 μ, surrounded by transparent shell and contains coiled tadpole-like larvae.

Life Cycle

The female worm when fully gravid passes down to migrate several inches outside the anus to deposit eggs. These eggs are transferred by fingers (autoinfection) and by contaminated food or fomites to the mouth and they are swallowed. On reaching the intestine, outer shell is dissolved by digestive enzyme thus liberating the larvae. In the presence of oxygen, larvae become infective.

Pathogenesis and Clinical Picture

The movement of adult worm (female) at the time of laying eggs causes intense itching inducing the patient to scratch the affected area (anal canal and perianal skin). The scratched area may become eczematoid.

Laboratory Diagnosis

❖ Detection of adult worm in the stools
❖ Demonstration of eggs in stool and finger nails, perianal skin scraping and washings from underwear.

Treatment

❖ Piperazine.

Dracunculus Medinensis (Guinea Worm)

In 1984, there were around 40,000 guinea worm cases in 12,840 villages in 89 districts of seven endemic states. However, only 371 cases of guinea worms were reported during the year 1994 which is a reduction of over 99% as compared to year 1984. Majority of these cases were from the states of Rajasthan (93%) followed by Madhya Pradesh 4% and Karnataka 3%. This is because of successful strategy adopted by Guinea Worm Eradication Programme including continuous detection and surveillance of guinea worm cases, prompt and free treatment, vector control through temephos application to drinking water sources, supply to fine nylon meshy stainers, etc.

The last case of guinea worm infection, Banwari Lal, 25 years old was reported in Jodhpur district of Rajasthan in 1996. The International Commission for the certification of Dracunculiasis Eradication has declared India to be free from guinea worm in the year 2000.

Geographical Distribution

India (especially Rajasthan), Burma, Arabia, Africa, West Indies, Russia and America.

Habitat

The adult female is usually found in subcutaneous tissue (legs, arms and back).

Morphology

Female adult worm is long, cord-like, measuring 60 to 100 cm × 1 to 1.5 mm. At blunt end there lies triangular mouth lined with thick cuticle. Male worm measures 2 to 4 cm in length. The body is cylindrical, smooth and milk white in color. The worm in viviparous and discharges embryo in successive batches. Body fluid is toxic. The life-span of female is one year and that of male is 6 months.

Embryos are coiled bodies with rounded head and long slender tapering tails. They measure 650 to 750 µ × 17 to 20 µ.

Life Cycle

Two hosts are required, man being definitive host and cyclops serve as intermediate host. Cyclops with larvae are swallowed in drinking water. The cyclops are digested in the stomach of man and larvae are liberated. They penetrate gut wall and enter retroperitoneal connective tissue where they mature into adult males and females. Male dies after fertilization of female. The gravid female reaches the skin of those parts of body which usually come in contact with water (feet, legs, shoulder, back). On reaching skin, toxin in secreted and blisters are produced. When blisters burst on coming in contact with water, embryos are discharged in water. Embryos reach cyclops and the cycle is repeated.

Pathogenesis and Clinical Picture

The worm produces a reddish papule (2 to 7 mm) which later on becomes vesicle. The central portion is necrosed to form ulcer with burning itch.

Laboratory Diagnosis

❖ Detection of adult worm
❖ Detection of embryo as milky fluid
❖ Intradermal test
❖ X-ray (calcified worm).

Treatment

❖ Extraction of worm
❖ Ambithus to kill worm.

Wuchereria Bancrofti

Geographical Distribution

It is confined to the tropics and subtropical regions. In India, endemic areas are along the sea coast and banks of large rivers.

Habitat

Adult worms are found in lymphatic vessels and lymph nodes of man only. Microfilaria are found in the blood.

Morphology

Adult Worm:
❖ Male and female worms remain coiled together
❖ Adult female worm is about 8 to 10 cm long and 0.24 to 0.3 mm wide
❖ Adult male is 4 cm long and 0.1 mm wide
❖ Anterior end is ventrally curved in case of male
❖ Life-span of adult worm is 10 to 15 years.

Microfilaria:
❖ 230 to 296 µ in length covered by delicate sheath
❖ Double row of nuclei are present all along the length except posterior end
❖ Life-span in human blood is 70 days.

Life Cycle

The man is the definitive host and mosquito (culex, aedes and anopheles) acts as intermediate host.

Adult worms live in the lymph nodes, lymphatics and body cavities of man. After fertilization the gravid female produces larvae (microfilaria) which are active and reach general blood circulation periodically.

When female mosquito bites the infected man microfilaria are sucked with blood meal and reach mosquito gut. There microfilaria shed their sheath and penetrate the gut wall to reach the thoracic muscles of mosquito where microfilariae develop into infective filariform larvae. After 2 moultings (4th and 6th days) the infective forms migrate from thoracic muscles to the mouth parts.

When such mosquito bites a healthy person the infective larvae migrate by process of chemotaxis to the wound produced by mosquito. They penetrate the skin through wound and reach subcutaneous lymphatics and then gradually migrate to various tissue. They undergo 2 moultings and mature to develop in adult worm in about one year.

Clinical Picture and Pathogenesis

Site of localization is according to the site of bite. It may be in lymphatic system of superior or inferior extremities.

The microfilaria in peripheral blood stream are harmless. However, it may cause eosinophilia, lymphangitis, choroid degeneration and granulomatous lesions in the tissues.

The adult worm may cause inflammatory lesion in the body tissues. Recurrent attacks of inguinal lymphadenitis, orchitis, funiculitis, epididymitis, etc. are caused due to mechanical irritation by parasite or by the action of toxins secreted by worms. Secondary bacterial infection may precipitate acute exacerbation.

Mechanical obstruction of the lymphatics by adult worms and inflammatory reaction in surrounding tissue causes localized edema, lymph, varices, hydrocele, chyluria, chylous ascites and chylous diarrhea. Recurrent attacks of lymphangitis leads to elephantiasis.

In occult filariasis microfilaria are absent in peripheral blood but they are present in lymph

Table 42.2: Differences between classical and occult filariasis.

Classical	Occult
• Due to adult worms	Microfilaria
• Lymphatics and lymph nodes are involved	Lymphatic vessels lungs, liver and spleen
• Microfilaria present in peripheral blood	Absent in blood but present in tissues
• Lesions produced are lymphangitis and lymphadenitis	Eosinophilic granuloma
• No therapeutic response	Responds to microfilaria killing drugs like DEC

nodes and other internal organs like lungs, liver and spleen **(Table 42.2)**. Occult filaria is also called tropical pulmonary eosinophilia. It is believed to be due to immune response. It is characterized by high eosinophil counts, high antibody titer to filariae, high IgE levels, nocturnal wheezing, cough and dyspnea, etc.

Laboratory Diagnosis

❖ Demonstration of microfilaria
    i. Direct unstained smear
    ii. Stained smear (Leishman stain)
    iii. Concentration techniques like membrane concentration
    iv. DEC provocation test
    v. Microfilaria may be demonstrated in lymph, chylous, urine, hydrocele fluid, etc.
❖ Demonstration of adult worm in biopsied lymph node and calcified worm in X-rays
❖ Serodiagnosis is done using IHA, ELISA, IFA and RIA tests. Other test like intradermal, CFT using *Dirofilaria immitis* antigens, are neither specific nor sensitive
❖ Xenodiagnosis.

Treatment

Diethylcarbamazine (DEC).

Brugia Malayi

Geographical Distribution

It occurs in India, Indonesia, Malaysia, Thailand, Vietnam, China, Burma, Korea, etc.

Habitat

Adult worm is found in the lymphatic system.

Morphology

Adult worms are slightly smaller otherwise resemble *Wuchereria bancrofti*. Microfilaria shows following peculiarities.

- Smaller in size and lies folded with head close to tail
- Possesses secondary kinks
- The nuclei are curved hence difficult to count
- Two distinct nuclei one at the tip of tail and another subterminal one
- Cephalic space twice as long as broad.

Life Cycle

It resembles *Wuchereria bancrofti*. Intermediate host is mansonia (Indian species *Mansonia annulifera*). Larval development is completed in 6 to 8 days. The microfilaria is nocturnal periodic.

Pathogenicity and Clinical Picture

Lymphangitis and elephantiasis are produced.

Treatment

Diethylcarbamazine (DEC).

Onchocerca Volvulus

Geographical Distribution

Africa, Central America and South Arabia.

Habitat

Adult worms reside in the subcutaneous connective tissue of man.

Morphology

Male adult worm is 3 × 0.13 mm with coiled tail. The female measures up to 50 × 0.4 mm. The gravid female may live up to 15 years. Cuticular oblique and annular thickening is more prominent in females.

Microfilariae are unsheathed and non-periodic found in skin. They measure 300 μ × 6 to 8 μ. The column of nuclei does not extend up to the tail.

Life Cycle

Man is the definitive host while day biting female black fly (simulium) is intermediate host. Development in black fly is completed in 6 days.

Pathogenicity and Clinical Picture

The incubation period is one year. The adult worm resides in subcutaneous connective tissues only. Following lesions are produced.

- Subcutaneous nodule formation due to adult worm
- Dermatitis, pruritis may be caused by toxin from larva or adult worm. Development of hydrocele, elephantiasis of leg and scrotum may occur
- Occular lesions are caused by microfilariae.

Laboratory Diagnosis

- Demonstration of microfilaria in shaved pieces of skin and adult worm inside excised nodules
- In ocular lesion, microfilariae are detected by means of slit lamp
- Eosinophilia.

Treatment

Enucleation of nodules and use of drugs like DEC or Surmic.

Loa Loa

Geographical Distribution

Occurs in Central and West Africa.

Habitat

Adult worms live in subcutaneous connective tissues of man often in subconjunctival tissues of eye.

Morphology

Male adult worm measures 3 mm × 0.35 mm. Female measures 6 cm × 0.5 mm. The life-span of adult worms may be 15 years or more.

Embryo measures 300 μ × 7 μ and is enveloped in a sheath. They are found in peripheral blood during daytime.

Life Cycle

It passes its Life cycle in man and chrysops. Larval form follows the same course as in other microfilariae. Loa loa is maintained in nature by interhuman transmission.

Pathogenicity and Clinical Picture

The incubation period is 3 to 4 years. With the bite of chrysops, embryo is introduced in man. It gets migrated rapidly to various parts of the body and in subdermal connective tissue. It shows predilection for creeping in and around eyes. The disease is named as loiasis.

Treatment

Diethylcarbamazine (DEC).

Mansonella ozzardi

Geographical Distribution

West Indies, Central America and South America.

Habitat

Adult worm lives in the mesentery of man.

Morphology

Adult worm (female) is 7 cm × 0.25 mm. The cuticula is smooth and the tail end possesses a pair of flaps like papillae.

Microfilariae are found in blood. They are small unsheathed and non-periodic. The tail end is sharply pointed.

Pathogenicity

Nonpathogenic.

Laboratory Diagnosis

By demonstrating microfilaria in blood.

Cestodes

It means girdles or ribbon. They are segmented tapeworm whose size vary from few mm to several meters. They do not have body cavity or alimentary canal. Nervous system and excretory system is rudimentary. They are hermaphrodite.

Medically important tapeworms are:

A. Pseudophyllidean tapeworms
- *Diphyllobothrium latum* (fish tapeworm)
- *Sparganum mansoni* and *sparganum proliferum*

B. Cyclophyllidean tapeworms
1. Genus *taenia*
   - *Taenia saginata* (beef tapeworm)
   - *Taenia solium* (pork tapeworm).
2. Genus *Echinococcus*
   - *Echinococcus granulosus* (dog tapeworm)
   - *Echinococcus multilocularis.*
3. Genus *hymenolepis*
   - *Hymenolepis nana* (dwarf tapeworm)
   - *Hymenolepis diminuta* (rat tapeworm).

Diphyllobothrium Latum (Fish Tapeworm)

Geographical Distribution

Central and Southern Europe especially in Scandinavian countries. Also occurs in Siberia, Japan, North America and South Africa. It has not been reported from India so far.

Habitat

Small intestine of man, dog, cat, fox, etc.

Morphology

The adult worm measures 3 to 10 meters in length and the life-span is 5 to 15 years. The

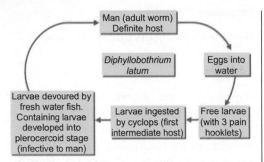

Fig. 42.1: Life *cycle of Diphyllobothrium latum.*

head (scolex) is elongated and spoon shaped with 2 slit-like grooves (bothria) measuring 2 × 3 × 1 mm³. It lacks rostellum or hooklets. The neck is thin and unsegmented. The body segments are 3000 to 4000 and are greater in breadth than length. Each segment measures 2 mm × 10 to 20 mm.

Life Cycle (Fig. 42.1)

There are two intermediate hosts, i.e., (i) fresh water cyclops and (ii) fresh water fish. Man is the definitive host.

Clinical Picture

❖ Gastrointestinal problem
❖ Macrocytic anemia
❖ Eosinophilia.

Laboratory Diagnosis

❖ Microscopic examination of stool for the demonstration of operculated eggs
❖ Examination of segments passed in feces.

Treatment

Niclosamides, quinacrine, praziquantel are useful drugs.

Prophylaxis Prevention

Proper cooking of fish, checking of fecal contamination of water and deworming of pet dogs and cats.

Taenia Saginata (Beef Tapeworm)

Geographical Distribution

Worldwide in distribution. In India, it is prevalent in Mohammadens who are beef eaters.

Habitat

The scolex of grown-up worm embedded in the mucosa of the wall of ileum and rest of worm extends through the lumen.

Morphology (Fig. 42.2)

Adult Worm:
❖ It is white transparent tape-like
❖ It measures 5 to 12 meters (up to 24 meters)
❖ Scolex is pear-shaped 1 to 2 mm in diameter with 4 round suckers without rostellum and hooks
❖ Neck is long and narrow
❖ Proglottids may be up to 2000 in number, terminal gravid segment 2 cm × 0.5 cm, genital pore is situated near the margin at the posterior end of each segment alternating irregularly in right and left margin, gravid uterus having 15 to 30 lateral branches

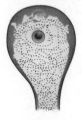
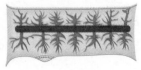
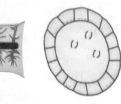

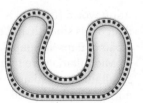

Scolex with 4 suckers   Mature segment   Egg   Cysticercus

Fig. 42.2: *Taenia saginata.*

❖ Gravid segments are expelled singly
❖ Adult worm is usually single in a host
❖ Life-span of adult worm is nearly 10 years.

Larvae:
❖ It is called *cysticercus bovis*
❖ It is found only in cattle
❖ It is eliptical in shape (7.5 mm × 5.5 mm).

Egg:
❖ Spherical and measures 30 to 40 µ in diameter
❖ Bile stained
❖ Thin outer transparent shell
❖ Embryophore is brown in color, thick-walled radially striated
❖ Contains an oncosphere with 3 pairs of hooklets
❖ Does not float in saturated saline solution
❖ About 80,000 eggs in a proglottid which are liberated by rupture of mature proglottid
❖ Eggs remain viable up to 8 weeks.

Life Cycle

Man is the definitive host whereas cow or buffalo acts as intermediate hosts.

Eggs are passed out with stools on the ground and cow or buffalo swallow these eggs while grazing in the field. The eggs are not infective to man. In the intestine eggs rupture with liberation of oncospheres which penetrate gut wall with the help of hooks, enter blood stream and are filtered into muscular tissues (tongue, neck, shoulder and cardiac muscles) where they settle and grow. In 8 days oncospheres are transformed into *cysticercus bovis*.

Man is infected by eating uncooked beef containing cysticerci (measly beef). In the intestine scolex exvaginates (stimulation by bile) and anchor to the gut wall by its suckers and slowly grows into adult worm. It attains sexual maturity in 2 to 3 months and starts producing eggs.

Clinical Picture

It is usually asymptomatic. It may cause abdominal discomfort, hunger pain, indigestion, diarrhea alternating with constipation, loss of appetite, pruritus ani, intestinal obstruction and appendicitis.

Laboratory Diagnosis

❖ Demonstration of proglottids or eggs.
❖ Serodiagnosis is done with the help of tests like indirect hemagglutination, IFA and ELISA.

Treatment

Niclosamide, mebendazole, praziquantel and bithional are the drugs used.

Taenia Solium (Pork Tapeworm)

Geographical Distribution

It is worldwide especially in pork eating persons.

Habitat

Adult worm lives in the small intestine.

Morphology (Table 42.3)

Adult Worm (Fig. 42.2):
❖ It measures 2 to 3 meters long
❖ Scolex is pinhead size, globular in outline with 4 suckers and head is provided with

Table 42.3: Differences between Taenia solium and Taenia saginata.

Taenia solium	Taenia saginata
• 2 to 3 meters	5 to 10 meters
• Below 1000 proglottids	Above 1000
• Nonpigmented suckers	Pigmented
• Hooklets present	Absent
• Gravid proglottid	2 × 0.6 cm
• 1.2 cm × 0.6 cm	
• Proglottids expelled in the chain of 5 to 6	Single proglottid crawls out of anus
• Uterine branches	15 to 30 dichotomus
• 5 to 10 dendritic	
• 150 to 200 testicular follicles	300 to 400
• Accessory ovarian lobe	Absent
• Vaginal sphincter absent	Present
• Neck of worm short	Long
• Life-span up to 25 years	10 years
• Scolex globular	Quadrate
• Rostellum present	Absent

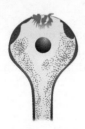
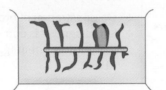
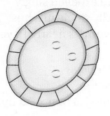
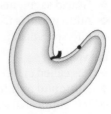

| Scolex with 4 suckers, rostellum having 2 rows of hooks | Mature segment (uterus with few branches) | Egg | Cysticercus cellulosae |

Fig. 42.3: *Taenia solium.*

rostellum with two rows (small and large) of hooklets
- ❖ Neck is short 5 to 10 mm
- ❖ Proglottids 1000, gravid segment longer than broader while immature segment broader than longer, genital pores lie laterally at middle of each segment (alternating left and right), testis with 150 to 200 follicles, ovary with two symmetrical lobes and an accessory lobe and gravid segments are passed passively in the stool.

Larva (Fig. 42.3):
- ❖ It is called *cysticercus cellulosae*
- ❖ Occurs in pig and man
- ❖ It is small, oval, milky white bladder measuring 8 to 10 mm in breadth and 5 mm in length
- ❖ Contains milky fluid rich in albumin and salts
- ❖ It lies parallel to muscle fibers as white spot which represents future head invaginated into bladder
- ❖ The pork containing cysticercus is usually named as measly pork.

Eggs (Fig. 42.3):
Morphological features resemble that of eggs of *Taenia saginata.*

Life Cycle

Similar to the Life cycle of *Taenia saginata.* However, larval stage (cysticercus cellulosae) occurs in man too. Man acquires infection by eating inadequately cooked pork (containing cysticercus cellulosae) or by ingesting eggs of

Taenia solium by consuming contaminated food and drinks.

Clinical Picture

As in *Taenia solium.*

Diagnosis

- ❖ Demonstration of proglottids or eggs.

Treatment

- ❖ Same as of *Taenia saginata.*

Cysticercus Cellulosae

Morphology
- ❖ Measures 10 mm by 5 mm.
- ❖ It has opaque invaginated scolex with 4 suckers, hooks and bladder filled with fluid.
- ❖ Development to the infective form usually takes 9 to 10 weeks.

Transmission

- ❖ By ingestion of eggs of *Taenia solium*
- ❖ By autoinfection (reverse peristalsis)
- ❖ External re-infection from anus to finger to mouth.

Clinical Features

- ❖ It may be asymptomatic
- ❖ Symptomatic picture includes involvement of eye, skin, viscera and muscles. Neuro cysticercosis involve CNS and spinal cord and presents as epilepsy, hydrocephalus,

encephalitis, diplopia, aphasia, amnesia, etc.

Laboratory Diagnosis

❖ Biopsy of nodule and study of its histological picture
❖ Radiology
❖ Serological tests like complement fixation test, indirect hemagglutination, ELISA and immunofluorescence using crude antigen (extracted from pig cysticerci) and purified antigen.

Treatment

Surgical excision or drugs like praziquantel is quite effective.

Echinococcus Granulosus (Dog Tapeworm)

Geographical Distribution

Worldwide more prevalent in temperate climate than tropical areas. It is quite common in cattle and sheep predominating places. From India, West Asia and Mediterranean countries, high incidences of hydatid cyst are reported.

Habitat

Adult worm is found in the small intestine of canines like dog. Larval form is found most commonly in liver, lungs, etc. of man.

Morphology

Adult Worm:
❖ Attached to the wall of intestine of canines like dogs
❖ It has scolex, neck and 3 to 5 segments
❖ It measures about 3 to 9 mm in length
❖ Scolex is spherical provided with rostellum carrying 30 to 40 hooks in 2 rows. There are four suckers
❖ First one or two segments are immature followed by segment sexually mature

❖ The last segment is gravid one containing about 400 to 500 eggs. The uterus bursts open before evacuation of gravid proglottides into the intestine. Thus, the process of release of eggs occurs
❖ Life-span is about 6 months.

Eggs:
❖ Spherical
❖ 31 to 40 μ
❖ The outer shell surrounds the inner embryophore.
❖ Oncosphere has 3 pairs of hooklets within embryophore
❖ Eggs resemble other taeniid species of dog
❖ Eggs survive in the soil for 6 to 12 months
❖ Eggs are infective to man, cattle and sheep.

Larval Form:
❖ It is found within hydatid cyst growing in the organs of sheep, cattle and man
❖ Future scolex of adult worm remains invaginated within vesicular body
❖ Larval form remains live and continues to develop for many years.

Life Cycle

Dogs, pigs, fox and jackal are definitive hosts. Intermediate hosts are sheep, goat, cattle, horse, pig and man.

As a result of disintegration of gravid proglottids in the intestine eggs are discharged through stools of definite host. Ingestion of contaminated food (with eggs of *Echinococcus granulosus*) by intermediate host results in hatching out of hexacanth embryo out of eggs (8 hours after ingestion). This liberated oncosphere penetrates the mesenteric blood vessels and gets distributed to various organs of the body like liver, lungs, etc. Wherever embryo settles it grows into hydatid cyst containing thousands of scolices.

The hydatids are ingested by definite host, e.g., dog and grow into adult worms in 6 to 7 weeks in the intestine and start laying eggs which are passed through stools. Thus, life cycle is repeated.

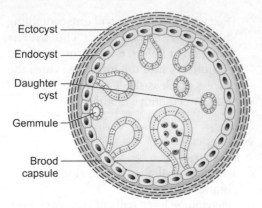

Fig. 42.4: Structure of hydatid cyst.

Hydatid Cyst (Fig. 42.4)

It grows very slowly. At the end of a year it is about 5 cm in diameter. Hydatid cyst consists of:

Ectocyst
* It is 1 mm thick.
* It is outer cuticular layer which is as matter of fact laminated hyaline membrane.
* It is elastic in nature and resembles the white of a hard boiled egg.

Endocyst
* It is an inner germinal layer
* It is cellular and consists of a number of nuclei dispersed in a protoplasmic mass
* It is about 1/4th of mm
* It has a role in the formation of outer layer, secretion of hydatid fluid and to form brood capsule with scolices.

Hydatid Fluid
* It is secreted by endocyst
* It is clear, colorless or pale yellow fluid, weakly acidic, of low specific gravity, containing sodium chloride, sodium sulfate, sodium phosphate, and calcium salts of succinic acid. It is antigenic, highly toxic and provides nutrition for developing scolices.

Hydatid Sand
* It is granular deposit
* It consists of liberated brood capsules, free scolices and loose hooklets.

Formation of Daughter Cysts

The endogenous daughter cyst develops inside the mother cyst and can also develop from detached fragment of germinal layer. On the other hand exogenous daughter cyst development results owing to increased intracystic pressure which may cause either herniation or rupture of germinal as well as laminated layers through weakened part of the adventia, e.g., bone hydatid disease.

Animal Model

They are golden hamsters and guinea pigs.

Immunology

Both humoral (IgG or IgE) and cell-mediated immune responses are involved. Immune unresponsiveness is reported in about 10% cases.

Clinical Features

Location of cyst and its stage of development give rise to particular signs and symptoms. It may remain asymptomatics for years altogether and is found accidentally. Rupture of cyst gives rise to allergic symptoms and signs, e.g., rupture in lungs causes chest pain, cough, dyspnea and hemoptysis. Cyst in cerebrum may give rise to epilepsy. A cyst in kidney may cause hematuria.

Laboratory Diagnosis

* DLC shows eosinophilia in many cases
* X-rays, CT scan, angiography, ultrasound and magnetic resonance imaging (MRI)
* Exploratory cyst puncture is dangerous because of accidental spilling of contents resulting to secondary spread or anaphylaxis
* Detection of scolex in stool, sputum or vomiting in cases where cyst ruptures into bile duct, intestine or bronchus
* Casoni test where 0.2 mL of hydatid fluid (filtered by Seitz or membrane) is injected intradermally in one ventral aspect of forearm and an equal volume of saline as a control in the other forearm. In positive

case, a large wheel about 5 cm in diameter with multiple pseudopodia-like projections appears in 30 minutes only at test side which fades away in 60 minutes. It is sensitive but not specific test.

Serodiagnostic tests are as under:

- Complement fixation test (CFT)
- Indirect hemagglutination (IHA)
- Counter current immunoelectrophoresis
- ELISA
- Radioimmunoassay (RIA)
- Dot ELISA
- Indirect immunofluorescence test (IFT).

Treatment

❖ Surgical extraction of hydatid cyst
❖ Albendazole and mebendazole are also reported as effected in treating metacestodes of *E. granulosus.*

Echinococcus Multiloculares

The salient features are:

❖ It is prevalent in Germany, Switzerland, North Vietnam, China, Russia, etc.
❖ Causes multilocular hydatid disease
❖ Adult worm is relatively smaller than *E. granulosus*
❖ Eggs are more resistant to cold
❖ Life cycle involves foxes and oriental rodent
❖ Major source of human infection is fruits and vegetable contaminated with feces of fox, etc.
❖ Liver is more commonly involved
❖ Cyst lacks fluid and there is no hyaline membrane and capsule. Cyst is sterile. Germinal layer is hyperplastic
❖ It has features resembling malignant neoplasm
❖ Metastasis occurs in blood and secondary lesions usually in the brain and lungs.

Hymenolepis Nana (Dwarf Tapeworm)

Geographical Distribution

It is cosmopolitan in distribution more predominantly seen in warm climate.

Habitat

It lives in the upper two-third of the ileum.

Morphology

❖ It is one of the small intestinal cestodes infecting man
❖ It is 1 to 4 cm long and 1 mm thick
❖ It has short lifespan (2 weeks)
❖ Scolex has 4 suckers and a single row of hooklets
❖ There are 200 segment and each mature segment measures 0.3 mm × 0.9 mm

Eggs:

❖ Spherical or ovoid measuring 30 to 45 μ
❖ There is thin colorless outer membrane and an inner embryophore
❖ Embryophore encloses hexacanth oncosphere
❖ The space between two membranes contains yolk granules and 4 to 8 polar filaments arising from two knobs of embryophore. Eggs are non-bile stained and float in saturated saline solution.

Life Cycle (Fig. 42.5)

The life cycle takes place in man. There is no intermediate host. *H. nana* undergoes multiplication in the body of host unlike other helminths.

A different strain of *H. nana* infects rat and mice. The eggs passed in rodent stools are ingested by rat flea *(Xenopsylla cheopis)* which act as intermediate host. The eggs develop into cysticercoid larvae in the hemocele of these insects. Rodents get infected when they eat these insects. Human strain may infect rodent

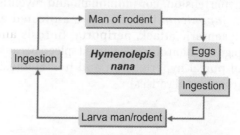

Fig. 42.5: Life cycle of *Hymenolepis nana.*

which constitutes a reservoir of infection for the human parasite.

Clinical Picture

Generally, it does not produce any problem. However, sometimes symptoms occur due to allergic response like abdominal discomfort, diarrhea, pruritus, weight loss, weakness, irritability and keratoconjunctivitis.

Laboratory Diagnosis

❖ Demonstration of eggs from the feces either in direct smear or formal ether concentration is useful in establishing the diagnosis.

Treatment

Niclosamide.

▌TREMATODES

Schistosoma

They are also called blood flukes. *Schistosoma hematobium* (bilharzia) involves predominantly genitourinary system, *S. mansoni* the gastro-intestinal tract and *S. japonicum* the small and large intestine, liver and central nervous system.

General Clinical Symptoms

Schistosoma hematobium causes urinary schistosomiasis characterized by painless terminal hematuria. In *S. mansoni* infection is manifested as dysenteric attacks, hepatomegaly, periportal cirrhosis, portal hypertension, cor pulmonale and myelitis. *S. japonicum* infection is manifested as dysenteric attack, periportal fibrosis and pigmentation of liver, enlarged spleen because of portal hypertension and hematemesis (esophageal varices).

Schistosoma hematobium (Bilharzia Hematobium)

Geographical Distribution

Nile valley, most parts of Africa and West Asia. Some endemic areas in Ratnagiri, south of Bombay were reported by Gadgil and Shah in 1952.

Habitat

The adult worm lives in urinary bladder and pelvic plexuses of veins.

Morphology

The male is 10 to 15 mm long and 1 mm thick. It is covered by finely tuberculated cuticle. There are two muscular suckers the oral sucker is small while the ventral sucker is large and prominent. There is gynecophoric canal in which the female worm is held. It begins behind the ventral sucker and extends to the caudal end. The adult female is 20 mm by 0.25 mm with cuticular tubercles confined to the two ends (**Fig. 42.6**).

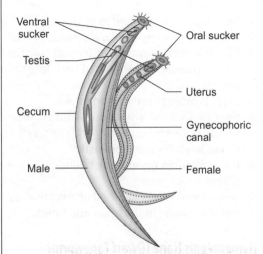

Fig. 42.6: Morphology of *Schistosoma hematobium*.

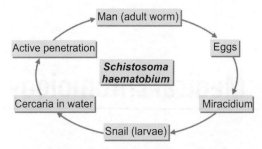

Fig. 42.7: Life cycle of *Schistosoma hematobium*.

The eggs are ovoid 150 μ by 50 μ with a brownish transparent shell having a terminal spine at one pole.

Life Cycle (Fig. 42.7)

Man is a definitive host. The infection is acquired from fresh water containing infective cercaria larvae. The intermediate host is snail. In India the species of snail is limpet *Ferrisia tenuis.*

Cercariae swim about in water after being released from infected snail. If within 1 to 3 days they come in contact with host (bathing or wading in water), they penetrate through the intact skin. Skin penetration is facilitated by lytic substances secreted by penetration glands present in cercaria.

On entering the skin, the cercaria shed their tails and become schistosomules which enter the peripheral venules. Through vena cava they enter right heart, lungs, left heart and ultimately go to systemic circulation finally reaching liver. About 20 days after skin penetration they become sexually mature and differentiated inside intrahepatic portal veins. Then they reach vesiate and peloic venous plexus via inferior mesenteric veins. They further gain maturity and start laying eggs. Eggs start appearing in urine 10 to 12 weeks after cercarial penetration. The lifespan of adult worm is 20 to 30 years.

Pathogenicity and Clinical Features

The clinical features during penetration are cercarial dermatitis (itching) and anaphylactic or toxic symptoms (fever, headache, malaise and urticaria).

The typical manifestation because of egg laying and extrusion is painless hematuria. Cystoscopy shows hyperplasia and inflammation of bladder mucosa with minute papular or vesicular lesion.

In chronic stage there may be generalized hyperplasia and fibrosis of the vesical mucosa with a granular appearance known as sandy patch. There is pseudoabscesses formation at the sites of deposition of the eggs with the infiltration of lymphocytes, plasma cells and eosinophils. To start with trigone is involved but later on inflammation of entire mucosa with thickening and ulceration occurs followed by secondary bacterial infection which ultimately leads to chronic cystitis. There may be deposition of uric acid and oxalate crystals around the eggs and obstructive hyperplasia of ureter and urethra. Schistosomiasis favors urinary carriage of typhoid bacilli and chronic schistosomiasis is associated with bladder cancer tentatively.

Laboratory Diagnosis

❖ Blood examination for eosinophilia and aldehyde test
❖ Eggs with terminal spine may be demonstrated by microscopic examination of centrifuged deposits of urine of the patient (urine especially at the end of micturition). Eggs are also seen in seminal fluid, feces, vesical or rectal biopsies, etc
❖ Intradermal allergic test (Fairley's test)
❖ Complement fixation test
❖ Bentonite flocculation
❖ Indirect hemagglutination test
❖ Immunofluorescence
❖ Gell diffusion
❖ ELISA
❖ Circumoval precipitation where there is globular or segmented precipitation around schistosome eggs incubated in positive sera.
❖ Cercarian Hullen reaction where there is development of pericercarial membrane around cercariae incubated in positive sera.

Treatment

Metrifonater or praziquantel are useful.

Medical Entomology

INTRODUCTION

Insects form the largest group of species in the animal kingdom and most important source of human diseases. Their medical importance lies to their capacity to cause morbidity and mortality and their extensive distribution over the face of the earth. In most instances, the microorganism were first of all the parasites of insects, and majority of microorganism are so well-adopted to the insects host that they produce no tissue damage.

Arthropods as transmitters of pathogens: As transmitters of various pathogens to man, insects vary in the intimacy of their association with the disease producing microorganisms. They may only be mechanical vectors of etiologic agent. Most important insect transmitted diseases employ the insect as biological vector, requiring a period of incubation or development in this host. For example, trypanosome or malarial parasite develop inside tsetse fly and female anopheles mosquito respectively before they become infective to man. Rocky Mountain spotted fever, scrub typhus, filaria infection are other examples of biological vectors.

Non-blood sucking flies may deposit a vomit drop containing pathogens on human food or drink, e.g., typhoid infection of man. Some non-blood sucking flies may ingest filth during their larval (i.e., maggot) stage and their associated pathogens may be retained in their intestine during the period of pupation, later to be deposited by the adult fly on human food or human tissues.

Blood sucking insects may introduce microorganisms into the human skin. They obtain parasite organisms in a blood meal from patient and later deposit them a vomit drop in the puncture wound (plague), or in fecal pellets near the puncture wound (typhus) made in the skin of uninfected person. Still others discharge, the organisms (malaria sporozoites) through hypopharynx in minute droplets of salivary secretion at the time they puncture, a blood meal or (filaria larvae) from proboscis sheath, thus, enabling the pathogens to migrate.

Bugs have thwarted human efforts to establish stable and safe environments throughout the past centuries. During sixth century BC, malaria and plague flourished in newly established cities.

Although various insects were known to live on the outer surfaces of mammals, untill 19th century little was known of the relationship between insects and disease agents. Towards, the end of the 19th century, scientists launched an intensive, systematic study of infectious diseases. One product of this work was the demonstration in 1893 by T Smith et al. that ticks transmit the protozoa *Babesia bigemina*, which causes Texas cattle, or red water fever.

The discovery of this insect microbial association provided a model that investigators could use to show the significance of other insects to disease epidemiology. Sir Ronald Ross applied the model in his way, demonstrating the importance of *Anopheles* spp. mosquitoes to malaria.

In recent years, knowledge of insects borne diseases has increased immeasurably. Along with several areas of related research this knowledge forms the specialization referred to as medical entomology. This field of study is concerned with the recognition and description of insects, the distribution of insect associated diseases, the effect of disease agents on the insect vector, the effect of disease agent on the host, and the control of insects.

Sources of Pathogens Transmitted by Insects

Man himself is the only source from which anopheles mosquito obtains the infection. Filaria worms which infect man are almost invariably derived from human sources. However, *Brugia malayi* may be derived from resevoir host strains. Bubonic plague is obtained by flea from the rat. Epidemic typhus passes from man to man, with the body louse as the transmitting insect.

Insect as Etiologic Agents of Disease

In addition to their role in transmission of pathogenic organisms to man, insects themselves play a significant role as disease producing organisms. Larval stage of the myiasis producing flies, the chigoe and the sarcoptic mite, invade the tissue of man and produce serious lesions. Trauma results when tick introduces its hypostome and chelicerate into the skin preparatory to obtaining a blood meal from man. Certain ticks produce paralysis in some persons, presumably due to toxins in their secretions. Venoms introduced into the skin by the bite of scorpion or black widow spider or bee at times produce both local reactions and profound systemic shock. Blood sucking flies, in depositing droplets of saliva in the skin, may provoke serious allergic reactions.

Physiology of Insects

The growth hormone of all insects is ecdysone, secreted by the prothoracic gland. It stimulates growth and differentiation of all tissue except muscle which requires a neurosecretory hormone.

Biology of Insects

The insects were originally aquatic which always breathe by means of gills. Many insects forms have to remain on land or to the air and, as a result, the gills have been sunk into the body to form back lungs, or have completely atrophied and have been replaced by a tracheal system of respiration. In aerial species wings have developed. Conquest of several of the most deadly human diseases has been or will be made possible only by control of insect transmitters.

Life Cycle of Insects

Life cycle of an insect starts when egg produced by female is inseminated by a spermatozoon from male. In some cases the egg proceeds with its development even without fertilization. Among the less highly developed groups of insect, the stages in development consist of egg followed by one or more larval stages (resembling the adults) and finally adult stage. However, in several groups of insects, there is a appreciable morphologic transformation between the last larval stage and the adult with a pupa or "resting stage" inbetween. Still between the simplest and most complex types of development, there are groups with partial metamorphosis.

Bed Bugs (Cimicidae)

❖ 13 mm long
❖ Broad flat reddish brown insects
❖ In males the abdomen is pointed at the tip
❖ In females abdomen is evenly rounded
❖ The greater part of the body is covered with bristles **(Fig. 43.1)**
❖ Eggs are pearly white and oval with lid
❖ Complete life cycle in 15 to 50 weeks
❖ Lifespan varies from many months to around one year

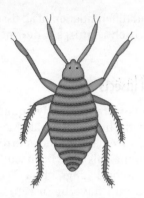

Fig. 43.1: Bed bug (female).

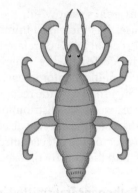

Fig. 43.2: Pediculus fumanus (male).

* Bed bugs, e.g., *Cimex hemipterus* and *Cimex lectularius* may be naturally infected with hepatitis-B virus which can transmit this virus mechanically or via feces
* Bed bugs may cause dermatitis or asthma, etc.
* Control includes:
  ▪ Pouring of boiling water to kill egg and nymph
  ▪ Use of kerosene, turpentine, benzene and petroleum, etc.
  ▪ Use of 5% DDT.

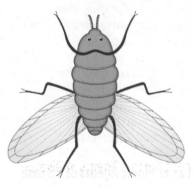

Fig. 43.3: Housefly.

Lice (Pediculus humanus corporis, and Pediculus humanus capitis) Pubic or Crab Louse

* Have dorsoventral flattened body
* Two to four mm in size; elongated and grayish white with piercing and sucking mouth parts
* Lack wings but have clawed legs
* Eggs are 0.8 mm long **(Fig. 43.2)**
* Principal habitats are body or hair
* Lifespan of adults up to 1 month
* May transmit typhus fever and cause irritating dermatitis
* May be responsible for transmission of *Salmonella* species
* Control includes:
  ▪ Use of benzyl benzoate, DDT, benzocaine
  ▪ Mixture of kerosene oil and olive oil
  ▪ Kerosene oil having 0.12% pyrethrins.

Housefly (Musca domestica)

* Male measures 5 to 6 mm and female 6 to 7 mm
* Dusky gray in color
* The head is broad, frons straw and dark brown, antennae brown
* Possess squarish ovoid thorax having 4 dark stripes
* Wings are transparent having straw colored base.
* Foot or terminal segment at the end of each leg is provided with a pair of horny claws, pair of ventral cushions, each with many glandular hair **(Fig. 43.3)**.
* Eggs are pearly white each one is 1 mm long.
* Completes life cycle in about 2 weeks.
* Responsible for transmitting pathogenic microorganisms mechanically, e.g., *Salmonella* tubercle bacilli *Yersinia pestis,*

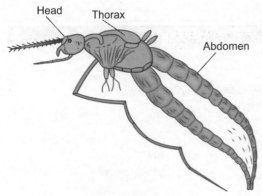

Head   Thorax

Abdomen

Fig. 43.4: Mosquito.

Bacillus anthracis, Brucella abortus, Chlamydia, etc.

❖ There is a close association between house flies and myiasis.

❖ Control includes:

■ Use of flypaper and flytraps

■ Garbage to be kept in close fly proof containers which is incinerated at frequent interval

■ Insecticidal spray, e.g., chlorinated hydro–carbon (1% water emulsion) to be sprayed twice a week over breeding area for fly ova.

Mosquitoes (Fig. 43.4)

❖ Slender, delicate forms with 3071 species all over the world

❖ Have elongated piercing sucking mouth parts adopted for sucking blood, especially in female mosquito

❖ Have long antennae feathery in male and hairy in females

❖ Scales on wings look spotted in anopheles mosquitoes and uniformly black in Culex **(Table 43.1)**

❖ Life-span of male mosquito is about 7 days and 1 month in case of female.

❖ Responsible for transmission of diseases, i.e., malaria (*Anopheles*), yellow fever (*Aedes*), Eastern equine encephalomyelitis (*Aedes*), Western equine encephalomyelitis (*Aedes*), Venezuelan equine encephalomyelitis (*Aedes, Anopheles, Culex*), chikungunya

fever (*Aedes*), dengue fever (*Aedes*), Japanese encephalitis (*Culex*), filariasis (*Aedes, Culex* and *Anopheles*), etc.

❖ Prevention and control includes:

■ Reduction of breeding places of mosquitoes like drainage, clearing or, filling of ditches and elimination of water containers

■ Use of insecticides

■ Use of mosquito repellant, e.g., residual sprays or lotion, gases or vapors

■ Diversion of mosquitoes from man to animals (cattles). This is called zooprophylaxis, a method hardly practised deliberately but often naturally effective

■ Genetic control is successful by introducing sterile male mosquitoes (by radiation or exposure to UV light) into natural population

■ Introduction of larvicidal fishes like gambusia and gold fish to breeding places of mosquitoes.

■ Many birds eat adult mosquitoes, e.g., swifts, night hawks, etc.

■ Wall lizards, frogs and spiders destroy mosquitoes

■ Many aquatic plants, e.g., chara, utricularia, etc.

■ Certain bacteria help of destroy larvae.

Fleas (Fig. 43.5)

❖ Adults are small, oblong, compressed, hard skinned, bristly, wingless and dark brown in color

❖ They have concealed antennae and long jumping legs

❖ The head is broadly joined to thorax

❖ The abdomen consists of 10 segments; the last 3 are modified for sexual purposes

❖ All parts of body are furnished with backward projecting bristles and spines which prevent it from slipping backwards and moving ahead between dense hair

❖ Male fleas are easily identified by rakish upward tilt of abdomen. In cases of female it is rounded

Table 43.1: Differentiating features of Culex, Aedes and Anopheles.

Anopheles	Aedes	Culex
1. Eggs		
• Boat shaped • Laid in flowing, fresh water	• Elliptical • Cavities of trees filled with water, domestic containers	• Cigar like • Stagnant dirty water
2. Larva		
• Lies parallel to water surface	• Hangs at an angle	• Hangs from water surface at an angle
• Surface feeder	• Bottom feeder	• Bottom feeder
3. Pupa		
• Green	• Colorless	• Colorless
4. Adults		
• Grayish, wings carry dark spots	• Blackish brown with white silvery stripes on thorax and abdomen	• Uniformly grayish body
• Resting posture inclined, head down at 45° angle.	• Horizontal to ground	• Horizontal to ground
• Body slender with delicate legs	• Well built with stout legs	• Well built with stout legs
• Abdomen with few or no scales	• Covered with scales	• Covered with scales
• Maxillary palp equal to proboscis (terminally pointed—females)	• Equal to proboscis in male but shorter in females	• Maxillary palp longer than proboscis in male but shorter in females

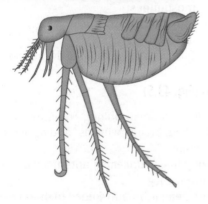

Fig. 43.5: Flea.

❖ The eggs are deposited in dark and dry places in the haunts of its host that takes about 70 to 75 days to mature

❖ Fleas may transmit plague (*Yersinia pestis*) endemic typhus fever, etc.

❖ Flea bite may cause flea dermatitis

❖ For control DDT, rotenone (1%), malathion (4%), pyrethrin (1%) may be used. In case of infested floor, rugs, carpet, pillows, etc. spray of kerosene solutions or emulsions of 3% malathion or 1% diazinon are useful. Rodent control can also check fleas.

Sandfly (Phlebotomus)

❖ Small about 2 mm long

❖ Humpbacked, fawny in color with prominent black eyes

❖ Body, wings and legs are hairy

❖ Wings veins do not cross with each other

❖ Oval lanceolate wings are carried erect

❖ Only the females feed on blood

❖ Feeding usually occurs at night and flies hide in dark, often damp places in day time

❖ Have long, slender antennae, long maxillary palpi and a proboscis longer than head **(Fig. 43.6)**

❖ The egg (long, ovoid) laying starts after 30 to 36 hours of blood meals and life cycle is completed in 60 to 65 days

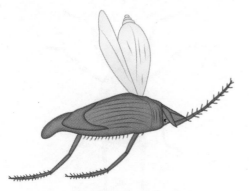

Fig. 43.6: Sandyfly.

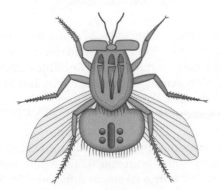

Fig. 43.7: Maggot fly (adult).

❖ May be responsible for transmitting cutaneous leishmaniasis, visceral leishmaniasis, viral 3 days fever, tularemia, loasis, etc.
❖ Control includes:
  ▪ Elimination of breeding grounds, cracks, crevices from walls and floors, etc.
  ▪ Use of insecticides like DDT, etc.
  ▪ Oiling pools of water can kill adult females who dive to lay eggs.

Fly Maggots (Fig. 43.7)

❖ The adult fly is dirty yellowish brown with the tip of abdomen rusty black
❖ The posterior respiratory openings of maggots consists of stigmatal plates. These are hardened, dark colored eye like spots surrounded by sclerotized ring and button like mark

❖ The position and shape of plates, the development of ring plus button and the forms of slit (straight, bent or looped) are of great importance in the identification
❖ The first stage maggots are recognizable by the absence of anterior as well as posterior spiracular plates
❖ The life cycle is completed in about 10 weeks. Eggs are transformed into larvae in 2 weeks. Larva take several weeks to become pupa and finally to adult
❖ May cause myiasis (infestation of living organs or tissue by maggots)
❖ Myiasis may be atrial (involving oral, nasal, aural, vagina, urethra, etc.), cutaneous (involving skin), intestinal, etc.
❖ There are numerous species of fly maggots but the only larva that sucks blood by puncturing skin of man is congo floor maggot *Auchmeromyia luteola*, found all over tropical Africa, etc. where people sleep on the floor. The larvae lie buried under the floor mat during day time and come forth during night to pierce skin with their mouth hook and suck blood
❖ Control includes:
  ▪ Proper disposal of carcases to prevent laying their eggs
  ▪ If feasible maggots are removed using forceps after spray of 5% chloroform in light vegetable oil and lesion dressed with antiseptics
  ▪ Adult fly of both sexes are attracted by swormlure-2, chemically defined bait and they are intoxicated by 2% dichlorvos
  ▪ A genetic control measure using mass reared, sterile male has also been tried successfully for species like *Cochiomyia hominivorax*.

Cockroaches

❖ Body is narrow elongated, symmetrical, smooth and flattened dorsoventrally
❖ Adult measures 2.5 to 5 cm in length and 2 cm in width

- ❖ The color is reddish brown
- ❖ The body is segmented into head, thorax and abdomen
- ❖ Body bears 2 pairs of wings (outer pair leathery and inner pair membranous)
- ❖ Development from egg through nymph to adult requires 32 to 90 days depending on species and temperature
- ❖ Domestic cockroaches are intermediate host of *Hymenolepis diminuta,* etc. They may transmit enteric viruses and many bacteria. About 40 species of pathogenic bacteria have been isolated from contaminated cockroaches. *Aspergillus fumigatus* and *Aspergillus niger* have also been isolated from cockroaches. Cysts of *Giardia* and *Entamoeba histolytica* have also been found. An interesting report proposes the transport of *Toxoplasma gondii* from feces of the domestic cat by cockroaches. They also serve as a potentially important source of contactant, inhalant, infectant, and ingestant allergens. Hence, they may cause itching, dermatitis, localized necrosis, asthma and hey fever
- ❖ Control measures are:
  - ■ Kerosene oil spray on cockroach hiding place. Care must be taken to protect food.
  - ■ Use of suitable insecticides, e.g., fenitrothion, propoxur or dioxacarb used at 1%.

Ticks (Fig. 43.8)

- ❖ It may be soft bodied ticks (Argasidae) or hard bodied ticks (Ixodidae)
- ❖ In the soft bodied ticks, there is no hard dorsal plate, the mouth parts are situated ventral to the anterior extremity, and the spiracles are usually located directly behind the third pair of coxal segments, e.g., *otobius, antricola,* etc.
- ❖ In Ixodidae, body is ovoid, dorsoventrally flattened and unsegmented. Capitulum projects from anterior end of body. Dorsal surface of body is covered by shield-like

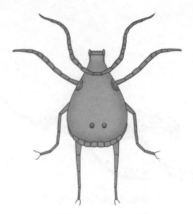

Fig. 43.8: Ticks (Ixodidae).

scutum bearing eyes. Walking legs are 4 pairs with adhesive pads and claws. Female is larger than male. They produce ixodin which acts as anesthetic agent and host does not feel pain.

- ❖ Ticks are responsible for causing human diseases. They also act as vectors of many human pathogens including rickettsiae, viruses and protozoa. Thus, responsible for tick-borne rikettsial infection (Rocky mountain fever, Queensland tick typhus, etc.), viral (encephalitis, hemorrhagic fever, severe myalgia with fever, etc.), protozoa (babesiosis), other diseases like Lyme's disease erythema chronicum migrans, etc.

Mites

- ❖ Usually a millimeter in greater length or breadth than ticks
- ❖ They have hypostome unarmed with tooth-like anchoring processes
- ❖ Parasitic form feeds on blood, lymph, digested tissues, or sebaceous secretions on near the surface of the skin
- ❖ Some tunnels subcutaneously causing an intense pruritus
- ❖ Certain mites may serve as both reservoir and vector of *Rickettsia tsutsugamushi*
- ❖ House dust mites either produce or concentrate potent allergens commonly found within the home.

Clinical Microbiology

SECTION 8

The Normal Flora

The collection of species found in the normal, healthy individual and which usually coexist peacefully in a balanced relationship with their host are known as indigenous or normal flora of body.

It is not possible to eliminate the normal flora of the skin and intestine. Antibiotics are capable of drastically reducing their number to a minimum. So, the pathogenic organism gets the opportunity to overgrow and cause lesions or diseases.

The normal flora is acquired during and shortly at birth and changes continuously throughout life. It is basically environmentally determined. Breastfed infants have lactic acid streptococci and lactobacilli in their gastrointestinal tract, on the other hand bottlefed children show a much greater variety of organisms.

The term flora is used because the majority of the organisms are bacteria. Man has about 10^{14} bacteria associated with him, most of them in the large intestine.

▇ LOCATION OF NORMAL FLORA

Normal flora are found in those parts of the body that are exposed to or communicate with the external environment, e.g., skin, nose, mouth, intestine and urogenital tracts. Internal organs and tissues are normally sterile.

Skin

Staphylococcus epidermidis is one of the most common species (90%) of aerobes occurring in densities of 10^3 to 10^4 per square centimeters. *Staphylococcus aureus* may be present in the moist regions of the body (axillae, perineum, between toes, scalp).

Anaerobic diphtheroids are found below the skin surface in hair follicles, sweat and sebaceous glands, e.g., *Propionibacterium acnes*. *Candida* may occur on scalp and around nails. They are infrequent on exposed skin, but can cause infection in moist skin folds (intertigo).

Nose and Mouth

They are heavily colonized by streptococci, staphylococci, diphtheroids and Gram-negative cocci. Some of the species found as a part of the flora in healthy persons are potentially pathogenic (*Staphylococcus aureus, Strepto-coccus pneumoniae, Streptococcus pyogenes, Neisseria meningitidis, Lactobaccillus, Candida* etc.). The microbial density of normal flora here is 10^{11} per gram wet weight of tissue. The surface of teeth and the gingival cervices carry a large number of anaerobic bacteria. Plaque is a thin film of bacteria attached with polysaccharide matrix which the bacteria secrete. When teeth are not cleaned regularly there is increased activities of certain bacteria like *Streptococcus mutans*, which may lead dental caries. Acid fermented by these organisms from carbohydrates, can invade dental enamel.

The pharynx and trachea carry their own normal flora, e.g., alfa and beta streptococci, staphylococci, neisseria and diphtheroids.

Gastrointestinal Tract

The stomach contents give shelter to transient organisms, the acidic pH providing unfavorable environment. Gastric mucosa may be colonized by acid tolerant lactobacilli and streptococci.

The upper intestine is colonized (10^4 organisms per gram) but density increases in the ileum. Here streptococci, lactobacilli, enterobacteria and bacteroids may all be present.

In the large intestine, bacterial numbers are quite high (10^{11} per gram) and many different species are found. The majority (95 to 99%) are anaerobes, bacteroides being common and major component of stool matter. A number of harmless protozoans occur in the intestine, e.g., *Entamoeba coli*.

Urogenital Tract

Urethra in males and females is lightly colonized with *Staphylococcus epidermides*, *E. fecalis* and diphtheroids. In females, before puberty, the predominant organisms are staphylococci, streptococci, diphtheroids and *Escherichia coli*. Subsequently lactobacilli predominates, its fermentation of glycogen being responsible for maintenance of an acid pH, which prevents overgrowth by other vaginal organisms. In case vaginal pH rises, *Candida* may overgrow causing a condition called thrush.

Advantages of Normal Flora

1. They prevent colonization of potential pathogen, e.g., skin bacteria produce fatty acids, gut bacteria release bacteriocin, colicin plus metabolic wastes and lack of oxygen, vaginal lactobacilli maintain acid pH, etc.
2. Gut bacteria release vitamin B and K.
3. Antigenic stimulation provided by intestinal flora is considered important in ensuring the normal development of the immune system.
4. Antibodies produced in response to normal flora cross react with pathogens thus raising immune status of the host. The endotoxin liberated by normal flora trigger alternative complement pathogen.

Disadvantages

1. The disadvantage of the normal flora lie primarily in the potential hazard for spread into previously sterile parts of the body, e.g., when intestine is perforated, skin is broken, extraction of teeth, *E. coli*, from perianal skin ascend the urethra to cause urinary tract infection.
2. Overgrowth by pathogenic members of normal flora may occur in conditions like after administration of antibiotics, increase in stomach or vaginal pH or when immune system becomes ineffective.
3. Isolation of normal flora may cause confusion in the diagnosis.

Collection and Transport of Clinical Specimens

INTRODUCTION

By and large, report from bacteriological laboratory can indicate on what has been found by microscopic and cultural examination. An etiological diagnosis is thus confirmed or denied. Failure to isolate the causative organism, however, is not necessarily the fault of inadequate technical method but it is frequently the result of faulty collection technique. The following points should be remembered in collecting the material for microbial examination:

1. Preferably specimen should be obtained before antibiotic or other antimicrobial agents have been administered. If the culture has been taken after initiation of antibacterial therapy, laboratory should be informed so that specific counteractive measures, such as adding penicillinase or merely diluting the sample may be carried out.

2. Material should be collected where the suspected organism is most likely to be found and with as little external contamination as possible. This is particularly true of draining lesion containing coagulase positive staphylococci.

3. The other important factor for successful isolation of causative agent is the stage of disease at which the specimen is collected for culture. Enteric pathogens are present in much greater number during acute or diarrheal stage of intestinal infections and they are most likely to be isolated at that time. Viruses responsible for meningoencephalitis are isolated from cerebrospinal fluid with greater frequency when fluid is taken during the onset of disease rather than at a time when the symptoms of acute illness have subsided.

4. Specimen should be of a quantity sufficient enough to permit complete examination and should be kept in sterile containers. A serious danger to the laboratory workers as well as to all others involved is the soiled outer surface of sputum container or a leaking stool sample.

5. If morning sputum sample collection is required then patient or attendant of patient should have full instructions.

6. Arrangement should be made for prompt delivery of specimens to the laboratory. It is often difficult to isolate *Shigella* from stool specimen that has remained in the hospital ward too long as it results in overgrowth of commensals and an increasing death rate of *Shigella*.

7. The laboratory should be provided with sufficient clinical information to guide the microbiologist in the selection of suitable media and appropriate techniques. It is essential that close cooperation and frequent consultation among clinician, nurse and microbiologist be the rule rather than the exception.

8. The collection of specimens for anaerobic culture, the use of double-stoppered collection tube gassed out with oxygen-free carbon dioxide and nitrogen is recommended. The specimen (pus, body

fluid or other liquid material) is injected through the sterilized rubber stopper while avoiding the introduction of air.

The following points must be kept in mind while collecting of samples from a patient suspected to have anaerobic infection:

❖ Avoid contamination with normal flora
❖ Avoid contact with oxygen
❖ Do not refrigerate the samples
❖ Process immediately after collection
❖ Transport media should be used only when delay in culturing specimen is inevitable.

Specimen Containers and their Transport

A sterile container should be used and specimen be plated as soon as possible. Apart from usual containers, the most useful piece of collecting equipment is cotton, calcium alginate or polyester tipped applicator stick. Collection of material from throat, nose, eye, ear, wound at operative site, urogenital orifices and rectum is done in a Pyrex test tube (20 × 150 mm) which is cotton plugged having applicator stick and small test-tube containing thioglycollate broth. The swab inoculated with material from the patient is placed in inner broth tube to prevent drying out and promptly sent to the laboratory.

In case significant delay is unavoidable between collection of specimen and culturing, transport media is required. Transport media prolong the survival of microorganisms, e.g. Stuart medium maintains a favorable pH and prevents both dehydration of secretions during transport as well as oxidation and enzymatic self-destruction of pathogen present in the specimen. Cary and Blair transport medium is used for fecal culture to isolate *Salmonellae*, *Shigellae*, *Vibrio*, etc. For anaerobic culture double stoppered collection tube gassed out with oxygen-free carbon dioxide or nitrogen are recommended for collection of specimen and transporting it to laboratory.

Some bacteria, such as *meningococcus* in cerebrospinal fluid are quite sensitive to low temperature and require immediate culturing. On the contrary, clinical material likely to contain abundant microbial flora may be held at 4°C in a refrigerator for several hours before culturing if it cannot be processed immediately, e.g., urine, feces, etc. Refrigeration will preserve the viability of most pathogens and also prevent the overgrowth of commensals.

If specimen is to be delivered by post, it must be sealed in such a way as to prevent the leakage of material and outer envelope must be marked "Microbial Specimen and Fragile—Handle with Care".

Handling of Specimen in the Laboratory

It is not always practical for many specimens to be inoculated as soon as they arrive in the laboratory. Refrigeration at 4°C–6°C offers a safe and reliable method of storing many clinical samples until they can be conveniently handled. However, some may require immediate plating.

Urine specimens for culture may be refrigerated for 24–48 hours without affecting the bacterial flora. Swabs from wound, urogenital tract, throat, rectum and samples of feces and sputum may be refrigerated for 24–48 hours without appreciable loss of pathogens. Gastric washings and resected lung tissue for the culture of *Mycobacterium tuberculosis* should be processed immediately after delivery as *Tubercle bacilli* may die rapidly in these specimens.

Sputum, bronchial secretions, bone marrow and purulent material from patients suspected of having systemic fungal infection should be inoculated as soon as possible, particularly when diagnosis of histoplasmosis is considered. However, pieces of hair or scraping from skin and nail submitted for fungal culture may be kept at room temperature for several days before inoculation. Specimen submitted for isolation of virus should be frozen immediately. Specimen of clotted blood for virus serology may be refrigerated but never frozen.

Selection of Laboratory Investigations

Diagnostic tests in infectious diseases fall into the following four groups:

1. The demonstration of an infectious agent (bacterial, viral, protozoal, helminthic or mycotic) in specimens obtained from the patient.
2. The demonstration of a meaningful antibody response in the patient. It requires two serum specimens usually obtained at an interval of 10–20 days or longer.
3. The demonstration of meaningful, cell-mediated responses or skin tests to antigens associated with a particular infectious disease.
4. The demonstration of deviation in a variety of clinical laboratory determinations that nonspecifically suggest or support a suspicion of infectious diseases.

Collection and Preliminary Processing of Specimens

Specimen Collection from Different Parts of the Body

It has two-fold objective: (a) to indicate the commensal organisms commonly found and pathogens of utmost importance in material from different parts of the body, (b) to indicate basic routine for collection and initial investigations of material. One should know that bacteriological examination is usually completed in 2 to 3 days' time whereas culture of *Mycobacterium tuberculosis* takes 3–8 weeks. Collection of specimen from particular parts of the body is as follows:

Skin: The commensals are *Staphylococcus albus* and diphtheroid bacilli. Many more bacteria and some fungi are also present on skin but only temporarily. The important pathogens are *Staphylococcus pyogenes* (boils), *Streptococcus pyogenes* (impetigo, cellulitis), *E. coli, Proteus, Pseudomonas, Candida albicans* (intertrigo), dermatophytes, pox and herpes virus.

Swab moistened with sterile broth or saline may be used for collection of specimen. Crust of scab in a sterile bottle is more useful especially in viral lesions. In fungal lesions, scraping from skin, hair and nail may be used. For bacteria Gram staining, culture on blood agar and MacConkey's media may be made, for *Candida albicans* culture on Sabouraud's medium and for dermatophytes wet preparation of scraping in KOH and culture on Sabouraud's medium is made.

Conjunctiva: The common commensals are staphylococci, diphtheroid, *Streptococcus viridans*, nonpathogenic *neisseriae*, etc. The important pathogens are *Neisseria gonorrheae, Staphylococcus aureus, pneumococcus, Haemophilus influenzae,* chlamydiae, adenovirus and herpes virus.

It is desirable to have microscopic slides and culture plates in clinics and wards. Alternatively, patient may be sent to laboratory. Smears are made and culture inoculated with material taken from conjunctival surface by sterile platinum loop. Otherwise, conjunctival swab is never taken as adequate specimen for bacteriological investigations like Gram-stained smear and inoculation on blood agar, chocolate agar, aerobically and in 5–10% CO_2.

Ear: Commensals of external ear are same as of skin. However, middle ear is sterile. The important pathogens are *Staphylococcus pyogenes, Streptococcus pyogenes, Pseudomonas aeruginosa, pneumococcus, Haemophilus influenzae,* etc. A swab may be used to collect specimen from external ear or from middle ear that is discharging through eardrum. Gram's staining and culture on blood agar, chocolate agar, MacConkey media may be done.

Throat swab: The commensals are *Staphylococcus albus, Streptococcus viridans,* nonhemolytic streptococcus, diphtheroids, lactobacilli, nonpathogenic neisseriae, etc. The important pathogens are *Streptococcus pyogenes, Staphylococcus pyogenes,* diphtheria bacilli, *Hemophilus influenzae,* Vincent's organisms and *Bordetella pertussis,* etc.

Throat swab taken from patient's mouth wide open and tongue depressed. Care is taken to touch only pharyngeal mucosa. Blood culture, although it does not provide information at once, is usually positive for *Haemophilus influenzae* and should be carried out as the best means of confirmation of diagnosis. In the presence of membrane, especially when diphtheria is suspected part of the membrane must be removed.

Initial investigation is done by doing Gram's staining, smears stained with dilute carbol fuchsin for Vincent bacteria and Albert staining for diphtheria bacilli. Media used are blood agar, Löffler's serum and tellurite (diphtheria), chocolate agar (*Haemophilus influenzae* and *Neisseria meningitidis*), Bordet-Gongou medium for *Bordetella pertussis*.

Alimentary tract: Commensals include lactobacilli, anaerobes of the bacteroides and clostridia, streptococci and certain protozoa. The pathogens are *Escherichia coli, Shigellae, Salmonellae, Vibrio cholerae, Staphylococcus aureus, Candida*, rotaviruses, etc. Stool specimens are collected in a screw-capped bottle which may be obtained from laboratory. If it is difficult to collect stool specimen then rectal swab may be taken. Naked eye inspection of the specimen is done for consistency, presence of blood or mucus. For culture inoculation is done on blood agar, MacConkey and DCA plates. Enrichment media like selenite broth may be used. Gram's staining should be done if staphylococcal or candida enteritis is suspected.

Blood culture: Essentially blood is sterile and hence no commensals are present. Detection of organism in blood is always abnormal finding. The important pathogens are *Staphylococcus aureus* (acute septicemia), *Neisseria meningitidis* (chronic septicemia), *Streptococcus viridans,* enterococci (subacute bacterial endocarditis), *Salmonellae* (enteric fever), *Brucellae* (undulent fever) and *Plasmodium* (malaria).

Blood may be collected strictly aseptically using autoclaved syringe. It is always best to obtain blood at a time when patient's temperature is rising as at this time patient is having highest number of bacteria in the blood. About 5–10 mL blood is transferred in 50 mL culture media in blood culture bottles. For *Salmonellae* organisms, bile glucose broth and for other organisms glucose broth is used. Bile broth is used in enteric fever since bile lyses WBCs and releases the intracellular organism.

In case of infective endocarditis, multiple cultures are required because of intermittent nature of bacteremia.

Sometimes, it may be necessary to use special medium, such as broth with 10% sucrose to recover the bacteria from blood.

In some laboratory sodium polyanethol sulphonate is used in broth culture media which prevents blood from clotting and inhibits bactericidal activity of blood. All cultures are incubated at 37°C. Subculture is done after 24 hours, 96 hours and 14 days' incubation at 37°C.

Some laboratories use blood culture media containing radiolabeled metabolic substrates. The gases in the culture bottles are monitored by automation to detect $_{14}CO_2$, a metabolic by product that indicates growth.

Urinary tract: Apart from skin commensals, urinary tract is sterile. The important pathogens are *Escherichia coli, Proteus, Citrobacter, Pseudomonas, Moraxella, Acinetobacter, Staphylococcus, Streptococcus fecalis, salmonellae, Mycobacterium tuberculosis*, etc. For nontuberculosis purposes, a midstream fresh urine is collected in an autoclaved cotton-swabbed test tube. In tuberculosis, patient first morning urine sample or 24-hour urine collection is required in clean and dry container. Specimen must be processed immediately after collection. In case 3 to 4 hours' delay is inevitable, then urine sample may be kept in refrigerator at 4°C. Urine samples are streaked on blood agar and MacConkey agar plates. Microscopic examination of urine should also be done especially for pus cell, RBC and bacteria.

Diagnostic Microbiology—
An Approach to Laboratory
Diagnosis

▮ INTRODUCTION

Microbiology is perhaps the least easy to codify in fixed routines. Every patient with the suspected infection is a new biological problem that both clinician and bacteriologist can solve. Only by following their noses wherever the investigations lead them, and any attempted identification of infecting microbe in the laboratory may lead the microbiologist along unexpected paths. Clinical microbiology is an explanatory art that demands flexibility of mind and technique. The latest methods are less important to the (would-be) practitioner than a set of uniformly good procedures with which to explore the common and not-too-rare infection of man with which he stands a reasonable chance of discovering new ones.

Etiology of microbial diseases may be established mainly by three methods: (1) Micro-scopy, (2) Culture and (3) Serology/skin tests. Unstained microscopic examination is useful to demonstrate trophozoites of protozoa, eggs of helminths, pus cells/red blood corpuscles in body fluids and motility of bacteria. Unstained wet preparations using dark ground illumination are useful for the demonstration of *Treponema pallidum*. Ziehl-Neelsen staining is useful for the demonstration of *Mycobacterium tuberculosis* and leprae bacilli. Gram-staining is useful in gonorrhea, Vincent's angina and infections caused by other organisms. Microscopy is also useful for diagnosis of fungal diseases and demonstration of inclusion bodies. However, fluorescent antibody technique is gaining momentum in establishing its place in rapid diagnosis.

Cultural examination includes isolation and identification of organism. For identification we need colony morphology, biochemical tests, pathogenicity or toxigenicity test and differentiation of types of bacteriocin, phage typing, etc.

Serology is useful in demonstrating antibodies in the serum of patients. Examination of single specimen of serum is not diagnostic. Four-fold rise in the levels of specific antibodies in patient serum during course of illness is usually diagnostic. The most common serological tests are: (i) agglutination, e.g., Widal's test for enteric fever, (ii) precipitation test, e.g., VDRL used for syphilis and (iii) complement fixation test, e.g., Wassermann test used for syphilis. New serological test like indirect hemagglutination (IHA), radioimmunoassay, and ELISA are currently in use.

Skin tests are not very reliable diagnostic procedures. The important examples of skin test are: Casoni test for the diagnosis of hydatid cyst (immediate hypersensitivity), tuberculin test for the diagnosis of tuberculosis (delayed type hypersensitivity) and Frei's test for the diagnosis of lymphogranuloma venereum (delayed type of hypersensitivity).

The other nonspecific tests like red blood cell count, total and differential leukocyte count, erythrocyte sedimentation rate (ESR), C-reactive proteins, etc. are also useful for establishing the diagnosis and determining the prognosis of disease.

Before proceeding for the laboratory diagnosis of a disease we must know the etiology (causative) agents, specimen required, collection of specimen, its transport to laboratory and processing of specimen, i.e. microscopy for morphological study, culture identification, serology to demonstrate four-fold rise in titer in paired sera and skin tests.

Some common problems concerning the laboratory diagnosis establishment are discussed as below:

PYREXIA OF UNKNOWN ORIGIN (PUO)

Peterson and Beeson defined PUO as illness of 3 weeks' duration temperature exceeding 38.3°C on several occasions. Invariably diagnosis is not established even after one week's stay in the hospital.

The causes of PUO are:

Acute (short duration):
1. Enteric fever
2. Amebic hepatitis
3. Urinary tract infections
4. Malaria
5. Subacute bacterial endocarditis
6. Brucellosis
7. Typhus fever.

Chronic (long duration):
1. Brucellosis
2. Pulmonary tuberculosis
3. Typhus
4. Subacute bacterial endocarditis
5. Kala-azar.

Investigations are done as below:

i. Urine for microscopic examination especially for pus cells. In case of presence of pus cells culture and drug sensitivity is done.
ii. Blood examination:
   a. **TLC** and **DLC** shows leukocytosis in urinary tract infection, subacute bacterial endocarditis and amebic hepatitis. Leukopenia is a feature of enteric fever and malaria. Lympho-cytosis may be observed in brucellosis.
   b. **RBC** count and hemoglobulin estimation indicates anemia.
   c. Peripheral blood film may show malarial parasite.
   d. Bone marrow may show **LD** bodies.
iii. Sputum examination is done for the demonstration of acid-fast bacilli by direct, concentrated and culture methods.
iv. Stool examination for trophozoites and cysts of *Entamoeba histolytica* is done. One may also look for Charcot-Leyden crystals.
v. Blood culture is done by collecting 5 to 10 ml of blood from the patient aseptically using autoclaved syringe. Blood culture bottles are used containing 50 mL of broth **(Fig. 47.1)**. Glucose bile broth is used for enteric fever, glucose broth for subacute bacterial endocarditis or other pyogenic organisms and liver infusion broth (Castaneda's media) for brucellosis. These bottles are incubated at 37°C and subcultured on solid media (blood agar and MacConkey agar plates) after 24 hours, 48 hours, 7 days and 14 days. For enteric look for nonlactose fermenter colonies (NLF) which are Gram-negative bacilli, oxidase negative, ferment glucose and mannitol, Indole and VP negative, and MR plus citrate positive. Final confirmation for enteric bacilli is done by slide agglutination with

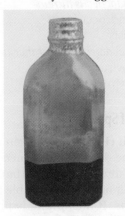

Fig. 47.1: Blood culture bottle.

specific antisera. For subacute bacterial endocarditis subculture is done on blood agar plate after 2, 7 and 30 days and study the colonies of *Streptococcus viridans, Staphylococcus albus*, and *Streptococcus fecalis*. For brucellosis incubation is done in 5–10% CO_2 and look for Gram-negative coccobacilli, nonlactose fermenter, nonmotile and oxidase negative bacilli. Confirmation is done by agglutination with specific antisera.

vi. **Serology:** Widal's test is done for enteric fever. Agglutination test for brucellosis may be done. Weil-Felix test using OX_2, OX_{19} and OXk antigen is done for typhus fever. Formal gel test can be done for kala-azar.

vii. Pus may be examined microscopically for trophozoites of *Entamoeba histolytica* and necrotic debris.

SORE THROAT

Etiology

a. Membranous
1. *Corynebacterium diphtheriae*
2. Candida
3. Vincent's angina

b. Nonmembranous
1. *Streptococcus pyogenes*
2. *Staphylococcus aureus*
3. Pneumococcus
4. Pertussis
5. *Corynebacterium diphtheriae*
6. Adenovirus
7. Rhinovirus

Collection of Specimen

Throat swab **(Fig. 47.2)** is taken aseptically using tongue depressor. It is necessary that collection of throat swab should be undertaken under proper light. It is advisable to take two throat swabs. If membrane is present one must make it a point to remove part of the

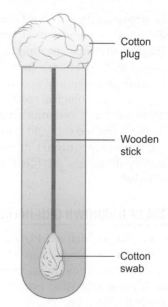

Fig. 47.2: Throat swab.

membrane because chances of recovery of causative organism are more from membrane.

Culture

Immediately after the collection of specimen, inoculate it on blood agar, blood tellurite and Löffler's serum slope. Incubate these plates at 37°C for 12 to 48 hours. In the meantime smears from throat swabs are prepared, then Gram's and Albert staining is done. In stained smear, look for Gram-positive bacilli, which are thin, slender, pleomorphic with metachromatic granules showing Chinese latter arrangement. These characters are suggestive of *Corynebacterium diphtheriae*, Gram-positive cocci in chains (*Streptococcus*), in clumps (*Staphylococcus*) and if in pairs (*Pneumococcus*). Budding yeast cells are found in candida. In Vincent's angina we find curved and spiralled organisms, i.e. fusiform bacilli.

In diphtheria cases, we may find small, convex colonies on blood agar plates. On Löffler serum slope, there is abundant growth which is moist, cream-colored or pigmented. Blood tellurite agar is selective and indicator medium (black colonies) showing differentiation among gravis, intermedius and mitis. Sugar sets are used. Sugar media is prepared in Hiss serum. In case of gravis, starch and glycogen are fermented without formation of gas. Pathogenicity tests are useful like Elek's test, animals inoculation test, e.g., rabbit and guinea pig in which material may be injected intradermally or subcutaneously.

In *Staphylococcus aureus* cases we find colonies 2–3 mm in diameter, smooth, glistening butyrous, opaque and golden yellow showing beta hemolysis on blood agar plate. They are catalase positive and Gram-positive cocci arranged in clusters. They exhibit pathogenicity tests like coagulase production, mannitol fermentation, lipase, DNase and phosphatase production.

The *Streptococcus pyogenes* is Gram-positive cocci arranged in chains. They are catalase negative. On blood agar plate they are small, low convex, semitransparent, discrete colonies showing beta hemolysis. They are matt to mucoid when freshly isolated. Biochemically they ferment lactose, glucose, sucrose and mannitol with only acid production. Most common Lancefield group responsible for throat infection is A.

Pneumococcus shows alpha hemolysis. The colonies are small, flat and transparent. They show positive bile solubility test, ferment insulin and optichin sensitivity test is positive. They may kill mice when injected intraperitoneally.

URINARY TRACT INFECTION

It is a common urological condition. Sometimes it is impossible to eradicate it because of development of drug resistant bacteria. So the wrong therapy is likely to make sensitive organism resistant to drugs. Hence prior isolation of causative organisms and their sensitivity to antimicrobial drugs should be done before any rational treatment is given to the patient.

Causes

1. *Escherichia coli*
2. *Klebsiella*
3. *Enterobacter*
4. *Serratia*
5. *Proteus*
6. Providentia
7. *Pseudomonas aeruginosa*
8. *Alcaligenes*
9. *Acinetobacter*
10. *Moraxella*
11. *Streptococcus fecalis*
12. *Staphylococcus pyogenes*
13. *Streptococcus pyogenes*
14. *Salmonella*
15. *Neisseria gonorrheae*
16. *Mycobacterium tuberculosis*
17. *Candida albicans.*

Collection of Specimens

Midstream urine is collected aseptically in a sterilized container. Two successive clean voided midstream urine specimens may be collected in order to have 95% confidence level when using a bacterial count of 10^5 per milliliter as an index of significant bacteriuria. It is necessary to process the urine in the laboratory within one hour of collection. In case of inevitable delay urine may be stored in refrigerator at 4°C. The technique of dividing voided urine from male patients into urethral, midstream and post-prostatic massage may help to increase the accuracy of localizing urinary tract infection. Since specimens of urine either clean voided or catheterized are frequently contaminated so the recovery of even pathogens does not necessarily establish urinary tract infection. Bacterial counts on fresh, voided urine from infected patient show more than 100,000 (10^5) organism per milliliter significant bacteriuria. However, bacterial counts of less than 10^5 per milliliter may occur in patient on antibacterial therapy or in patients who are excessively hydrated causing dilution of urine (**Fig. 47.3**).

Cultural Procedure

Flame sterilized and cooled, about 4 mm, platinum loop (standardized) charged with

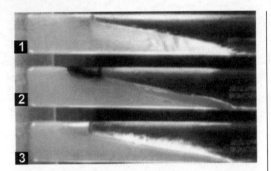

Fig. 47.3: Nitrate agar; 1. Control, 2. *Escherichia coli*, 3. *Acinetobacter calcoaceticus*.

uncentrifuged urine is streaked on blood agar and MacConkey agar plate. A bacteriological loop of 4 mm diameter holds 0.01 mL of urine which should be inoculated on to the medium, growth of more than 100 colonies is considered significant. Incubate both plates at 37°C and study the plates next morning. Estimate the total count from blood plate and Gram-negative bacterial count from MacConkey agar plate. After determining the plate bacterial count, proceed with the identification of the organisms present and then find out their susceptibility to antibiotics. If no growth occurs after 24 hours, hold the plates at 37°C for another day and if negative, report it as "no growth after 48 hours."

The other quantitative methods of estimation of bacteriuria in urine are:

1. Blotting paper strip method where two blotting papers (12 × 6 mm) are dipped in urine and impressed—one on blood agar and the other on MacConkey plate. After 37°C incubation colonies are counted. Twenty to thirty colonies represent significant bacteriuria (10^5/mL).
2. **Uricult**: It is dip slide with nutrient agar on one side and MacConkey's medium on other side. Viable count is determined by comparing density growth on each medium and matching with manufacturer's chart.
3. **Microstik**: These are strip-like uricult and used as per instructions of manufacturer.
4. **Tri-phenyl tetrazolium chloride test**: 2 mL urine with 0.5 mL of reagent is incubated at 37°C for 4 hours. Appearance of red precipitate in solution means 10^5/mL bacterial count.
5. **Nitrite test**: Nitrites are not found in normal urine. Its presence means coliform bacteria in urine **(Fig. 47.3)**.
6. **Catalase test**: The presence of catalase as evidenced by frothing on addition of hydrogen peroxide indicates bacteriuria, although positive result is obtained also in hematuria.

MENINGITIS

Causes

❖ *Bacterial:*
  ▪ Meningococci
  ▪ Pneumococci
  ▪ *Hemophilus influenzae-b*
  ▪ Streptococci
  ▪ Staphylococci
  ▪ Coliform organism
  ▪ *Mycobacterium tuberculosis*
  ▪ *Treponema pallidum*
  ▪ *Leptospira*
❖ *Viral:*
  ▪ Mumps
  ▪ Coxsackie
  ▪ Echo
  ▪ Herpes simplex
  ▪ Lymphocytic choriomeningitis
  ▪ Poliomyelitis
  ▪ Arbovirus
❖ *Fungal:*
  ▪ *Cryptococcus*
  ▪ *Coccidioides*
  ▪ *Histoplasma capsulatum*

Collection of Specimen

Specimen required for investigation of meningitis is cerebrospinal fluid. It is collected aseptically in an autoclaved container by performing lumbar puncture and specimen should be arranged to be transported to laboratory quickly. If delay is inevitable then specimen may be kept at 37°C for not more than 4 hours. It should never be kept in refrigeration or icebox.

Processing and Culture of Specimen

In the laboratory, gross examination of cere-brospinal fluid is done to note color, turbidity and any deposit or clot. Microscopic examination is also done for white cell count. Some fluid is immediately transferred into glucose broth. Fluid left behind is centrifuged. Supernatant may be used for biochemical test like protein, sugar and chloride. Smear is prepared from deposit and stained by Gram's method. Deposit is also used for culture on blood agar plate. Similarly, subculture from glucose broth may be done on blood agar plate. After 37°C incubation for 48 hours plates are studied and colonies are identified by various biochemical reactions. Drug sensitivity is also determined.

In tuberculosis cases, cerebrospinal fluid frequently contains clot (cobweb or spiderweb). Smear and then Ziehl-Neelsen stain from this clot may show acid-fast bacilli. Löwenstein-Jensen medium may be used for the culture of *Mycobacterium tuberculosis* and for animal inoculation. Cerebrospinal fluid deposit may be injected into guinea pig.

For demonstration of fungus microscopic examination is done. Subsequently for cultural purposes Sabouraud's agar media may be used. Some serological tests may be helpful in diagnosing fungal etiology.

For the demonstration of virus as etiological agent electron microscope, tissue culture and serological techniques may be undertaken.

▋ INFECTIVE DIARRHEA

Causes

❖ Bacterial:
  ■ *Escherichia coli* (O_4, O_{29}, O_{55}, O_{80}, O_{111}, O_{124}, O_{130}, etc.)
  ■ *Shigella*
  ■ *Salmonella*
  ■ *Vibrio cholerae*
  ■ *Vibrio parahemolyticus*
  ■ Staphylococcal infection
  ■ *Campylobacter*
  ■ *Clostridium difficile*
  ■ *Clostridium perfringens*
  ■ *Bacillus cereus*
  ■ *Pseudomonas*
  ■ *Proteus*
  ■ *Klebsiella.*
❖ Viral:
  ■ Rotavirus
  ■ Norwalk agent
  ■ Adenovirus
  ■ Asteroid virus
  ■ Echo virus (11, 14, 18 types)
  ■ Coxsackie virus.
❖ Parasitic:
  ■ *Entamoeba histolytica*
  ■ *Giardia lamblia*
  ■ *Ascaris lumbricoides*
  ■ Whipworm
  ■ Tapeworm
  ■ Alkylostoma (hookworm)
  ■ Plasmodium (rare cause).
❖ Fungal:
  ■ *Candida albicans.*

Collection of specimen: Stool specimen is preferably collected aseptically in screw-capped water tight container provided with small plastic spoon **(Fig. 47.4)**. This spoon may be used to transfer safely into the container small amount of stool specimen. From young children where collection of specimen is difficult rectal swab may be obtained. If culture of stool is required and delay in transporting the stool specimen to microbiology laboratory is inevitable, transport media (glycerol saline) may be used. If *Vibrio cholerae* is expected, it is advisable to use at least alkaline peptone water.

Further Processing and Culture Procedure

Naked eye examination for consistency, presence of blood, pus and mucus is done. Wet microscopic (both saline and iodine) preparations are used for detection of ova and

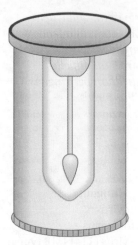

Fig. 47.4: Container used for collection of stool specimen.

cysts. Plasmodium may cause diarrhea and so peripheral blood film should be scanned for plasmodium.

Aerobic culture on blood agar for pathogenic strain of *Escherichia coli* and *Staphylococcus aureus* is done. MacConkey or DCA medium may be used for Shigellae and Salmonellae. Selenite F broth may be used if salmonellae is suspected which may be subcultured subsequently on MacConkey or DCA media. Just reporting of *E. coli* without serotyping is not sufficient. *Pseudomonas, Proteus* and *Klebsiella* are not always normal flora of intestine and their presence in stool may be abnormal especially when associated with diarrhea.

Virus culture is tedious and difficult job in ordinary laboratories and is difficult to obtain. However, where electron microscope facilities are available, rotavirus may be identified by virtue of its characteristic cart-wheel appearance. Of course serological techniques are also helpful in establishing viral etiology.

Further, we may proceed blood culture for septicemia, Widal test of salmonellae infection, Chinese hamster cell culture or rabbit ileal loop assay for enterotoxigenic strains of *Escherichia coli* and mycological culture for *Candida albicans* can be done. If feasible, detection of parenteral infection and immunological deficiency may be made out.

■ WOUND INFECTION

Etiology

Aerobes

1. *Staphylococcus aureus*
2. *Streptococcus pyogenes*
3. *B. proteus*
4. *Pseudomonas*
5. Coliform bacilli.

Anaerobes

1. Streptococci
2. Bacteroides—Nonspore former
3. *Clostridium perfringens*
4. *Clostridium tetani*—Spore former
5. *Clostridium septicum*
6. *Clostridium edematiens.*

Fungi

1. *Candida*
2. *Aspergillus.*

Source of infection may be exogenous (from environment) or endogenous (from commensal of body). Open wound may be infected with multiple organisms whereas closed undrained wound is usually infected with single organism like *Staphylococcus aureus, Streptococcus pyogenes* and so on.

Collection of specimen: Specimen should be collected aseptically in an autoclaved container. Pus specimen is comparatively better than swabs. If swab is present over the wound peel it off and then swab is well-soaked in wound material. If abscess is there then aspirate it with sterilized needle. It is always advisable to obtain two swabs, one for smear and second for culture.

Chemicals like liquid (sodium polyanethole sulfonate) can be used to neutralize the toxic substance present in blood.

Processing of a tissue in broth is more useful than taking a swab. The swab should be moist. Specimen should be taken from margin of the ulcer.

Direct anaerobic culture can be performed on exudates which do not show squamous cells under microscope and also on fluids showing bacteria in smears where organisms morphologically resemble anaerobic bacteria.

The material collected is sent to laboratory. First of all material is examined grossly for especially bluish green color (*Pseudomonas*), and presence of gas (*Clostridium, Klebsiella, Escherichia coli*).

Smear stained with Gram's stain shows whether organism is Gram-positive or Gram-negative. Gram-staining also provides the information if the organism is cocci or bacilli. If Gram-positive cocci are arranged in cluster (staphylococcus), or in chains they are streptococcus. Gram-positive bacilli (spore bearer) may be *Clostridium tetani* or *Clostridium perfringens*. Gram-negative bacilli may be *pseudomonas, proteus, klebsiella, Escherichia coli*, etc.

Specimen may be cultured on blood agar plate (aerobically and anaerobically) and Robertson cooked meat medium (anaerobic culture). Aerobically specimen may be cultured on blood agar plate and MacConkey medium **(Fig. 47.5)**. Now colonies or growth on these media may be studied and smears also be prepared:

1. *Staphylococcus aureus* shows golden-colored, beta hemolytic colonies which are catalase and coagulase positive.
2. *Streptococcus pyogenes* shows pin-point, beta hemolytic colonies which are catalase negative. 99% belong to Lancefield group A.
3. Pseudomonas colonies are bluish green in color. They are oxidase positive and use glucose oxidatively (Hugh Leifson media).
4. Proteus colonies show characteristic swarming character. PPA and urease tests are positive. Species identification depends upon H_2S production, indole and citrate.
5. Coliform colonies are pink in color on MacConkey (lactose fermenter). Identification of species is based on biochemical tests (IMViC).

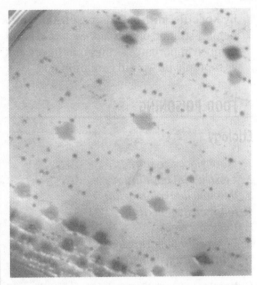

Fig. 47.5: MacConkey Agar; *Escherichia coli* (large pink colonies), *Salmonella typhi* (colorless colonies), *Staphylococcus aureus* (small pink colonies), *Streptococcus faecalis* (pin-point colonies).

Clues to the development of anaerobic infections are as follows:
1. Foul smell
2. Gas formation
3. Black exudate
4. Presence of granules (sulfur)
5. History of aminoglycoside therapy without any improvement.
6. Treatment with cytotoxic and immuno-suppressive drugs.

For anaerobic culture, inoculation is done immediately in Robertson cooked meat medium or thioglycollate medium and blood agar plates. If delay is inevitable we may use Stuart transport medium.

1. *Clostridium perfringens* is identified on the basis of morphological characters, demonstration of capsule and biochemical reactions (litmus milk stormy clot, Nagler's reaction positive and strongly sacchrolytic activity).
2. *Clostridium tetani* shows characteristic drumstick appearance. Demonstration of production of toxin and its neutralization

by specific antitoxin is essential. Only demon-stration of *Clostridium tetani* is not of much importance as they may be present as saprophytic wound contaminants.

FOOD POISONING

Etiology

1. *Staphylococcus aureus*
2. *Clostridium botulinum*
3. *Salmonella typhimurium*
4. *Salmonella enteritidis*
5. *Bacillus cereus*
6. *Clostridium perfringens*
7. *Vibrio parahemolyticus.*

Collection of specimen: Stools are collected aseptically in an autoclaved container. In case of any delay in sending the stools to laboratory stools may be collected in glycerol saline.

If isolation of causative organism is to be made from food then macerate food in Ringer's solution and then proceed for culture.

It is worthwhile to discuss collection and cultural method of each individual organism.

1. *Staphylococcus aureus* may be cultured from food or even from feces. Food is macerated in sterile Ringer's solution and inoculated on blood agar and 10% salt agar plates. Incubate at 37°C for 24 hours and look for golden colored colonies showing beta hemolysis with coagulase test positive.

2. *Clostridium botulinum* may be demonstrated in food by preparing smear and doing Gram-staining. Presence of spore bearing Gram-positive bacilli is suggestive of proceeding further. Food is macerated, centrifuged and filtered through filter paper. Now it may be injected into mice and guinea pig. The mice may show paresis of hind gut and difficulty in breathing. Similarly, guinea pig shows difficulty in breathing, flaccid abdominal muscles, salivation and congestion of internal organs. Further extensive thrombosis and hemorrhages may be noted at necropsy.

For isolation of *Clostridium botulinum*, food is macerated in sterile saline which is heated at 65–80°C for ½ hour to get rid of nonsporing bacteria. However, unheated samples should also be processed as spores of type E strains may be inactivated by heat. Inoculate the material on Willis and Hobb's medium containing neomycin and incubate at 32°C for 24 hours anaerobically. *Clostridium botulinum* is identified on the base of biochemical tests like fermentation of glucose, fructose and maltose with production of acid and gas.

Fluorescent antibody test is of great diagnostic aid. Smear of food sample is prepared and stain it with fluorescent tagged antibody and study it under fluorescent microscope.

3. *Salmonella:* Fecal matter is streaked on MacConkey, DCA, bismuth sulfite agar, selenite F, and tetrathionate broth. Incubate them at 37°C for 24 hours. Now study the colonies and do biochemical and serological tests for confirmation of salmonella.

In case isolation from food is desired then 25 gm of food may be taken in two sterile screw capped bottles. Now add 25 mL of 25% of Ringer's solution in each bottle. Incubate them at 37°C for 2 hours and add 50 mL double strength tetrathionate broth to the other. Now incubate at 37°C for 24 hours and subculture from each on MacConkey, DCA, and bismuth sulfite agar. If culture is negative repeat subculture after three days and then after 24 hours. Colonies are picked up and processed for biochemical and serological tests.

4. *Clostridium perfringens* may produce nonhemolytic colonies on horse blood agar plate. They are markedly heat resistant spores which are characteristically associated with mild form of food poisoning. However, intermediate heat resistant spore may also produce food poisoning. Heat resistant spores strain may be isolated by inoculation of feces in Robertson cooked meat medium. Heat it at 80 to 100°C for

1 hour, cool it and incubate at 37°C for overnight. Subculture it on Willis and Hobbs medium and incubate it anaerobically at 37°C for 24 hours. They show positive Nagler's reaction (if done) and are Gram-positive bacilli with squarecut ends.

Isolation of typical food poisoning strain of *Clostridium perfringens* from food is difficult as spores of it are rarely abundant in food. Food is macerated in broth, subcultured on Willis and Hobbs's medium containing neomycin and horse blood agar plate. Incubate them at 37°C for 24 hours anaerobically. Identify Nagler positive, nonhemolytic (horse blood), Gram-positive bacilli with square-cut ends. Heat resistance of spore is demonstrated by first growing spore bearing bacteria in Ellner medium. Final identification may be done by slide agglutination test with series of agglutinating antisera prepared against different food poisoning strain of *Clostridium perfringens*. For heat sensitive and moderate heat resistant spores, the food and stool may be processed like food as described above.

5. *Bacillus cereus* may be isolated from food by macerating food in saline and inoculating it on blood agar and nutrient agar media. Identification is done by colony characters. They are large Gram-positive bacilli, motile, noncapsulated and show low pathogenicity for mice. They are usually associated with fried rice. Their spores withstand cooking and then germinate later with production of toxin. This toxin is responsible for food poisoning.

6. *Vibrio parahemolyticus* is associated with food. Feces may be collected and inoculated on bile salt agar medium. After 37°C incubation for 24 hours, the colonies are identified by virtue of colony characters and biochemical reactions like fermentation of glucose, oxidase positive, catalase positive, indole positive, VP negative, urease negative, lysine, orinithine, decarboxylase positive and arganine dehydrolase negative.

PULMONARY TUBERCULOSIS

Sputum

Collection of specimen: Patient should be advised to brush his teeth, rinse his mouth with water and then cough up the specimen in a wide-mouthed clean container. It is usually desirable to collect 24 hours' collection of sputum. Nowadays first morning sputum sample is preferred. The most purulent or necrotic or hemorrhagic portion is removed by sterile forceps, platinum loop or Pasteur pipette for further processing.

Smear preparation and stainings: It is prepared by squash method, by keeping small portion of selected material on the slide and keeping the other slide over it. Now draw the slide apart. Two smears are ready. Dry them in the air and fix them by passing over the flame two or three times. Now stain them by Ziehl-Neelsen method and look for acid-fast bacilli. If negative repeat the specimen for two more occasions.

Concentration method (Petroff's method): Mix equal portions of sputum and 4% sodium hydroxide. Incubate at 37°C for 15 minutes to half-an-hour. Centrifuge it at 3000 revolutions per minute for half-an-hour. Now decant the supernatant and neutralize the deposit by adding N/10 HCl drop by drop. Again centrifuge it and discard the supernatant. From deposit prepare smear; do Ziehl-Neelsen stain and look for acid-fast bacilli. For quicker demonstration of acid-fast bacilli auramine O stain may be done and study under fluorescent microscope. Löwenstein-Jensen media may be used for culture by rubbing the deposit over it.

Laryngeal Swab

It is obtained by using sterilized nichrome or brass wire. Patient is asked to sit comfortably and with one hand pass laryngeal mirror while with the other hand pass the swab wire and collect the specimen in duplicate. Put the swab into the test tube containing 10% sulphuric acid for 5 minutes. Now transfer it to another tube containing 4% sodium hydroxide for 5 minutes. Drain each swab of excess of fluid and inoculate two bottles of Löwenstein-Jensen media.

Gastric Lavage

It is usually done in children who have the habit of swallowing sputum. Gastric juice is having harmful effect on acid-fast bacilli. So, it becomes necessary to process it as soon as possible. If delay is inevitable then neutralize it with N/10 sodium hydroxide and keep it in refrigerator till processed.

The specimen is collected before breakfast with Ryle's tube. Specimen is allowed to stand in a refrigerator. Supernatant is discarded and sediment centrifuged at 3000 revolutions per minute for 15 minutes. Smears are made and stained by Ziehl-Neelsen or auramine O. The remaining deposit is treated with equal amount of 4% sodium hydroxide. Incubate, centrifuge and discard the supernatant. Now neutralize the deposits with N/10 HCl and culture on Löwenstein-Jensen medium. Material is also used for inoculation in guinea pig, rabbit or mice.

Culture on Löwenstein-Jensen medium appears in 10–14 days at the earliest. It may take more than 8 weeks. Human strains grow luxuriantly than bovine strains. The addition of glycerol in the medium enhances the growth of human strain. However, two tubes of Löwenstein-Jensen media are used for each specimen. Every week media is inspected for any evidence of growth, aeration and removal of water of condensation. Growth of typical human strain is raised, irregular, wrinkled and creamy white in color. On liquid medium (Dubos') growth appears on the top as wrinkled pellicles. However, diffused growth may be obtained by adding Tween-80.

Animal inoculation: Guinea pig may be used for human as well as bovine strain. However, it is resistant to atypical mycobacteria. Rabbit is more susceptible to bovine than human strain whereas mice is susceptible to atypical mycobacteria.

About 0.5 mL each of concentrated material is injected intramuscularly into two guinea pigs. Local swelling appears in 10 days' time involving neighboring lymph nodes. Tuberculous nodules appear subsequently in other organs like spleen, liver, lungs and kidney. Death of animal may occur in 8 weeks' time.

Animals are examined weekly for the appearance and progress of lesion. One animal is killed as soon as lesion appears. If no lesion appears then the other animal is killed after 8 weeks and autopsy is performed to record the lesions. Smears are prepared from lesions and Ziehl-Neelsen stain is done to demonstrate acid-fast bacilli.

INFECTIVE ENDOCARDITIS

Causes

❖ *Streptococcus viridans*
❖ *Enterococcus fecalis*
❖ *Staphylococcus epidermidis*
❖ *Staphylococcus aureus*
❖ *Haemophilus influenzae*
❖ *Coxiella burnetti*
❖ *Chlamydia psittaci*
❖ *Bacteroides*
❖ Members of Enterobacteriaceae
❖ *Candida albicans*

Collection of Specimen

About 5 mL of blood is drawn by venepuncture aseptically and in to blood culture bottle containing 50 mL of 1% glucose citrate broth. The ratio of blood to broth should be about 1:10. The dilution of blood in broth helps in inhibiting the action of antibodies, antibiotics and leukocytes on bacterial growth. It is recommended that 3 to 6 samples of blood (10 mL each) may be collected over 24 hours. Samples of blood preferably should be collected at the height of fever.

Culture Procedure

Culture bottles are incubated at 37°C and after 48 hours subcultures are made on blood agar, MacConkey agar or any other suitable media. If this subculture is negative further subculture on 7th, 14th and 21st day are necessary, before declaring the culture as negative. Castaneda's bottle can also be used.

Enzymes like penicillinase may be added to inhibit the action of chemotherapeutic agents on bacteria and p-amino benzoic acid may be used for sulfonamides.

Infection with *C. burnetti* is diagnosed by animal inoculation and demonstration of antibodies in serum.

For anaerobic organisms thiol broth with added CO_2 under marked vacuum may be used. A dilution 1:17 of blood in broth is used.

Thus, the organisms grown are identified by usual methods.

▌SEPTICEMIA/BACTEREMIA

It is a condition where there is actively multiplying microorganism in the blood stream and formation of toxic products in the blood with manifestations (sign and symptoms).

Laboratory Diagnosis

Etiology of Septicemia

❖ *Salmonella typhi*
❖ *Salmonella paratyphi A*
❖ *Salmonella paratyphi B*
❖ *Salmonella paratyphi C*
❖ *Brucella*
❖ *Hemophilus influenzae*
❖ *Escherichia coli*
❖ *Klebsiella pneumonia*
❖ *Enterobacter*
❖ *Proteus*
❖ *Bacterioides*

❖ *Pseudomonas*
❖ *Streptococcus mitis*
❖ *Staphylococcus aureus*
❖ *Staphylococcus epidermidis*
❖ *Streptococcus pyogenes*
❖ *Pneumococcus*
❖ *Neisseria meningitidos*
❖ *Listeria monocytogenes*

1. Blood culture (1:10) is done with glucose broth. For anaerobic culture, thioglycollate borth is used. Alternatively, RCM may be used. Sodium polyanethol sulfonate (SPS) may be added which acts as anticoagulative, antiphagocytic, anticomplementory etc. It interferes with certain antibiotics, e.g., aminoglycosides and thus enhances growth rate and increases the rate of isolation

2. Castaneda method

3. Automated blood culture system, e.g., bacteria (detection of CO_2 by radiometric or optical methods)

4. Culture of other specimen:
   a. I/v catheter tips
   b. Swab from infected burn
   c. Swab from wound or abscess
   d. Urine in urinary tract infection
   e. Sputum in respiratory tract infection.

5. Nonculture method to detect circulating antigens and other microbial products.
   a. Latex agglutination test, e.g., *H. influenzae*-b antigen, *N. meningitidis*, *Streptococcus pneumoniae* and yeasts, etc.
   b. Counter current immunoelectrophrosis (CIEP) used to quickly identify *pneumococcus*, Klebsiella, *H. Influenzae* etc.
   c. Limulus ambocyte lystate assay tests may be used to detect circulating lipopolysaccharide (endotoxin) of Gram-negative bacteria in blood.

6. Gas liquid chromatography detects metabolic end products of anaerobic micobacterial activity in serum.

■ INTRODUCTION

Various serological techniques are used to demonstrate antibodies in the serum of patients. The formation of these antibodies in the serum of patient is the result of provocation by microbial infection. Their demonstration is of great diagnostic value especially in conditions where isolation of causative organism takes quite a long-time. In the interpretation of these tests following points should be kept in mind.

1. The duration of antibody responses to various organisms differs. Evidence in support of fresh infection is rising titer of antibodies. It can be demonstrated by collecting two serum samples at a week's interval. Four-fold rise of antibody titer is considered significant.

2. It is important to know basal titer of normal healthy individuals of the same age, habitat and social habitat of the patient. This is important before attaching any significance to antibody titer measured by particular test.

3. Antibody responses are not detectable for a week's time after onset of infection. So, the serum sample collected within a week of a disease is not expected to give appreciable or significant antibody titer.

4. Anamnestic reactions is defined as rise in the level of previously formed antibody in response to nonspecific stimulus of quite different infection. It is recognized with Salmonella H agglutinins showing increase in titer following unrelated febrile illness.

5. Detectable antibodies may not be formed in a patient suspected of suffering from illness in which antibodies are mostly formed. Hence, antibodies are not detected in patients' blood even weeks after the onset of disease. This may be explained on the basis of derangement of antibody forming mechanism.

6. Antibodies are not necessarily protective in nature and so not related to person's immune status.

Here we will discuss important serological tests like widal test, serological test for brucellosis, antistreptolysin O (ASO) antibody test, cold hemagglutination test, Paul-Bunnel test, Weil-Felix test and streptococcus-MG agglutination test.

1. **Widal test:** This investigation is done for the diagnosis of enteric fever or other Salmonella infection. Conventionally, H and O suspensions of *Salmonella typhi* and paratyphi are used. For the test serial dilutions of patient's serum (1 : 10, 1: 20, 1: 40, 1: 80, 1: 160, 1: 320....) are pipetted in small amounts (0.3 mL) into special small tubes. One complete set of dilutions is prepared for each bacterial suspension used in the test. An equal volume (0.3 mL) of appropriate bacterial suspension is added to each tube of particular row. Control tubes are also set up containing saline and bacterial suspension but no patient serum. Control is set up to ensure that the bacteria do not agglutinate spontaneously. Now these tubes are incubated at 37°C in water bath for overnight. Floccular

agglutination of H suspension and granular agglutination of O suspension are noted after 12 to 24 hours' incubation. However, in H suspension after 55°C incubation for 2 hours, floccules become apparent. The results of the test are expressed as antibody titer.

Low levels of antibodies that agglutinate Salmonella suspension may be detected in the blood of patient without history or relevant illness or of immunization. Hence, it may be taken as normal. Anamnestic reaction is more common in H agglutinin than O agglutinin. The most reliable serological evidence of Salmonella infection is a four-fold or more increase in O agglutinin levels between first and second or later weeks of illness. However, absence of antibodies response does not exclude the possibility of typhoid as patient may fail to produce detectable levels of antibodies.

2. **Serological test for brucellosis:** Brucellosis may cause persistent pyrexia. For brucellosis agglutination test may be done using suspension of *Brucella abortus.* Demonstration of rising titer of 1:100 or more indicates active brucellosis. In chronic cases, we may find low agglutination titer or prozone phenomena (failure of serum to cause agglutination until serum is further diluted). Prozone phenomena may be because of blocking action of nonagglutinating IgG antibodies. Coomb's test or complement fixation test with a titer of 1:32 or more in either test points towards active brucellosis.

Patient's serum is inactivated at 56°C for 30 minutes. Serial dilution of serum, i.e., 1:10, 1:20, 1:30, 1:40, 1:80 and so on are prepared. Now equal quantity of bacterial suspension is added in each tube. After 37°C incubation for 48 hours agglutination of each tube is noted.

3. **Antistreptolysin O (ASO) antibody titer:** ASO titer is expressed in Todd unit. One todd unit is the amount of serum (antibodies) neutralizing 2½ MHD of standard hemolysin. A titer of 400 units or higher is considered highly significant and diagnostic, i.e., streptococcal infection.

Patient's serum is inactivated and double dilution is prepared. 0.5 mL of diluted antigen (streptolysin O) is added to each serum dilution. Mixture is incubated in water bath at 37°C for 15 minutes. To each tube 0.5 mL of rabbit blood cells are added. Now incubate the mixture at 37°C for another 45 minutes. ASO titer is represented by the last tube in which hemolysis has not occurred.

4. **Cold hemagglutination test:** This test is used for the diagnosis of primary atypical pneumonia caused by mycoplasma. Prepare serial dilution of the serum of the patient. In the tube add 0.5 mL of human RBC of blood group O (1%). Shake the rack and keep in refrigerator at 4°C overnight. Reading is taken immediately after taking out the rack from refrigerator. Clumping of RBC is labeled as positive reaction.

5. **Paul-Bunnel test:** It is used for the diagnosis of infectious mononucleosis. Serum of the patient is inactivated at 56°C for half an hour. Serial dilution of this inactivated serum is prepared. Now 1 mL of sheep red blood cells (1%) are added to each tube. After incubation at 37°C for 4 hours, tubes are examined for any evidence of clumping of red blood cells. Titer of 1:100 is suggestive of infectious mononucleosis. If positive, then the test is further done using guinea pig kidney suspension and ox red cell for removal of Forssman antibody.

6. **Weil-Felix test:** This test is used for the diagnosis of typhus fever. In this test, sera of the patient is tested for agglutinins to O antigens of certain nonmotile proteus strains: OX_{19}, OX_2 and OXk. The basis of test is the sharing of an alkali stable carbohydrate antigen by some rickettsiae and by certain strain of proteus, i.e., *P. vulgaris* (OX_{19} and OX_2) and *P. mirabilis,* i.e., (OXk). The test is mostly done as tube agglutination

test. However, rapid slide agglutination methods have also been employed for rapid screening. The antibody appears rapidly during the course of disease. Peak titer is 1:1000 to 1:1500 in second week and decline rapidly during convalescence. The test is of no value in the diagnosis of rickettsial pox, trench fever and Q fever. False-positive reaction may occur in cases of urinary or other infection caused by proteus, typhoid fever and liver disorders. Hence, rising titer should be demonstrated.

7. **Streptococcus MG agglutination test:** This test is used for the diagnosis of primary atypical pneumonia caused by mycoplasma. Here unheated patient serum is used. Serial dilutions of patient serum are prepared. 0.5 mL of diluted heat killed suspension of MG streptococcus antigen is added to each dilution. After 2 hours' incubation of mixture at 37°C, it may be refrigerated overnight. Reading is taken as in Widal's test. A titer of 1:20 or more is suggestive of this infection.

8. **Skin tests:** The following skin tests are commonly used as diagnostic aid for detecting immune status and for detecting hypersensitivity:
   a. Schick test is used to find out immune status against diphtheria. Small amount of diphtheria toxin injected into the skin of nonimmune person causes erythema which begins to appear 1–2 days after injection, reaches maximum in 4 days and persists for about a week or two. There may be small swelling at the site of injection. In persons whose level of diphtheria antitoxin is sufficient to protect him against an attack of diphtheria the toxin is neutralized and hence no reaction.
   b. Dick test may be used to determine the need of immunization against scarlet fever. Reaction is more rapid and is transitory.
   c. Tuberculin test is based on type IV hypersensitivity. The test material used may be old tuberculin or purified protein derivative. Positive tuberculin test indicates past tuberculous infection and also probable immunity. In positive reaction, we find palpable induration (10 mm or more) which is maximum in 2-3 days after injection. Erythema may be there but is in part nonspecific and so difficult to interpret. The purpose of tuberculin test is: (i) diagnostic for individual patient, (ii) to find out foci of infection, i.e., in the absence of vaccination high incidence of active tuberculosis is encountered meaning active dissemination of disease, (iii) survey of population to find out the frequency of tuberculosis in the community, (iv)selection of subject for BCG vaccination, i.e., negative tuberculin test indicates the requirement of BCG vaccination, (v) assessment of the efficacy of BCG vaccination.
   d. Brucellin test may be used for the diagnosis of brucellosis but this test is of little diagnostic importance.
   e. Lepromin test is used in leprosy patients.
   f. Frei's test is used for the diagnosis of lymphogranuloma venerium.
   g. Skin test may be used in cat scratch fever. Pus from active cases diluted 1:5 and heated 60°C for 10 hours can be used as skin antigen. It gives positive reaction in some individual with a clinical picture.

The other skin tests are for the diagnosis of chanceroid *(H. ducreyi),* tularemia and Schultz-Charlton reaction (streptococci Group A), herpes simplex, mumps, etc.

Microbiology in the Service of Human Being

Microbes have positive contribution in day-to-day activities of human being. Some microbes are useful in souring milk, ripening of cheese, production of antibiotics, fermentation, acetic acid, butanol and so on. Some organisms are capable of killing mosquitoes and can be useful in the control of disease like malaria, commensals microorganisms are useful in maintaining health and normal functions of the body. Normal flora of intestine is also responsible for production of vitamins. They also maintain balanced and favorable atmosphere for other forms of life by releasing carbon, nitrogen, oxygen in the environment, etc. They are used in research and study and understanding of genetics. Microorganisms are also used in genetic engineering for the production of hormones, vaccines, etc. On the other extreme organisms exhibit affinity for ores and may be used to locate ores like gold, sulfur, etc. Microorganisms are at the same time harmful too especially in causing infectious diseases and their proposed use in bioterrorism.

Microbiology is the branch of science dealing with study of microbes like bacteria, viruses, fungi and parasites. There are other branches of microbiology like medical microbiology, industrial microbiology, food microbiology, soil microbiology, plant microbiology, etc.

▓ MEDICAL MICROBIOLOGY

Medical microbiology is closely associated with diagnosis, epidemiology, control of infections and treatment. One needs to understand that disease producing capacity of microorganism may be enhanced by environmental and host factors, e.g., contaminated food, drinks, air malnutrition, tissue damage and overcrowding. Medical microbiology has the constitution as a model in structure of genetics, molecular biology, diagnostic, prevention and control of various microbial diseases.

Medical microbiologist may plan out various steps likely to be effective to control infections as below:
1. Microorganisms can be eliminated from its source or breeding places. Thus, transmission to new host is checked.
2. Securing clean hand and edibles, drinks with control of house files and cockroaches. This checks intestinal infections like typhoid, cholera, dysentery, food poisoning, etc.
3. Seeking proper disposal of hospital wastage and sewage which is a health hazards.
4. Use of insecticides killing vectors and hence checking malaria, dengue, louse-borne disease.
5. Prophylactic vaccination.
6. Surveillance of communicable diseases by keeping track of source and spread of infecting agent and study of conditions that may favor the spread of infection in the community. Overall, it gives prognostic predictions about future trends and assessment of deliberate control measures.

▓ ROLE OF MICROBIOLOGY

Role of medical microbiologist may include as follows:
1. Diagnosis is made by isolating the causative agent from pathological lesions. Serological

methods and latest techniques like PCR, probes, etc. are of great help.

2. Prognosis of disease may be reviewed by microbiologist, e.g., Widal test. Rising titer is interpreted as active disease. Declining titer means curing and that treatment is effective.

3. Guidance in treatment is provided by antibiotic sensitivity test report.

4. Medical microbiologist can also help in finding out source of infection, e.g., in a sudden outbreak of typhoid disease in a hospital ward, one can find out carrier of Salmonella (kitchen workers) by subjecting their stool samples for bacteriological culture.

5. Microbiologist is engaged in the preparation of vaccine against outbreak of infection around.

IMPORTANCE IN DIAGNOSIS OF INFECTIOUS DISEASE

Medical microbiologist are enthusiastic to confirm diagnosis by making smears, preparing cultures from lesions (boil, cellulites) to demonstrate microorganisms and suggesting effective antibiotics. Each investigation of a patient is as a matter of fact a challenge and thrill. It is dealt as a research project in miniature. In a way, a clinician by requesting an investigation is asking a questions and microbiology laboratory attempts to reply in a realiable and rapid way.

Adequate clinical management of microbial diseases depends on accurate identification of involved organism and antimicrobial sensitivity. Molecular biological techniques have increased the speed and sensitivity of detection methods as well as allowing laboratories to identify organisms that do not grow or grow slowly in culture. These techniques also allow microbiologists to identify genes that result in resistance in antibiotics and to fingerprint individual isolates for epidemiological tracking.

Infections diseases still remain a major cause of morbidity despite decades of progress in diagnostic front, preventive measures and treatment. Every now and then new antimicrobial agents are introduced with the hope that infectious diseases would be eliminated. Emergence of resistance of enterococci to vancomycin, pneumococci to penicillin and so on are clinical problems and matter of concern. In a way that is how microorganisms are developing the ability to elude activities of antibiotics. Result is ever increasing antibiotic resistance. Further, the emergence of unique infectious disease or novel mechanisms of resistance will always cause us to haul the old tools out of closet until these agents have been identified and characterized.

Smallpox is completely eradicated from the world since 1977. We have progressed towards conquering over many infectious disease like anthrax, plague, etc. Some infectious diseases are re-emerging, e.g., malaria, influenza, dengue cholera, tuberculosis. Many infectious agents have been discovered recently, i.e., HIV, Marburg virus, Ebola virus, Hunta virus, Nipah virus, Hendra virus, etc. Of course campaign is in progress with vaccines and other effort on war footing to deal with these infectious challenges.

Community Microbiology

ROLE OF MICROBIOLOGY IN COMMUNITY

Microbiology is closely concerned with the epidemiology and control of infection in any community where the transmission and disease producing capacity of the infecting microorganisms may be enhanced by environmental or host factors like contaminated food, drink or air, malnutrition, tissue damage and overcrowding.

Epidemiology is concerned with etiological factors and it has had conspicuous successes in their elucidation among both infectious and noninfectious diseases, e.g., cholera, typhoid fever, pellagra, lung cancer, etc. Improved public health measures like safe water supply, proper disposal of sewage, good housing and nutrition of citizen are major factors in the decline of epidemic infectious diseases.

Certain infections are due to opportunistic invasion of tissues by commensal microorganisms previously resident elsewhere in the body. These are called endogenous infection (originating from within). They are not ordinarily transmissible from one person to another, e.g., urinary tract infection, subacute bacterial endocarditis, etc. On the other hand, measles, whooping cough, chickenpox, etc. are infectious and communicable. They are transmissible from one person to another and are called exogenous (originating from without) infections. Yet there is another group of infections that are transmissible from vertebrate animals, animal hosts to man and not communicable ordinarily from man-to-

man. They are called zoonosis, e.g., bubonic plague, brucellosis, rabies, etc.

No one can deny the importance of carriers in the study of sources and modes of spread of infections. Both bacteriological and epidemiological studies brought to light the convalescents and more persistent stool excreter of typhoid fever thus confirming the hypothesis of Koch that in typhoid fever, the acute or convalescent patient was a common source for subsequent infection. After sometime it was shown that carriers (individual with no clinical disease but carry and disperse a pathogenic microorganism) were important links in the chain of dissemination of various infections in the community. Antibodies titer to specific pathogens or their toxin has shown that inapparent infections may have a role in raising the resistance of a community to epidemic outburst of disease.

Microbiologists and health officers with sound knowledge of the epidemiology of communicable disease can plan out various steps likely to be quite effective for its control. Even in the field of prophylactic immunization microbiologist can be a valuable partner.

The main causes of death, among the infections a century ago were tuberculosis, pneumonia, bronchitis, typhoid fever, diarrheal diseases and scarlet fever. Only recently AIDS, pneumonia and bronchitis took a heavy toll of life. The death rate from tuberculosis, and diarrheal disease have started declining. Rheumatic heart disease still has high death rate. New infections are emerging all over the world like HIV, campylobacter, *Helicobacter pyloridis,* etc.

The extraordinary reduction in deaths from infections is due to improvement in nutrition, environmental sanitation and living conditions and use of antimicrobial drugs. Still infection remains the major cause of sickness especially children, e.g., respiratory infections (cold, sore throat, catarrh bronchitis, etc.), specific fevers (measles, whooping cough, chickenpox, mumps, etc.), diarrheal diseases and staphylococcal infections. There is no doubt to the fact that infections if not treated promptly and effectively may lead to impairment of physical or mental development or death. Laboratory services for general practitioners are therefore quite essential and so collaboration between the practitioner and microbiologist will definitely help to improve the quality of patient care in the community.

A community infection of special kind occurs among patients admitted in hospitals (nosocomial infection). However, many infectious diseases are being controlled by good environmental sanitation, by the destruction of insect vector like louse, flea, mosquitoes or by prophylactic vaccination, e.g., typhus, plague, etc. Smallpox is completely eradicated from the world since 1977. At the same time many infections like AIDS, malaria, tuberculosis, leprosy, diarrheal diseases, pneumonia, viral hepatitis, etc. take a heavy toll of life and health in most of the developing countries.

Control of community infections: It may be achieved as below:
1. Pathogen can be eliminated from its source or breeding ground and hence transmission to a new host is checked, e.g., syphilis, gonorrhea, mycobacterial infections
2. Securing clean hands, water, milk and food with control of flies. Thus, intestinal infections like typhoid, dysentery, cholera and food poisoning can be controlled
3. Proper disposal of sewage
4. Prophylactic vaccination
5. Use of insecticides thus killing vectors and hence control of malaria, yellow fever, dengue, louseborne typhus, etc.

Surveillance: Broadly, it means natural history of disease associated with continuous observation of its occurrence. Surveillance of communicable disease connotes the active follow-up of specific infections in terms of morbidity and mortality in time and place, keeping track of the source and spread of infecting agent and the study of conditions that may favor or inhibit the spread of infection in the community. Of course, it requires teamwork with the obvious involvement of the microbiologist. It permits prognostic predictions about future trends and objective assessment of deliberate control measures.

Surveillance in the control of infections is quite effective, e.g., campaign against poliomyelitis, first with killed and later with live vaccine resulted in the virtual disappearance of paralytic polio. It has been followed by an intense epidemiological surveillance at both laboratory and clinical levels in order to monitor the effectiveness and safety of vaccine and to detect viruses other than polio virus which may cause infantile paralysis.

It may be concluded that use of antimicrobial drugs in acute infections, isolation of patients, blocking of channels of spread and protection of susceptible host allows the microbiologist and workers of other disciplines, to reduce the load of infection and control its spread whether locally within the family, hospital or within the general community.

Microbiology influences the community infection as below:
❖ Collection of exact data
❖ Laboratory investigation
❖ Spread of infection
❖ Zoonosis.

Hospital Infections

INTRODUCTION

Infections which are acquired from hospitals are called nosocomial infections. If the organisms come from another patient it is called cross infections and if the patient himself carries the infection to some other site then it is autoinfection. Infection may become apparent during the stay of the patient in the hospital or after his discharge from the hospital. There is actual increase in the frequency and severity of infection especially due to antibiotic resistant enterobacteria, *Staphylococcus aureus* and *Pseudomonas aeruginosa*. Thus, prolonged stay of the patient in the hospital is undesired and may be a serious matter for the patient and his family. Moreover, his maintenance in hospital and treatment is quite expensive. At the same time prolonged undesired stay of the patient in the hospital means occupation of bed which might otherwise be used for another needy patient.

HOSPITAL INFECTION AND PREVENTION

We should be aware of some important hospital infections and about their prevention:

1. **Wounds and burns**: It is important to remove all tissue debris from accidental wounds and burns as bacteria can establish more easily in damaged tissue. A careful and aseptic technique for dressing of wound preferably in dressing room reduces chances of cross infection.

2. **Urinary tract infection**: Catheter or other instruments into the bladder may cause urinary tract infection. Used catheters are difficult to sterilize and may be the cause of cross infection also, hence disposable sterilized catheter should be used aseptically. Continuous bladder drainage with indwelling catheter becomes necessary and so receptacles of the catheter should not be open to ward air (ascending infection) but should preferably be kept in disposable plastic bag.

3. **Alimentary tract infections**: Outbreak of *E. coli* gastroenteritis in children and of *Shigella sonnei* dysentery do occur quite oftenly in hospital. Isolation, general hygiene and exclusion of carriers are important preventive measures.

4. **Baths as means of cross infections**: It is commonly seen that series of babies are made to have bath in a same sink thus resulting in dispersal of pathogenic organisms especially *Staphylococcus aureus* through nursery. Hence, it is emphasized that if newborn babies need to be bathed, this should be done in stainless steel bowls which can easily be autoclaved after the bathing of each baby.

Patients Requiring Isolation

Some patients really need isolation. Patients of tuberculosis, typhoid, diphtheria, Lassa fever or smallpox should not be treated or nursed in open ward as these diseases are serious and easily transmissible. Similarly, infants with measles or whooping cough should not be nursed in general ward but may be treated at home. *Staphylococcus aureus* infection cases especially resistant to many antibiotics belonging to phage types (80/81 or 75/77) capable of causing serious epidemic of hospital sepsis, certainly require isolation. Isolation is also desirable for babies with *Escherichia coli* gastroenteritis and for many patients with *Pseudomonas aeruginosa* or diarrheal diseases infections. Isolation cubicles are suggested for these purposes which should be so designed, equipped and managed that no microorganism can pass from them to a ward. Attendant should use gown on entering the cubicle and remove on leaving. Washing facilities for the patient and attendant of the patient must be provided in the cubicle. Dressings should be discarded into paper bags which may be removed to incinerator. Beddings and clothings should be kept in disinfectant solution before sending to laundry. Excreta should also be treated with disinfectant and crockery should not be permitted to return to kitchen without sterilization. When the patient finally leaves the cubicle, it must be thoroughly washed with disinfectant and all equipment must be sterilized as far as possible.

Epidemiological Markers Useful in Investigating Hospital Infection

❖ Antibiogram and resistogram
❖ Biotyping
❖ Phage typing
❖ Bacteriocin typing
❖ Serotyping
❖ Serum opacity factor (analysis of marker proteins, analysis of enzyme production, e.g., *Staphylococcus aureus*)
❖ RNA electrophoresis as is done in rotavirus
❖ Cytotoxicity assay, e.g., *Proteus mirabilis*
❖ Reverse phage typing, e.g., *Staphylococcus aureus*
❖ Plasmid profile.

Prevention of Nosocomial Infections

❖ Proper washing of hands
❖ Isolation of patients, e.g., plague, influenza, measles, etc
❖ Careful and appropriate use of instruments
❖ Use of antibiotics only if required. It may be given to carrier staff or patient
❖ Use of blood transfusion only if must. Disinfectant of excreta and infected material
❖ Surveillance of infection properly and regularly
❖ Use of vaccine, e.g., tetany gas gangrene, hepatitis B, etc.

Factors Responsible for Hospital Infections

❖ Neonates and aged patients have risk of getting hospital infection because of long stay and decreased immunity
❖ Impaired defense mechanisms of patients due to disease or treatment
❖ Hospital environment contains relatively heavy load of microorganisms
❖ Major invasive diagnostic or therapy procedures
❖ Advance treatment of cancer, organ transplantation, etc
❖ Presence of multidrug resistant bacteria, etc.

The incident of hospital infection in developed countries is 2–12%. These are the hospitals where people suffering from various health problems are cured. Surprisingly, the hospitals are also responsible for transmitting diseases (especially infectious) to the patients being treated in the hospitals. One cannot forget what Florence Nightingale once said that hospitals should do no harm to the patients. Unfortunately, in spite of best efforts microorganism free environment in hospitals has never been achieved.

Sources of Hospital Infection

❖ Infecting microorganisms from fellow patients which may be multidrug resistant
❖ Infecting organisms from hospital staff
❖ Infecting organisms from instruments, blood products, intravenous fluid, etc.
❖ From patient's normal flora, etc.
❖ Insects are also the source of multidrug infection
❖ Organism may be present in air, dust, water, antiseptic solution, food, etc.
❖ Surfaces contaminated by patient's secretions, blood fluid, etc.

Mode of Infection

❖ Airborne
❖ Contact, e.g., hands, clothing, etc.
❖ Food and water
❖ Hospital equipment and instruments
❖ By parenteral route.

Outline of Investigative Approach of Hospital Infection Outbreak

It includes number of patients involved with their distribution in wards, times of onset, their symptoms, whether all or majority of cases followed operation if so whether they were operated in same operation theater and other clues as to the way in which they became infected. If their infection is by identical bacteria, effort should be made to trace human carrier or other sources of infection. Outbreak of infection in the hospital is generally because of defective ventilation in the ward or theater, in aseptic technique or in sterilization of dressings or instruments and improper cleanliness of hospital kitchen plus its workers.

▌MICROBES CAUSING NOSOCOMIAL ▌INFECTION

Gram Positive

❖ *Staphylococcus aureus*
❖ *Streptococcus pyogenes*

❖ *Staphylococcus epidermidis*
❖ *Streptococcus pneumoniae*
❖ *Clostridium difficile*
❖ *Clostridium perfringens*
❖ *Clostridium tetani*

Gram Negative

❖ *Escherichia*
❖ *Klebsiella*
❖ *Citrobacter*
❖ *Serratia*
❖ *Proteus*
❖ *Enterobacter*
❖ *Pseudomonas*
❖ *Legionella*

Viruses

❖ *Hepatitis B*
❖ *Hepatitis C*
❖ *Hepatitis D*
❖ *HIV*
❖ *Herpes virus*
❖ *Cytomegalovirus*
❖ *Influenza virus*
❖ *Enteroviruses*

Fungi

❖ *Aspergillus*
❖ *Candida albicans*

Parasites

❖ *Toxoplasma gondii*
❖ *Entamoeba histolytica*
❖ *Pneumocystis carinii*
❖ *Cryptosporidium*

▌BUNDLES IN INFECTION PREVENTION AND ▌SAFETY

Care bundles means a set of evidence-based points use of lengthen inpatients. They are much more useful than that of their use in individual patients. Bundle help to create reliable and consistent care system in hospital setting as they are simple clear and concise and they help to reduce and prevent infection, reduce use of antibiotics, limit the development of antibiotics resistant.

Specific care bundles include bundle for prevention:

1. Central lane associated blood stream infection.
2. Catheter associated urinary tract infections.
3. Ventilator-associated pneumonia.
4. Surgical site infection (SSI).

Central Line Associated Bloodstream Infection)

It occurs when bacteria or other microbes enter central line of patient and ultimately enter the bloodstream. Infection occurs this way is quite serious, catheter is placed veins of neck (internal jugular vein), chest (subclavian of axillary vein) or thru vein in arm [peripherally inserted central catheter (PICC)] line.

Causes

- *Staphylococcus aureus* (1%)
- *Pseudomonas aeruginosa* (3%)
- *Bacillus* species
- *Micrococcus* species
- Proploni bacteria
- Fungi
- Mycobacteria
- *Candida* (11%)
- *Enterobacter* (3.1°A)
- *E.coli* (2.7%)
- *Acinetobacter bacteria* (2.2%)
- Staph (coagulase negative) (34%)
- Enterococci (16%)
- Klebsiella (5.8%)

Prevention

- Use appropriate hand hygiene. Hand must be washed before and after palpating insertion site, dressing, etc.
- Maximal barrier precaution.
- Antiseptic of skin with chlorhexidine

- Optimal catheter site selection
- Daily assessment of central line is must
- Change of administration sets for continuous infusion after every four days.

Complications

- Infection
- Thrombosis
- Catheter malposition
- Phlebitis at insertion site
- Embolism
- Hematoma
- Arrythmia

Ventilators-associated infection

Causes

- *Pseudomonas aeruginosa*
- Methicilin-resistant *Staphylococcus*
- *Acetobacter* species
- *Enterobacter* species
- Vancomycin resistant *Enterococcus*
- *Klebsiella* pneumoniae
- *Legionella pneumophila*
- *Aspergillus*
- *Haemophilus influenzae*
- *Serratia*
- *Streptococcus* species

Preventive Measures

- Prevention of microbial multiplication in aerodigestive tract
- Avoid unnecessary antibiotic
- Oral rinse with chlorhexidine
- Short course infectible prophylactic antibiotic in high risk patients
- Prevention of aspiration of contaminated secretion by resign oral intubation
- Shorten the duration of mechanical ventilation
- Semirecumbent position minimizes gastric distention
- Subglottic suction

Surgical Site Infection

It is the infection of incision or organ or space that occurs after surgery. SSI may cause usually preventable death.

Prevention

- ❖ Antibiotic may be administered by infection about 1 hour before incision.
- ❖ In prolonged surgical procedures or major blood loss antibiotic may be continued in proper dose.
- ❖ Shave the part to be operated
- ❖ Use alcohol-based disinfectant for skin preparation in the operating room
- ❖ Maintain blood glucose less than 200 mg/dL
- ❖ Administer increased fraction of inspired oxygen during surgery
- ❖ Other measure includes hand hygiene, use of sterilize surgical instrument and equipment, etc.

Catheter-associated Urinary Tract Infection

It is catheter associated urinary infection with significant bacteriuria in a patient with catheter for last 48 hours.

Prevention

- ❖ Aseptic insertion and maintenances of catheter like proper hand washing, use of sterilized catheter, etc.
- ❖ Early removal of catheter
- ❖ Avoiding the use of urinary catheter by considering other alternative methods, e.g., condom catheters, intermittent catheterization, use of nappies, etc.
- ❖ Daily assessment of the presence and need for indwelling catheter.

BLOOD TRANSFUSION INFECTION

Infectious agents responsible for blood transfusion are as under:

Viruses

- ❖ HIV
- ❖ Hepatitis B
- ❖ Hepatitis C
- ❖ Hepatitis D
- ❖ Cytomegalovirus
- ❖ Human lymphotropic virus

Bacteria

- ❖ *Treponema pallidum*
- ❖ *Leptospira*
- ❖ *Borrelia burgdorferi*

Protozoa

- ❖ *Plasmodium* species
- ❖ *Leishmania donovani*
- ❖ *Toxoplasma gondii*
- ❖ *Trypanosoma cruzi*
- ❖ Babesia species

Helminthes

- ❖ *Wuchereria* species

INFECTION CONTROL COMMITTEE

It includes as under:
1. Hospital Director/Dean/Principal: Chairman
2. Microbiologist/Epidemiologist: Infection control officer
3. Chief of medical services: Member
4. Quality control/assurance officer: Member
5. Head of clinical/assurance officer: Member
6. Head of support system: Member
7. Head of pharmacy: Member
8. Chief nurse: Member
9. Infection control nurse: Member

Responsibilities of Infection Control Committee

1. Production and implementation of disinfectant policy

2. They must review microbiology record regularly to identify more than usual incidences of species of microorganism.
3. Conduction of outbreak investigation and act control measures.
4. They must arrange a meeting at least once in a month to formulate and reupdate policy of hospital for infection control and to manage outbreak of hospital infection.
5. It includes surveillance, control, monitoring of hygiene practice and education of all staff in the microbiologically safe performance of procedure.
6. To establish close working links between microbiology laboratory, different clinical department and support services like sterile services, laundry, pharmacy, etc.

Infection Control Team

The infection control team consists of:
❖ The director of infection control and prevention.
❖ An infection control doctor
❖ A microbiologist
❖ An antimicrobial pharmacist
❖ A lead nurse in infection control
❖ Infection control nurses
❖ An infection control nursery
❖ An infection control nursery service and administration

Responsibilities of Infection Control Team

❖ This team is responsible for advising and education staff at all levels on hoe to prevent and reduce cross infection in the hospital.
❖ They have the responsibility for advising the hospital administration which an infection outbreak occurs in a ward.
❖ Data collection, anaiyzing, communicate among staff etc
❖ Action plan

STANDARD ROUTINE PRECAUTIONS TO PREVENT HOSPITAL INFFECTION

Following precautions must be observed while dealing with patients, specimens, sharp, etc.
1. Hand hygiene
2. No touch technique
3. Use of gloves to avoid contact with blood, body fluid, secretion, etc.
4. Use of mask, gown, shoes, eye glasses, etc.
5. Sharp handling carefully.
6. Spoilage cleaning e.g., spills of infectious material immediately.
7. Disinfection of linen, equipment used by patient. They must be sterilized or discarded between each patient use.
8. Ensure appropriate biomedical waste separation and disposal.
9. Patients should be confined to restricted area.
10. If required nasal carriers must be treated with mupirocin.

PERSONAL PROTECTIVE EQUIPMENT

Personal protective equipment (PPE) includes gloves, mask, gown, shoes, eye cover and so on.

WHO needs PPE

1. Patients with confirmed COVID-19 infection should were facemask when being evaluated medically.
2. Healthcare workers should observe standard precautions when attending COVID-19 infection.

How to use PPE Gear

1. Ensure choice is gown size is correct. Tie all ties on the gown.
2. Perform hand hygiene using hand sanitirer.
3. Use N 95 fillering facepiece respizator

4. Put on face shield or goggles when wearing N95 respirator
5. Put on gloves that must cover wrist of gown.
6. Healthcare worker can enter patient room.

How to take off PPE Gear

1. Remove glove carefully

2. Remove gown
3. Healthcare personnel may now leave patient room
4. Perform now hand hygiene
5. Remove now face shield or goggles
6. Remove and discard respirator or facemask
7. Perform on hand hygiene after removing respirator or facemask.

INTRODUCTION

Hands have key role in patient care, e.g. touching the patients, using the equipment, furniture and even greetings. Nurse to patient and doctor to patient contacts occur through hands. At the same time, hands are also responsible in transmitting disease through microorganisms. Hence, nurses and other workers should keep their hands thoroughly clean before makng contact with patients.

Ignaz Semmelwers identified hands in transmission of infection by the hands. He observed that hand washing actually reduced the incidence of infections. Lord Lister used carbolic acid to wash the hands before and after attending the patients.

As a matter of fact, skin over the hands contain resident flora. Resident flora usually consists of:

1. *Staphylococcus epidermidis*
2. Micrococci
3. Gram-positive bacilli

Resistant flora is difficult to remove by simple washing or scrubbing. However, they are temporarily inactivated with antiseptic lotions, creams or antibiotic preparations. Inspite of all this, significant growth occurs within 24 hours of treatment. Microbial flora capable of causing diseases comprises of:

1. *Staphylococcus aureus*
2. Streptococci

3. Gram-negative bacilli like *Escherichia coli*, Pseudomonas etc.
4. Viruses.

Transient flora is loosely attached to upper layer of the skin and may be removed by washing with soap and water.

FACTORS INFLUENCING HANDWASHING

1. Alcohol or iodine or chlorohexidine can be used in high risk areas. When these compounds are used for hand washing the instruction given on the label must be followed strictly.
2. Frequency of handwashing with soap and water up to two per hour is alright. If frequency is more antimicrobial soap should be used instead of ordinary soap.
3. Amount of soap or antiseptic solution should be around 1 mL liquid soap for removing dirt. Alcohol containing antiseptic solutions need moisture to be effective, e.g., 3 mL antimicrobial soap solution for 10 seconds duration and 25 mL alcohol is required for 5 minutes to surgical scrub of hands and arm
4. Duration of wash should be atleast 10 to 15 seconds. For surgical purposes washing may be adequate for 1–2 minutes.
5. In washing hands along with palm and back side of the hands, area between fingers and nails should be cleaned thoroughly. It is desirable to keep the nails trimmed and short.

HAND HYGIENE

Methods of Hand Hygiene

There are two types of hand hygiene:
1. Hand rub:
   - Use 70% alcohol
   - Chlorhexidine 2 to 4% may be used
   - These solution (alcohol/chlorhexidine) must be in contact for 25 to 30 seconds.* Here drying of hand is not needed as solution gets evaporated very soon.
2. Hand wash
   - Washing of hands can be done using medicated soap or ordinary soap.
   - Contact time may be about one minute
   - Hand washing is a must if they are soiled with blood, pus, etc.

STEPS TO WASH HANDS

1. Wet hands and apply soap. Rub palms together until soap is bubbly
2. Rub each palm over the back of the other hand
3. Rub between your fingers (interlocked)
4. Rub between your fingers on each hand
5. Rub around each of your thumbs
6. Rub both palms with finger tips then rinse and dry your hands.

WHEN TO WASH HANDS

The hands are one of the most important cause of cross infection and spread of flu. To avoid spread of infection, signs must be posted at each and every sink instructing when and how staff, volunteers, etc., should wash hand. Handwashing is required as below:
- First thing one should do while arriving for duty
- Before and after eating food, feeding a child, administering medication
- Applying diapering and toileting
- Attending patients (before and after)
- After handling body fluids, e.g. blood, mucus, vomit, urine, etc.
- Wiping noses, mouth, sores, etc.
- Handling uncooked food (raw meat, poultry and vegetables)
- When leaving for the day
- After cleaning
- When hands appear dirty.

HOW TO WASH HANDS

Following methods should be followed:
- Make sure a clean, disposable paper (or single use) towel is available
- Turn on water (15.6–48.9°C) temperature
- Moisten hands with water and apply liquid soap to hands
- Rub hands together until soap lather appears and continue for 10–15 seconds
- Finally, wash hands with clean water and dry them.

Hospital and Laboratory Wastes

Hospital and laboratory waste includes all waste biological as well as nonbiological which is discarded and unlikely to reuse it in the hospital in future. Mainly hospital waste is of two following types:

Infectious waste: This type of waste of the hospital is harmful and may cause infectious diseases. In fact this type of waste may be microbiological waste, blood, body fluids, contaminated laboratory waste, sharps, pathological waste, soiled dressing, cotton plasters contaminated with blood or body fluids, cotton plugs, etc. Infectious waste is about 10–15% of total hospital waste.

Noninfectious waste: It is the waste of the hospital that is noninfectious. It comprises of 80 to 85% of total hospital waste. This category of hospital waste does not cause any harm.

Since we are facing diseases like AIDS, Hepatitis B, etc. It is necessary to follow universal precautions which are as below:

1. Consider all patients and clinical specimens potentially infectious especially for AIDS, Hepatitis B, etc.
2. All specimens especially blood must be dispensed in leak proof impervious bags for transportation.
3. Use of gloves, face mask with glasses while handling blood or fluid specimens.
4. Wear proper laboratory coats while working in the laboratory.
5. Pipetting by mouth must not be done.
6. Decontaminate the laboratory working surface with decontaminant after completion of laboratory procedures

7. In case of spillage of blood or other specimen, treat the surface with appropriate disinfectant.
8. Biological safetyhood must be used for laboratory procedures.
9. All potentially contaminated material should be decontaminated before disposal or reuse.
10. Remove all protective wearing/clothing before leaving the laboratory or attending the patients in operation theater or OPD.

INFECTIOUS WASTE OF HOSPITAL AND LABORATORY

1. Microbiology waste
2. Blood and body fluids
3. Used sharps
4. Pathological waste, i.e., samples and tissues
5. Bandages and cotton swabs
6. Animal carcasses
7. Beddings.

INFECTIOUS MICROORGANISMS ASSOCIATED WITH HOSPITAL OR LABORATORY

1. HIV
2. Hepatitis B
3. *Brucella*
4. *Mycobacterium tuberculosis*
5 *Bacillus anthracis*
6. *Francisella tularensis*
7. *Shigella*

8. *Salmonella*
9. *Coccidioides immitis*

SEGREGATION OF HOSPITAL WASTE

Hospital waste is segregated and disposed of as below:

1. Yellow plastic bags and containers with human anatomical and pathological waste are directly dispatched for deep burial or incineration.
2. Red plastic bags and containers having infectious waste material are quickly sent for sterilization by autoclavation. Thereafter, they are disposed-of by land filling.
3. Blue plastic bags and containers with plastic and rubber disposable material are first of all cut into small pieces to prevent reuse followed by treatment with sodium hypochlorite solution. Now they are autoclaved and disposed of by land filling or burial. If feasible treated material as mentioned above may be transported to reputed plastic industry for further reuse. By no means should it be allowed to incinerate or burn as they contain halogenated polyvinyl chloride. It emits dioxin gas into the air which is highly carcinogenic.
4. Blue or white transparent puncture proof containers need a little different treatment before disposal. Sharps must be destroyed, disinfected with 1% sodium hypochlorite solution and then finally disposed of in sharp pit that is covered and protected and not accessed to rag pieces for reutilization.

    However, noninfectious waste can be collected in any appropriate container and dispatched to municipal garbage bins.

TECHNIQUES FOR WASTE TREATMENT

Chemical Method to Dispose of Hospital Waste

Formaldehyde 6–8%, glutaraldehyde, hydrogen peroxide 6–30% or sodium hypochlorite 0.1% are in common use.

Incinerator

Advantages

❖ Ensures complete and safe disposal of waste
❖ Volume of waste is reduced considerably.

Disadvantages

❖ Sharps cannot be disposed of
❖ Not suitable at all for PVC plastic material because of possible emission of harmful gases
❖ It is quite expensive to operate and maintain.

Autoclave

Uses

❖ Microbiological and pathological waste
❖ Blood and its products
❖ Sharps
❖ Plastic waste
❖ Body fluids.

Advantages

❖ Quite economical
❖ Easy to operate
❖ Waste is transformed into noninfectious form
❖ Waste is disinfected without hazardous emission.

Disadvantage

In fact, there is no reduction of volume of waste at all.

Microwaving

Uses

❖ In real sense, it involves the use of radiations produced by microwave to break down molecular chemical bonds and as a result disinfect waste.
❖ This process may require preshredding the waste and injecting it with steam treatment

chamber. Thus, they evenly heat it for 25 minutes at 97–100°C under series of microwave units (radiation spectrum between frequencies of 300–300,000 MHz).

Advantage

It disinfects waste without any harmful emission.

Disadvantage

As it requires pretreatment of shredding of the waste, it is full of risks for infectious waste. Further, it cannot be used for cytotoxic hazardous and radioactive waste.

Hydroclaving

Advantages

* It is used to dispose of microbiological and pathological waste, sharps, etc
* No pretreatment is needed
* Perfect fragmentation and dehydration is done
* It is ideal for infectious waste
* Volume as well as weight reduction makes its transportation and land filling easy and less expensive
* There is no emission of toxic gases, etc.

* It is quite simple, cheap to operate and maintain.

There is hardly any disadvantage of hydroclaving.

Plasma Technology

It allows a complete and satisfactory destruction of waste.

Advantages

* It does transformation of all hydrocarbonated products into combustible gases without leaving behind any solid remnant
* Here there is no need of segregation of waste.

DISPOSAL OF HOSPITAL AND LABORATORY WASTE

* Land filling
* Burial
* Sewage draining.

Infectious hospital and laboratory material after treatment may be disposed of by land filling or deep burial. Waste in fluid form can be discarded in sewage drains. Apart of this treatment incineration is also a vital method of disposal.

54 Infection Control Measures for Nursing Staff

INFECTION CONTROL CHECKLIST FOR NURSING STAFF

Standard precautions should be used at all times with every patient. Use the following checklist to guide you.

Have you washed your hands?

❖ Single most important step in reducing infections. Use the seven-step technique before/after any activity that contaminates the hands
❖ Dry thoroughly afterwards, using disposable towels.

Do you need to use personal protect equipment?

❖ Use disposable gloves, aprons, masks, goggles:
  ▪ If potential contamination by blood or body fluid is likely
  ▪ While handling hazardous chemicals and some pharmaceuticals.

Are you preventing sharps injuries?

❖ Keep handling to a minimum and never re-sheath.
❖ Dispose of sharps carefully in a special container at the point of use.

Are you disposing of waste safely?

❖ Ensure disposal of waste safely, including the color coding of bags used for different types of waste.

Do you deal promptly with spillages?

❖ Spillages must be dealt with quickly using appropriate chemical disinfectants
❖ Ensure thorough knowledge of chemical disinfectants and their concentration.

Do you scrupulously decontaminate equipment?

❖ Clean, disinfect reusable items to make it safe for future use.

Appropriate use of indwelling devices

❖ Use the correct technique when using devices, follow work place policy for devices.

Do you know what to do in the event of an accident?

❖ If bodily fluids have splashed into eyes irrigate with cold water.
❖ If into mouth don't swallow rinse with cold water. Report incident to senior at once.

ARE YOU PREVENTING SHARPS INJURIES?

❖ Sharps include needles, scalpels, stitch cutters, glass ampoules and any sharp instrument.
❖ The main hazards of a sharps injury are hepatitis B, hepatitis C and HIV.

Handling syringes and needles

Do	Don't
• Pass syringes and needles in a tray. ALWAYS dispose of your own sharps • Preferably cut it with needle Cutters. • Put needle and syringes in 2% hypochlorite solution if needle cutter is not available. • Sharps containers are not filled by more than two thirds • Remove cap of needle near the site of use. • Pick up open needle from tray/drum with forceps. • Sharps are disposed of at the point of use	• Never pass syringe and needle on directly to next person. • Do not bent/or break used needle with hands. • Never test the fineness of the needle's tip with bare or gloved hand. • Never pick up open needle by hand. • Never dispose it off by breaking it with hammer/stone.

DO YOU DEAL PROMPTLY WITH SPILLAGES?

❖ If blood is spilled either from a container or during procedure, this should be cleaned as soon as possible.

Type of spill	Cleaning recommendations
Spot cleaning	• Wipe up spot immediately with a damp cloth, tissue or paper towel or with alcohol wipe. Discard contaminated materials. Wash hands
Small spills (Up to 10 cm)	• Collect cleaning materials and equipment • Wear disposable cleaning gloves • Wipe up spill immediately with absorbent material (e.g., paper hand towel) • Place contaminated absorbent material into plastic bag for disposal • Clean the area with warm water and detergent using a disposal cleaning cloth or sponge • Where contact with the bare skin is likely disinfect the area by wiping with sodium hypochlorite 10,000 ppm available chlorine or other suitable disinfectant solution) and allow to dry • Discard contaminated materials (absorbent toweling, cleaning cloths, disposable gloves and plastic apron)
Large spills (> than 10 cm diameter)	• Collect cleaning materials and equipment • Wear disposable cleaning gloves/eye wear and plastic apron should be worn if there is a likelihood of splashing • Cover area of the spill with paper towel, blotting paper, newspaper • Cover area of the spill with granular chlorine releasing agent or similar product in which 10,000 ppm available chlorine) and leave for 30 minutes or depending on formulation labeling and instructions • Use disposable scrapper (e.g., cardboard) scraper to scope up granular disinfectant • Discard contaminated materials (absorbent toweling, cleaning cloths, disposable gloves and plastic apron) in infectious waste bag • Wipe area with absorbent paper towel to remove any remaining blood. Wash hands • Mop area with warm water and detergent • Clean and disinfect bucket and mop, dry and store appropriately • Wash hands

DO YOU USE PERSONAL PROTECT EQUIPMENT AND KNOW STANDARD PRECAUTIONS

Standard Precautions

Certain standard precautions are needed to be followed in all health care settings. These are:

❖ Wash hands before and after all patients or specimen contact
❖ Handle the blood of all patients as potentially infectious
❖ Wear gloves for potential contact with blood and body fluids
❖ Place used syringes immediately in nearby impermeable container. Do not recap or manipulate needle in any way
❖ Wear protective eyewear and mask if splatter with blood or body fluids is possible (e.g., bronchoscopy, oral surgery, etc.)
❖ Wear gowns when splash with blood or body fluids is anticipated
❖ Handle all linen soiled with blood and/or body secretion as potentially infectious
❖ Process all laboratory specimens as potentially infectious
❖ Wear mask for Mycobacterium tuberculosis and other respiratory organisms (HIV is not airborne).

Selection of protective barriers

Type of exposure	Protective barriers	Examples
Low risk: Contact with skin, no visible blood.	• Gloves only	Injections, minor wound dressing
Medium risk: • Probable contact with blood • Splashing unlikely	• Gloves • Gowns and apron may be necessary	Vaginal examination, insertion or removal of intravenous cannula, handling of laboratory specimens, large open wounds dressing, venepuncture spill of blood.
High risk: Probable contact with blood splashing likely	• Gloves • Waterproof gown or apron • Eye wear • Mask	Major surgical procedures particularly orthopedic surgery and oral surgery, vaginal delivery.

Additional precaution for isolation of patients

Type of precautions	Airborne	Contact	Droplet
Room type	Negative pressure room preferred	Private room preferred or else cohort patient with similar pure illness	Private room preferred or else cohort patient with similar pure illness ensure 3 feet of spatial separation between patients
Other precautions for staff	• For chicken pox, measles, only immunized staff to enter the area • For patients with open tuberculosis wear mask before entering the room • Limit patients movement, patient to wear mask if transported outside his room	• Wearing gloves mandatory prior to contact with patient or any item of the patient • Do not touch environmental surfaces fomites after removing the gloves/gowns • Limit patient transport	• Wear mask at all times when delivering care or when within 3 feet space around patient • Limit patient transport if unavoidable ensure patient wears a mask
Common conditions	Tuberculosis, measles, and chicken pox	Patients infected with Clostridium difficile, rotavirus, etc.	Influenza and meningococcal meningitis

DO YOU SCRUPULOUSLY DECONTAMINATE EQUIPMENT?

Equipment	Frequency of change	Recommendation
Oral thermometer	Long-term patients weekly or after each patient discharge	• After each use, the thermometer is disinfected by wiping with a swab saturated with 70% isopropyl alcohol. Each thermometer is kept in a separate dry holder
Sphygmomanometer cuffs	As required	• Change covers regularly (1x/week) and wash inflatable section in detergent and water dry thoroughly

Equipment	Recommendation
Bed ends and frames	• Clean with detergent and water.
Bowls-bedpans/ urinals	• Bed pans, urine pots, and kidney trays are to be kept in 7% Lysol for 24 hours or 3–5% sodium hypochlorite solution for 30 minutes, then they are washed with soap and water and dried in sunlight
Hand basins	• Clean with detergent and water
Mattresses and Pillows	• All should be covered with an impervious plastic cover and are to be wiped over with detergent and water if visibly contaminated. Mattresses should be cleaned regularly and if possible kept in sunlight for 24 hours. Plastic and rubber covers of mattresses and pillows, they are washed with soap and water, cleaned with a suitable disinfectant, e.g.,7% Lysol
Mop heads	• Daily cleaning of mops. At the completion of each task of floor mopping, the mops should be thoroughly washed in a bucket containing HOT water and detergent. Squeeze as much water out of mop as possible and shake strands loose; leave hanging to dry in the sun if possible, or alternative, in the cleaner's room. The bucket is to be turned upside down to allow overnight drainage • Detachable mop heads are to be sent to the laundry, while reusable mops are to be cleaned in hot soapy water, then left to dry ideally in the sun
Walls	• Remove visible soiling with detergent as necessary
Clinic Trolleys	• Clean with a cloth dampened with detergent and water

DO YOU KNOW WHAT TO DO IN THE EVENT OF AN ACCIDENT?

Accidental exposure to blood and body fluids can occur by:

❖ Percutaneous injury—for example, from needles, instruments, injuries that break the skin
❖ Exposure of broken skin—for example, abrasions, cuts or eczema
❖ Exposure of mucous membranes, including the eyes and the mouth.

Action to be taken immediately following accidental exposure to body fluids

❖ Encourage bleeding of the wound by applying gentle pressure—do not suck
❖ Wash well under running water
❖ Dry and apply a waterproof dressing as necessary
❖ If blood and body fluids splash into eyes, irrigate with cold water
❖ If blood and body fluids splash into your mouth, do not swallow. Rinse out several times with cold water
❖ Report the incident to your occupational health department
❖ Complete an accident form
❖ In the case of an injury from a clean/unused instrument or needle, no further action is likely
❖ If the injury is from a used needle or instrument, risk assessment should be carried out with a microbiologist, infection control doctor
❖ Consent is required if a patient's blood needs to be taken.

APPROPRIATE USE OF INDWELLING DEVICES

Ventilator-associated respiratory infections	Prevention
Risk factors Duration of intubation Invasive ventilation	Limit duration Noninvasive ventilation is preferred
Ventilation procedures • Intubation and suction • Filters Disposable • Water for oxygen and aerosol therapy • Tracheal toilet • Tubing, respirators, and humidifiers • Suction tubes • Humidifier bottles	 • Aseptic technique should be used • Disposable filters should be used • Water should be sterile and changed regularly • Aseptic technique should be followed • Appropriate cleaning and disinfection to limit contamination and subsequent infection • Sterile, with aseptic technique should be used • Should be sterilized between use, should not be topped up

Hospital Associated Urinary Tract Infections

Risk factors	Prevention
Risk factors • Invasive urological procedures • Urinary catheter • Duration of catheterization **Catheter care** • Selection of catheter size • Insertion technique of catheter Aseptic "no touch" technique • Drainage system • Training of healthcare workers • Traumatic insertion of catheter	**Prevention** • Aseptic technique should be maintained. • Catheterization to be avoided unless compelling indication • Prolonged catheterization should be avoided • The smallest size which fits should be used to avoid urethral trauma • Use sterile gloves, hygienic hand and perineal disinfection prior to insertion • Closed system of drainage prevents infections • Education and training helps to avoid infections • Recommended technique should be followed

Intravascular Catheter Related Infections

Infection risks with IV catheters	Prevention
• Catheter system	• To be avoided unless indicated; Closed system to be maintained
• Duration	• Prolonged catheterization to be avoided
• Skin preparation	• Strict aseptic technique to be used
• Dressing change	• Frequency of dressing change to be limited
• Type of catheter	• Antibiotic coated catheter for short-term is preferred

Surgical Site Infections

Risk factors for surgical site infections	Prevention
Patient • Age • Nutritional status • Diabetes control • Smoking • Obesity reduce weight prior to surgery • Coexistent infections in a remote body site • Colonization with microorganisms • Altered immune response • Length of preoperative stay	• Avoid operating on very old or very young as they are at higher risk for developing infections • Build a good nutritional status • Maintain blood sugar levels • Cessation of smoking at least one month prior to surgery • Reduce weight prior to surgery • Treat adequately before operation • Screen and treat carriers; avoid preoperative shaving • Boost immunity if possible • Avoid long stay in hospital

Contd...

Contd...

Risk factors for surgical site infections	Prevention
Operational procedures	
• Duration of surgical scrub	• 2 minutes as effective as 10 minutes
• Skin antisepsis	• Use povidone-iodine/ chlorhexidine gluconate
• Preoperative shaving	• Avoid if possible or shave immediately prior to operation
• Preoperative skin preparation	• Allow drying of antiseptic
• Duration of operation	• Keep procedures as short as possible
• Antimicrobial prophylaxis	• Give suitable antimicrobial cover
• Operating room ventilation	• Adhere to specifications
• Inadequate sterilization of instruments	• Monitor central sterile supply department (CSSD) processes
• Foreign material in the operative site	• Maintain high-level of asepsis
• Surgical drains	• Avoid unless really necessary
• Tissue trauma	• Maintain good surgical technique and ensure minimal tissue trauma

HAVE YOU WASHED YOUR HANDS?

It is known that hand hygiene reduces the carriage of potential pathogens on the hands. Eighty percent (80%) of nosocomial disease transmission is thought to be via hands.

Indications for Handwashing and Hand Antisepsis

A. **When hands are visibly dirty or contaminated** with proteinaceous material or are visibly soiled with blood or other body fluids, wash hands with either a non-antiseptic soap and water, OR an antiseptic soap and water.

B. If hands are not visibly soiled, use an alcohol-based hand rub OR wash hands with an antiseptic soap.

Routinely decontaminating hands in the following situations:

❖ Before having direct contact with patients
❖ Before inserting indwelling urinary catheters, peripheral vascular catheters, or other invasive devices that do not require a surgical procedure
❖ After contact with a patient's intact skin (e.g., when taking a pulse or blood pressure, and lifting a patient)
❖ After contact with body fluids or excretions, mucous membranes, non intact skin, and wound dressings if hands are not visibly soiled

❖ After removing gloves
❖ Wash hands with non-antimicrobial soap and water or with antimicrobial soap and water if exposure to Bacillus anthracis is suspected or proven. The physical action of washing and rinsing hands under such circumstances is recommended because alcohols, chlorhexidine, iodophors, and other antiseptic agents have poor activity against spores
❖ After using the toilet
❖ After cleaning up any spillage
❖ Before handling food
❖ Before and after aseptic procedures
❖ After handling laundry and waste
❖ Before and after administering medication.

A seven—step handwashing technique should be followed:

Steps are:
Step 1: Palm to palm.

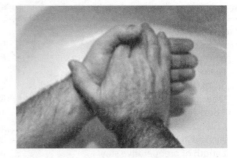

Step 2: Right palm over back of left hand. Change hands and repeat.

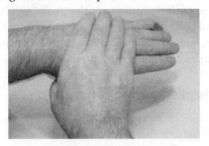

Step 3: Interlace fingers of right hand over left. Change hands and repeat.

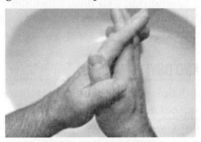

Step 4: Rotational rubbing backwards and forwards with clasped fingers of right hand in left palm. Change hands and repeat.

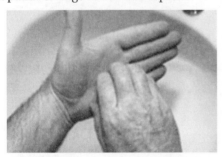

Step 5: Rotational rubbing of right thumb clasped in left palm. Change hands and repeat.

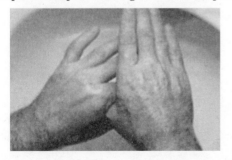

Step 6: Grasp left wrist with right hand and work cleanser into skin. Change hands and repeat.

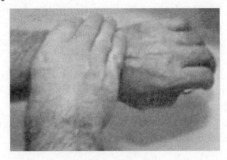

Step 7: Rub hands and wrists for 30 seconds, then rinse and dry thoroughly.

Other Aspects of Hand Hygiene

❖ Keep natural nails tips less than 1/4-inch long
❖ Wear gloves when contact with blood or other potentially infectious materials, mucous membranes
❖ Remove gloves after caring for a patient. Do not wear the same pair of gloves for the care of more than one patient, and do not wash gloves in between when using with different patients
❖ Change gloves during patient care if moving from a contaminated body site to a clean body site.

▮ FACILITIES

All clinical areas including consultation chambers, nursing stations and critical care areas should have:

❖ Handwashing facilities appropriate to the area
❖ Clear unobstructed access to the handwashing sink
❖ Handwashing sinks for that purpose only and clear of inappropriate items
❖ Liquid soap and alcohol hand rubs available at every sink
❖ Hand drying facilities with disposable paper towels must be readily available at every sink

❖ Handwashing posters should be placed by each sink
❖ All critical areas should have alcohol-based hand rubs installed at entry points for use by visitors
❖ All critical areas should have alcohol-based hand rubs by each patient bedside.

The Infection Control Council should be consulted before any new construction or refurbishment work is planned to advice on sink type, number and placement of handwashing facilities.

HANDWASHING AGENTS

There are three types of agent, which can be used to remove microorganisms from hands: soap, alcohol, hand rubs and antimicrobial agents.

Soap

Will mechanically remove transient micro-organisms but has little effect on resident microorganisms.

Alcohol-based Hand Rubs

❖ Can be applied quickly without access to water. However, they are not effective in removing soiling and should only be used if hands are visibly clean.

Recent studies advocate the use of alcoholic hand rubs between each patient contact as a measure, which reduces the rate of hospital-acquired infect.

Antiseptic Agents

These are designed to remove transient and reduce resident skin microorganisms. Chlorhexidine-based preparations have been found to be more effective than iodine-based solutions as they have a residual effect, which influences the survival times of many organisms on hand surfaces.

HAND DRYING AGENTS

Drying hands with paper products is preferable to using hot air or linen towels.

Drying with a high absorbency paper towel will remove some of the transient organisms that remain after handwashing. Paper towels should be wall mounted.

Types of hand decontamination; handwashing and hand antisepsis

Type	Purpose	Indication	Technique	Comment
Routine hand wash (soap and water for 15 seconds)	• Remove soil • Remove transient flora	**Before** • Significant contact with a patient, e.g., emptying a catheter bag, injection, venipuncture, changing a nappy, assisting to eat • Eating, smoking **Between** • Procedures on the same patient **After** • Activities likely to cause significant contamination: e.g., direct contact with body secretions, mucous membranes, wounds • Removing gloves • Personal ablutions	• Remove hand and wrist jewellery • Wet hands • Apply agent • Thoroughly rub all surfaces of hands together, (pay attention to nails and thumb of dominant hand) • Rinse under running water	• Applying the agent after the hands are wet may prevent undue stripping of hand oils • Transient flora, e.g., rotavirus, *Staphylococcus aureus* may live for hours on unwashed or improperly washed hands
Antiseptic hand rub (70% alcohol for 15 seconds)	• Destroy transient flora • Reduce resident flora • Note: will not remove or denature soil	• As for routine hand wash • May be performed in lieu of routine hand wash, but only if hands are free of visible soil • May be performed in emergency situations where there is insufficient time/facilities (water)	• Remove hand and wrist jewellery • Apply for 3–5 minutes to hands • Thoroughly rub all surfaces of hands together (pay attention to nails and thumb of dominant hand)	• Alcohol is not a good cleaning agent and is not recommended in the presence of dirt (soil) • Alcohol is an excellent antiseptic and works well on soil free hands • Preferred preparations contain moisturizer
Clinical handwash (antiseptic soap and water for 60 seconds)	• Remove soil • Remove transient flora • Reduce resident flora	• Nonsurgical procedures which require aseptic technique, e.g., peripheral venous cannulation, insertion of a urinary catheter, wound dressings	• Pat dry • Paper towel • Single use	
Surgical scrub (antiseptic soap and water for 2–6 minutes)	• Remove soil • Remove transient flora • Reduce resident flora for duration of surgery in case of glove tears	• All surgical procedures including insertion of all CVC lines • Used in conjunction with sterile gloves	• Keep hands above elbows • Pat dry • Sterile towel	• Brushes are not recommended as they abrade the skin and may liberate deep resident flora

Emergency Microbiology

Almost daily clinicians and microbiologists come across clinical situations where rapid detection and characterization of an infection are essential for the diagnosis and effective treatment of infectious diseases. Only a few techniques in clinical microbiology laboratory can be performed within 1–2 hours. Hence, they can be of much use in patients with overwhelming sepsis, e.g. meningococcemia. Other cases with meningitis or other life-threatening acute infections may benefit greatly by emergency laboratory procedures. In general, emergency procedures rely upon:

1. The visualization of the agent causing disease.
2. The detection of specific antigens of the offending organisms.
3. The detection of substances produced by the organisms while infecting the patient.
4. The detection of substances produced by the host to the infectious process.

While each of these approaches is valuable, results obtained by any of these techniques do not eliminate the need to submit specimens for conventional studies culture and antibiotic sensitivity test.

VISUALIZATION OF THE AGENT OF DISEASE

Microscopic detection of stained or unstained microorganisms is of great value for the detection of infection. Microscopic methods like phase contrast, Darkfield, light and electron microscopy have been employed to detect agents of infection. Phase contrast microscope may be employed for visualizing fungal elements in clinical specimen, Darkfield microscope is quite helpful in the diagnosis of early syphilis and electron microscope for visualizing viral particles from clinical specimen like stool. Light and ultraviolet microscopes are widely employed especially for Gram and acid-fast stain. Acid-fast bacteria are detected in clinical specimens by Ziehl-Neelsen, Kinyoun and auramine/rhodamine stain.

When appropriately applied to clinical situations, Gram stain is of immense use. Table 55.1 presents a list of diseases and specimens that may assist in the rapid diagnosis of infections.

Recently, application of fluorescent acridine orange stain to clinical specimens such as urethral exudate is recommended as it is more sensitive than visible microscopy. An additional benefit is that the smears stained with acridine orange can later be Gram-stained without previous decolorization.

ANTIGEN DETECTION

The detection of antigens and substances associated with the intact infecting agent or of antigens that are dis associated from the agent is an alternate means of rapidly detecting the presence of an infecting agent.

Its application is in the use of specific antiserum to serologically identification of pneumococci in clinical specimen by Quelling reaction. Use of fluorescein conjugated antibody reagents is helpful in rapid detection of organisms like *Bordetella pertussis, Corynebacterium diphtheriae, Legionella pneumophila*, viral, and rickettsial infections.

Table 55.1: Relation of Gram's smear from clinical specimens and diseases.

Diseases	Specimens	Results
• Septicemia	• Buffy coat	• Intracellular/extracellular bacteria
• Endocarditis	• Skin lesion	• Intracellular/extracellular bacteria
• Meningitis	• Sediments of spinal fluid	• Intracellular/extracellular bacteria
• Wound infection	• Biopsy aspirate	• Presence of predominant type(s) of organisms present
• Urinary tract infection	• Midstream urine	• Presence of >1 organism/oil immersion
• Pneumonia	• Expectorated sputum	• Predominance of sputum polymorphonuclear leukocytes and general absence of squamous epithelial cells Predominant organisms present

Increased sensitivity in detecting microbial antigens has been achieved by the use of more sensitive serologic tests like indirect particle agglutination, counter immuno-electrophoresis, radioimmunoassay and ELISA. The later test for cryptococcal antigen has proven to be of significant value in detecting cryptococcal infections in man. Counterimmunoelectrophoresis has been successfully used for rapid detection of antigens like *Neisseria meningitidis, Pneumococcus, Haemophilus influenzae* type b, streptococci, *Escherichia coli* with K or capsular antigen in CSF and other clinical specimens. This method is not very sensitive but is quite useful in identifying the causative agent in meningitis quickly. Radioimmunoassay and ELISA are more sensitive and used for the detection of hepatitis virus, rotavirus and many other microbial antigens.

An exciting development is the serological detection of microbial antigens using monoclonal antibodies. Antibodies produced this way are more sensitive, specific and more active and so no false-positive results. The Limulus Amebocyte Lysate test (LAL test) is shown to be very useful for rapid diagnosis of Gram-negative meningitis, Gram-negative bacteriuria and gonococcal urethritis.

Detection of Substances Produced by the Infecting Organisms in Specimens

A classic example is the detection of *Clostridium botulinum* toxin in serum and stool specimens obtained from patients with botulism. A more recent example is the diagnosis of antibiotic associated colitis by detecting *Clostridium difficile* toxin in stool specimen.

Infectious process may be detected by identifying the presence of microbial enzymes in clinical specimen, e.g. aminopeptidases, propanediol oxidoreductase, and β-lactamase.

One method of detecting microbial activity is by the detection of microbial metabolites in clinical specimens. Rapid diagnosis of invasive candidiasis is by detection of D-arabinitol, a fungal metabolite.

Detection of Substances Produced by the Host in Response to Infection

Classic examples are serodiagnostic tests employed to diagnose syphilis which measure treponemal and reaginic antibodies. However, these tests are of little value in first week of disease and more useful in late primary, secondary and tertiary disease. Detection of IgM antibody is of proven value in the rapid diagnosis of toxoplasmosis, rubella and many viral infections.

Concentration of lactic acid in cerebrospinal fluid and joint fluid may be of value in diagnosing infectious meningitis and infectious arthritis. Lactic acid concentrations in excess of 30–50 mg/dL have proven helpful in identifying the patient with bacterial meningitis.

A very important and useful aspect of control of spread. It requires:

1. **Vaccination:** Early vaccine was introduced by Edward Jenner to prevent smallpox. Smallpox was globally eradicated in 1975. Now we have vaccines for almost all infectious disease except very few like leprosy. Nurses must be vaccinated against hepatitis B and other infectious diseases. Also available other vaccines like typhoid, tuberculosis, cholera, rabies, Japanese encephalitis, mumps, rubella, measles etc.

2. **Balanced diet:** We need adequately nourished diet. Malnourishment may cause many indections diseases, e.g., tuberculosis. Balanced dite compromises of:
   i. Protein (20% of intake energy)
   ii. Fat (20% of daily food consumption)
   iii. Carbohydrate
   iv. Micronutrients, e.g., vitamins, calcium, manganese, zinc, phosphorus, etc.,
   However, children and pregnant ladies require more calories that means more quantity and quality. In other words a well balanced diet means less infectious diseases.

3. **Safe drinking water**: Safe drinking water must not contain microbes. Even one fecal *Escherichia coli* (present in stools) make the water unsafe for drinking. It may cause diarrhea, dysentery, poliomyelitis, jaundice etc. Drinking water must be subjected to laboratory bacteriological examination periodically. It assures safe drinking water.

BIOMEDICAL WASTE MANAGEMENT

Biomedical waste is:
1. The waste generated during diagnosis in laboratory
2. The waste of treatment and vaccination
3. Research work, etc.,
   Biological waste may be infection or noninfectious:

Infectious Waste

It includes infectious material:
❖ Tissues, organs, body fluids
❖ Syringes, blood bags, intravenous tubings, etc.
❖ Items mixed with blood, pus and contaminated with body fluid
❖ Microbiology waste from laboratory, e.g., culture media, swabs, serum samples, needles, cannulas, etc.

Noninfection

❖ Kitchen waste
❖ General office waste

Classification of Biomedical Waste

Category 1	Human anatomical waste
Category 2	Animal waste
Category 3	Microbiological waste
Category 4	Sharp (needles, scalpeis)
Category 5	Discarded medicine

Category 6	Solid waste
Category 7	Solid waste (kitchen and general)
Category 8	Liquid waste
Category 9	Incineration ash
Category 10	Chemical waste

Category of Waste

Yellow	Plastics	Incineration and burial
Red	• Disinfected • Plastic bags	• Autoclaving • Autoclaving • Chemical treatment • Microwave oven
White	Puncture proof	• Autoclave • Microwave oven • Chemical disinfectant
Black	Plastic bags	Landfill

USES OF SEPERATION OF WASTE

❖ Risk of infection to medical staff is reduced
❖ Cost of treatment becomes cheaper
❖ Spread of infection to community is reduced
❖ Formaldehyde used in operation theatres may be reused for autopsy and in pathology laboratory.

DISPOSAL OF THE WASTE

❖ Emptying of bins twice a day. Plastic bag in the bin must be tightly closed. The waste handler must were, apron, mask, gloves, gumboots and cap.
❖ Liquid waste should be treated with disinfectant (e.g., 2-3% sodium hypochlorite or phenol)
❖ Sharps e.g., scalpel needles must be put in puncture proof container. They may be sent for autoclavation or incineration
❖ Needles sharp may be cut into pieces with needle cutter.
❖ Intravenous tubing, gloves must be cut into pieces and put in yellow container.

❖ Record of waste disposed from the ward must be maintained.

DISINFECTION SUGGESTED PROCEDURES

Airways and endotracheal tube
❖ Single use or autoclaved should be used
❖ Disinfection with 2% glutaraldehyde is used

Ampoules

Neck of ampoule is wiped with 70% alcohol and allow to dry before opening ampoules.

Bedpans

❖ Must wear apron and gloves before handling bedpans
❖ They may be emptied using disposable wooden spatula and paper.
❖ May be washed bedpan with tap water
❖ Disinfect bedpans using 2% phenol for 10 minutes. In case of stools disinfection with 2% phenol is for one hour is done. Then wash bed pan with tap water.

Urinals

❖ Empty the urinals
❖ Wash with water
❖ Put urinals in drum of water kept at 80°C for 10 minutes
❖ Alternatively urinals may be treated with 2% phenol for 15 minutes.

Bedding

Every week blanket must be changed and used blanket may be sent to laundry.
❖ Bedsheet must be changed daily or whenever spoiled.
❖ Bedframe is to be cleaned with detergent and water after patients is discharged.

Mattresses

❖ Mattress are covered with impermeable cover.
❖ Wipe mattress cover with detergent before bed making
❖ Wipe mattress cover with 2% phenol or 5% savlon or 1% hydrogen peroxide after wash.
❖ If heavily contaminated then it must be fumigated
❖ Pillows are also treated like mattress as described above.

Blood Spill

❖ Cover blood spill area with absorbent
❖ Now pour 1% hypochlorite or 2% carbolic acid
❖ Leave it for 10 minutes
❖ Remove with gloves
❖ Wash the area with disinfectant

Blood-stained linen

❖ Soak in fresh bleach solution (14 Grams bleaching powder in one liter) for 3 minutes
❖ Now send linen to laundry.

Bowls

❖ Bowls need 2% carbolic acid or 5% lysol or 5% hypochlorite. After rinsing with water keep them inverted
❖ Surgical bowls may be autoclaved.

Cheatle Forceps

❖ They may be autoclaved or boiled.
❖ Forceps may be stored in 2% savlon.

thermometers

❖ Clean thermometer with 70% alcohol or 2% savlon. It is for thermometer used auxiliary.

❖ Keep the thermometer 2% savlon when not in use. Savlon solution should be changed daily.
❖ Before use clean the thermometer with clean water, dry it and use it. This is done for rectal thermometer.

Buckets

❖ They may be washed and dried.
❖ They should be kept inverted before use.

Catheter

❖ Must be discarded after use
❖ Can be autoclaved

Mops

❖ Use disposable mops
❖ Mops must be changed daily especially for operation theater
❖ For other mops must be washed with detergent thoroughly and dry before use
❖ In cases there is heavy contamination they may be immersed in 2 to 3 percent phenol.

Cystoscope

❖ It may be kept in 2% glutaraldehyde.
❖ It may be used after keeping in glutaraldehyde for 9 to 10 hours.

Endoscope

❖ It can be kept in 2% glutaraldehyde.
❖ It needs 10 to 30 minutes treatment with glutaraldehyde in between.

Practical Microbiology

SECTION OUTLINE

❖ **Microscope**

Microscope

■ MICROSCOPE

Human eye can see an object up to 30 mm only. Undoubtedly, microscope is one of the most important equipment in the hospital laboratory. It makes small objects appear larger than they actually are, so that details of the objects can be seen, which otherwise is not possible. It does so by the use of lenses like the ordinary magnifying glass.

Construction

The laboratory microscope has three main parts: microscope stand, mechanical adjustments and the optics or lenses **(Fig. 57.1)**.

The microscope stand: It provides metal support for all other parts of microscope. It consists of: (i) the tube which holds the objectives and the eyepiece; (ii) the body

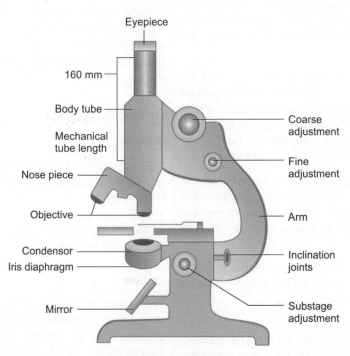

Eyepiece

160 mm

Body tube

Mechanical
tube length

Nose piece

Objective

Condensor

Iris diaphragm

Mirror

Coarse
adjustment

Fine
adjustment

Arm

Inclination
joints

Substage
adjustment

Fig. 57.1: Microscope.

which is concerned with their focusing; (iii) the arm which support all these; (iv) the stage on which specimen lies; and (v) the foot or base on which the whole instrument rests. These are discussed as under:

The tube: It supports at its lower end the objective and at its upper end the eyepiece. It holds these in line and the correct distance apart. The objective is screwed into the lower end of the tube. Usually, for laboratory work about 30 objectives are screwed into revolving nose piece, which allows any of the objectives to be quickly adjusted into place. The eyepiece is inserted loosely into the upper end of the tube. Eyepiece also has standard diameter so that eyepieces are interchangeable. Also eyepieces are moveable up or down in a sliding draw tube at the upper end of the tube.

The body: The tube is attached to the microscope by the body. The body is a block of metal containing the focussing mechanism.

The arm: The body of the microscope and the tube attached to it are supported at the correct height and tilted to required angle by firm arm which usually provides a lifting handle for the microscope.

The stage: This is a flat plate lying below the objective, on which specimen or object to be examined, is placed. It carries a pair of spring stage clips which hold it in place. In the center of the stage, there is a circular hole for the light to pass upward through it from below.

Mechanical stage: The stage may have attached to its upper surface of may incorporate a mechanical stage for the controlled movement of the specimen. In this case, stage clips are absent.

The substage: It lies just below the stage. It holds a condenser lens, iris diaphragm and holder for light filters and stops.

The foot: It may be of different forms, i.e., horseshoe, tripod, etc. As a matter of fact, microscope rests firmly on a foot upon the laboratory bench.

Mechanical Adjustments

It includes focusing of the objectives, adjustment of the mirror, condenser, iris and also the use of the drawtube and other movements.

Focusing adjustment: The quality of operation of microscope depends also on the perfect movement of its focusing mechanisms (coarse, fine). These focusing adjustments operate by a strip of metal sliding up and down in a matching slot carefully machined and lubricated to give smooth and easy movements.

The coarse adjustment is driven by a rack and pinion mechanism. It is generally controlled by a pair of large knobs, lying one on each side of the body. By rotating it, the tube with lenses moves. In some microscopes, the stage moves up and down rapidly. As a matter of fact, coarse adjustment is the focusing of low power lenses.

The fine adjustment is brought about by a micrometer thread. Here, high power lens requires fine adjustment, the knobs move the objectives or the stage up or down extremely slow. The two smaller knobs on each side of the body, may be graduates in micron to show the distance moved.

The Microscope Optics

Objectives

The objective is most important part of microscope. Usually, there are three objectives **(Fig. 57.2)**:
1. 10X (low power)
2. 45X (high power)
3. 100X (oil immersion)

Eyepiece

The most common form of eyepiece is Huyghens' eyepiece. Huyghens' eyepieces are available in a range of magnifications 4X, 6X, 7X, 8X, 10X, 15X and sometimes 20X. The higher, the power, the greater is the total

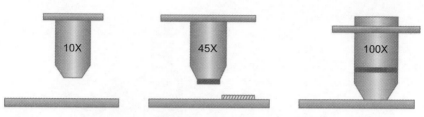

Fig. 57.2: Objectives.

magnification of microscope. The lower the power of eyepiece, the brighter and sharper is the image. 10X eyepiece is a good average lens, giving sufficient magnification and details for routine work **(Fig. 57.3)**.

Condenser and Iris

The condenser is a large lens mounted below the stage with an iris diaphragm **(Fig. 57.4)**. This lens receives a beam from light and passes it into the objective. The angle of beam can be adjusted by iris.

Mirror

Below condenser and iris is the mirror which is circular and mounted so that it can be turned in any direction and will stay in place. It reflects the light from source of light (sunlight, electric light, etc.) upwards through the iris into the condenser. It consists of two mirrors, mounted back to back. One of these, two mirrors is plane or flat and the other is concave. The flat mirror is used with condenser whereas plane mirror is used without condenser **(Fig. 57.5)**.

Drawtube

The tube length is adjusted simply by sliding the drawtube with its eyepiece up or down. The drawtube is usually 160 mm. Objectives work best at this tube length.

Inclination

The arm can be tilted upon the foot by hinge, which may have a clamping screw, to allow the tube and the stage to be inclined together to an angle as required.

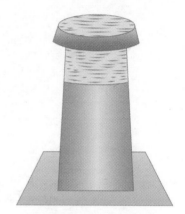

Fig. 57.3: Eyepiece.

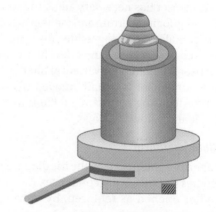

Fig. 57.4: Condenser.

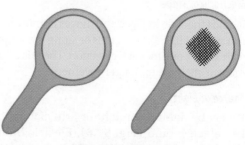

Fig. 57.5: Mirror.

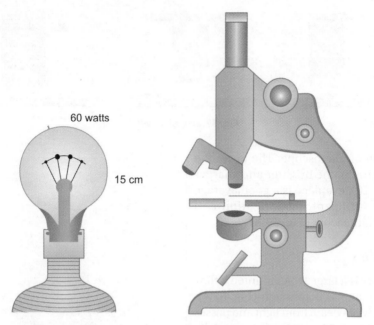

60 watts

15 cm

Fig. 57.6: Light source.

Condenser Adjustment

The condenser has necessary adjustments for its focusing, for its aperture and for its centering too. It can also be swing aside (for removal or to exchange it by a new one). Just below condenser is a holder for variety of filters.

The condenser is usually moved up and down for focusing by rotating a knob to one side of it and below the stage.

Aperture Adjustment

The aperture is adjusted by the iris diaphragm which lies just below the condenser. It can be closed or opened as required, by moving a small projecting knob.

Mechanical Stage

It holds the slide in place and moves it smoothly in a straight line either across or along the stage with knobs, one for each direction. There is also measuring scale for each movement.

Source of Light

It may be natural sunlight or artificial light, i.e., electric bulb **(Fig. 57.6)**. Electric bulb should be of 60 watt placed 18 inches away from microscope.

Routine Use of Microscope

❖ Place the microscope on firm bench so that it does not vibrate.
❖ If source of light is sun, flat side of mirror is used to reflect the light up through the condenser.
❖ Place the specimen on the stage and examine under low power (10X) and then under high power (45X). Specimen to be examined under oil immersion lens (100X) should be examined after placing a drop of cidar wood oil.
❖ Focus the objective using coarse focusing knob until the lens (objective) is near the specimen. Now use the fine focusing knob until sharp image comes into view.
❖ Turn the mirror until the illumination of image is at its brightest.
❖ Adjust and condenser, aperture of condenser and iris. Usually for stained specimen on slide, wide aperture is used. Reduced aperture is used to increase the contrast for usually unstained preparation on slide mounted in saline and under a coverslip.
❖ Now examine the slide moving it by mechanical stage.

Glossary

Abscess: A localized collection of pus.

Acid fast: Resistant to decolorization by acid after staining with hot carbol fuchsin and hence retaining a red color when stained by Ziehl-Neelsen method.

Accessory: Something added which helps.

Active immunity: Dependent upon stimulation of person's own immunological mechanisms.

Active: To make something work.

Adenine: A purine constituent of nucleic acid.

Adenosine triphosphate (ATP): Compound in which energy is stored in high energy phosphate bonds; its components are the purine adenine, D-ribose and three phosphoric acid groups.

Adjuvant: Insoluble materials which act to keep antigens in tissues for longer period, thus cause a longer stimulation of antibody production.

Aerobe: An organism which requires oxygen to live and reproduce.

Agglutinate: To join together to form clump.

Allele: One of a group of genes which can occupy a given place on a pair of identical chromosomes.

Allergy: An abnormal sensitive reaction.

Anaerobe: A microorganism not requiring oxygen to live or reproduce.

Anamnestic reaction: A rise of an existing antibody level in response to irrelevant stimulus.

Anhydrous: Containing no water.

Anode: A positive electrode.

Antagonism: Impairment of the efficacy of drug in the presence of the other.

Antibiotic: A substance used to kill micro-organisms. It is a product of microorganism.

Antibody: A globulin produced in the body in response to the antigen or foreign bodies.

Antigen: Any substance which can cause the production of antibodies.

Antiserum: A serum containing antibodies against particular organism.

Antitoxin: An antibody against particular toxin.

Asepsis: Without infection.

Atmospheric pressure: The pressure of air on earth.

Attenuated: Reduced virulence but retaining antigenecity for host.

Atypical: Unusual.

Autoinfection: Infection of oneself.

Automatic: Doing something by itself.

Bacilli: Stick-like or rod-like bacteria.

Bacteria: Single-celled organisms containing both RNA and DNA which reproduce by binary fission.

Bacteriology: The study of bacteria.

Bacteremia: Presence of bacteria in blood-stream.

Bacteriocide: A chemical used to kill bacteria.

Balantidium coli: A protozoan ciliate causative agent of balantidiasis, a type of dysentry.

Beaded: Staining at intervals along the length of bacillus.

Binary fission: Simple cell division by which the nucleus and cytoplasm divides into two.

Biologic oxidation: Any chemical reaction occurring within a cell that results in the release of energy respiration.

Biologic oxygen demand (BOD): A measurement of the amount of oxygen required for the microbial decomposition of the organic matter present in water.

Biopsy: The removal of small piece of tissue during life for examination.

Biotype: A classification or a group of genetically similar organisms.

Bipolar: The staining of bacillus at both ends.

Blepharoplast: Basal body structure in hemoflagellates from which axoneme arises.

Blister: A small swelling in the skin filled with serum.

Bovine: Associated with cattle.

Booster dose: Additional infection of antigen to maintain antibody production at its peak.

Brittle: Easily broken.

Brownian movement: Passive to-and-fro movement of bacteria suspended in a fluid, due to irregular bombardment of molecules in fluid.

Budding: An asexual form of reproduction of unicellular organisms, e.g., yeast cells.

Buffer: A solution, the reaction of which is not easily altered by adding an acid or alkali.

Candling: Inspection of an unbroken egg by holding it in front of bright light source to know whether embryo is alive or dead.

Capsid: The protein coat surrounding the genome of virus.

Capsomere: One of the units of which virus capsid is composed.

Capsule: A coating outside cell walls of some bacteria and fungi.

Carrier: One who is harboring but not currently suffering any ill-effect from pathogenic organism.

Cathode: A negative electrode.

Cell: A microscopic mass of protoplasm containing nucleus.

Cell line: An *in vitro* culture of cells of known origin.

Cellulitis: The result of a spreading infection of pyogenic bacteria in the subcutaneous tissues.

Characteristic: A quality which distinguishes something, i.e., typical.

Chemotherapeutic agent: A synthetic chemical suitable for systemic administration and effective in treatment of microbial infections.

Chitin: Polysaccharide containing glucosamine, characteristic of cell walls of some fungi and also found in insects.

Chromatin: Darkly staining nuclear material.

Chromosomes: Thread-like structure in the cell nucleus which contains genes carrying inherited characteristics.

Chronic: Slowly developing.

Clone: Cell derived from single cell.

Clinical disease: The ways by which a disease shows itself in a patient.

Clue cells: These are epithelial cells covered with large clumps of coccobacilli. They are good markers of infection.

Coccus: A rounded or ovoid bacterium.

Colony: A number of organisms living or multiplying together on culture media and they result from multiplication of a single organism.

Commensal: Deriving nourishment from a host without causing any harm or benefit to host.

Complement: A group of substances present in fresh serum and necessary for completion of some processes like lysis that result from anti-antibody interactions.

Control: A check.

Constitutive enzyme: Produced under all circumstances, not dependent upon the presence of appropriate substrate.

Conjugation: Exchange of genetic material between bacteria.

Culture: The growth and multiplication of microorganism.

Culture media: The material used in a culture to nourish the growth of microorganism.

Cytopathic effect: Degenerative changes occurring in tissue culture cells as a result of microorganism infection.

Cytoplasmic streaming: Continuous movement of cytoplasm within the cell which results in constant distribution of intracellular contents. It provides amoebic motility to some types of cells.

Darting: A fast jerky movement.

Decolorize: To remove color.

Deaminase: An enzyme which catalyzes the removal of an amino group from a molecule with liberation of ammonia, the process is called deamination.

Delicate: Fragile, which can be damaged easily.

Deposit: The sediment at the bottom of tube.

Desiccation: Drying or removal of water.

Detergent: A surface active agent used in cleaning.

Diplococci: Cocci which occur in pairs.

Disinfectant: A substance of chemical nature used for destroying pathogenic microorganisms.

Distorted: Altered or changed.

Effective: Producing a result.

Electrolyte: A chemical which helps to keep correct water balance between the fluid in the cell and that which surrounds it.

Elementary bodies: Single chlamydiae particle visible by ordinary microscope after staining.

Embed: To penetrate into tissue.

Emergency: A serious situation requiring immediate attention.

Encapsulate: To surround with a capsule.

Endemic: A disease constantly present in an area.

Endogenous: Originated by organisms or factors already present in the patient's body before onset of disease.

Endotoxin: A toxic component of microorganism (Gram-negative), largely dependent on the death or disruption of the organism for its release.

Enriched medium: A culture medium to which an extra nourishing substance is added.

Enrichment medium: A liquid medium used to encourage preliminary growth of an organism so as to enhance the chances of growing it on subsequent plate culture.

Enzyme: A chemical produced by living organism to help some particular reaction.

Epidemic: A disease that temporarily has a high-frequency in a given community.

Eradicate: To get rid of.

Excision repair: An enzyme system which can repair DNA by the elimination of ultraviolet light induced thymine dimers.

Exogenous: Originated by organisms or factors from outside the patient's body.

Exotoxin: A toxin released by living micro-organisms into the surrounding medium or tissues.

Exudate: A fluid, often from formed elements of blood, discharged from tissue to a surface or cavity.

Factor: A substance with a special purpose, e.g., blood clotting factor.

Facultative: Able to behave in a specified way, with the implication that is not, however, the usual behavior.

Fermentation: The slow decomposition, for example by microorganisms, of organic material, such as the decomposition of a sugar solution by yeast to form alcohol.

Filament: A fine thread-like structure.

Fimbria: Hair-like protrusion from bacterial cells.

Flagellum: Whip-like organ of motion.

Flocculant: A mass of cells floating or settled to the bottom in a liquid medium.

Flocculation: Precipitation in small cloudy mass.

Fluctuation test: It is to determine the development of mutants in culture. The test is based on the concept that mutation is a completely random event, and spontaneous mutation would result in the number of mutants in a series of identical cultures.

Fluorosis: Mottling of tooth enamel due to excessive amount of fluoride in water.

Fomites: Objects contaminated with pathogenic microorganisms.

Fragment: A piece broken off.

Fungus: A simple unicellular or multicellular structure which reproduces by forming spores.

Fusiform: Spindle-shaped.

Gel: To become solid, to set.

Gene: A unit of inheritance found on chromosomes.

Genetic: The study of inheritance.

Genome: The total genetic material of an organism.

Genotype: The inherited characters of a particular individual.

Genus: A group of closely related species of plant, animal or microorganism.

Globulin: A plasma protein divided into the alpha, beta and gamma fraction.

Gram-negative: Staining red by Gram's method.

Gram-positive: Staining violet by Gram's method.

Growth factor: An ingredient of which at least small amount must be present in a culture medium so that it supports the growth of given organism.

Granules: Small grains or particles, e.g., metachromatic granules of diphtheria bacilli.

Halophilic: Salt loving.

Hapten: A substance which acts as an antigenic stimulus only when combined with protein but capable of reacting with resultant antibody in uncombined state even.

Hemolysis: The destruction of red cells with the release of hemoglobulin.

Hereditary: Transmitted from one generation to the other.

Hetero: Different.

Heterologous: Related to different kind of organism.

Hfr strain: A high frequency mating strain.

Homologous: Related to same kind of organism.

Host: The organism from which a parasite takes its nourishment.

Hypertonic: A condition in which the fluid surrounding a cell is more concentrated than that within it.

Hypotonic: A condition in which the fluid surrounding a cell is less concentrated than that within it.

Identical: Exactly same.

Immune: Protected from disease by the presence of antibodies.

Immunoglobulin: Globulins which act as antibodies.

Inactive: The heating of serum at 56°C to destroy its complement and inhibitory factors.

Inclusion: Something which is enclosed.

Incubate: To keep at the same temperature for a given length of time.

Infection: The entry and multiplication of pathogenic organisms within the body.

Inoculate: To introduce a living organism into a culture medium.

Intra: Inside.

In vitro: In laboratory apparatus.

In vivo: In a living animal or human being.

L-form: Cell wall deficient mutant.

Ligases: Enzymes that catalyze the linking together of two molecules.

Locus: The definite place of a gene on a chromosome.

Lyophilization: Combined freezing and desiccation (freeze drying).

Lysis: Disruption.

Lysogenic conversion: Alteration of the property of bacterium as a result of lysogeny.

Lysogeny: A temporary stable relationship between bacteriophage and its bacterial host, in which the phage is reproduced in step with the bacterium and, thus, handed on to succeeding generation of bacteria.

Macrophage: A large mononuclear phagocytic cell.

Medium: A nutrient substance used to grow microorganisms.

Metabolism: The process of building up chemical compounds in the body and their breaking down during activity.

Microaerophile: An organism which grows best in subconcentration of oxygen.

Misense mutation: A change in cell's DNA with the effect that a wrong amino acid has been put into essential protein.

Molecule: The smallest part of an element or compound which can exist in normal way.

Monolayer: A sheet of tissue culture cells one cell thick.

Morphology: A study of the form of cells and organisms.

Motile: Capable of movement.

Moult: The shedding of skin.

Mutation: An alteration in genetic material.

Neutral: Neither acidic nor alkaline with pH of 7.0.

Nodule: A small rounded swelling.

Normal: Usual or ordinary.

Normal solution: A solution in which the equivalent weight in grams of a chemical is dissolved in one liter of solution.

Nucleoid: Genome.

Nucleocap: The genome and capsid.

Nucleus: An essential part of the living cell, containing the chromosomes and controlling cell activity.

Nutrition: Food.

Obligatory anaerobe: An organism which cannot live in oxygen.

Occult: Hidden.

Opaque: Not allowing light to pass.

Optimum: The most suitable.

Oxidation: Combination with oxygen.

Pandemic: World-wide epidemic.

Parasite: An organism which takes its food from another organism without giving anything in return.

Passage: Administration of microorganism to a host and its subsequent recovery from the host. This way pathogenicity of organism is modified.

Passive immunity: Dependent upon injection of readymade antibodies and not upon the subject's own immunological mechanisms.

Pathogen: An organism which can cause disease.

Petri dish: A shallow circular flat-bottomed glass or plastic dish used as a container for solid media.

Phage type: The identity of a bacterial strain as indicated by its sensitivity or resistance to the lytic action of bacteriophages.

pH: The symbol that indicates the acidity or alkalinity of a solution. pH less than 7 is acid and more than 7 is alkali.

Phagocyte: A cell which ingests microorganisms.

Phenotype: The expression of genotype.

Pigment: A coloring substance.

Pilus: Fimbria.

Plasmid: An extrachromosomal portion of genetic material.

Polymerase: General name of enzymes concerned with synthesis of nucleic acid.

Prophage: Bacteriophage in a lysogenic relationship with its host.

Prophylactic: A medicine to prevent disease.

Prozone: The occurrence of an antigen-antibody reaction only when serum is adequately diluted but not when it is used at higher concentration.

Protoplast: A bacterium deprived of its cell wall.

Puerperal fever: Acute infection following child birth due to introduction of infectious agent into the uterus.

Purulent: Containing pus.

Pus: A thick yellowish green fluid containing phagocytic cells collecting in tissues infected with pyogenic bacteria.

Pyogenic: Pus forming.

Rack: A stand for holding tubes.

Rash: A skin reaction, usually seen as small reddened or raised area.

Reaction: An action which takes place in response to something.

Reagin: Antibodies associated with certain types of hypersensitivity reactions. It may be contained in serum causing Wassermann reaction and related reactions.

Recombinant: A cell or clone of cells resulting from conjugation.

Reduction: The removal of oxygen from a chemical compound.

Replication: Virus reproduction.

Reticuloendothelial system: The system of phagocytic cells in the body.

Retraction: Shrinking.

Ribonucleoprotein: Material in the cytoplasm and nucleus of cell.

Rodent: A gnawing animal, e.g., rat, mouse.

Room temperature: Usually, 18–20°C.

Routine: Carried out regularly.

Sanitize: To reduce microbial number to safe levels.

Saprophytic: Living on dead organic matter.

Saturated solution: A solution which has dissolved as much as it can of a substance.

Satellitism: Enhancement of bacterial growth on a solid medium around a source of growth factor.

Selective medium: A solid culture medium on which all but the desired organisms are wholly or largely inhibited.

Septicemia: Presence and multiplication of bacteria in blood stream resulting severe disease.

Serology: The study of serum especially antibody contents.

Serotype: Antigenic type.

Specific antibody: An antibody which react with one particular antigen only.

Spheroplast: Similar to protoplast with the difference that cell wall damage is partial and reversible.

Spirochete: Genera of spiral bacteria.

Sterilization: The process of killing all living microorganisms including spores.

Symbiotic: Living in mutually with the host.

Technique: The method by which something is done.

Temperate phage: A phage capable of a lysogenic relationship with its bacterial host.

Thermostat: An instrument to control the temperature.

Tissue: A group of similar cells.

Titer: The highest dilution of antibody in a serum which will react with its specific antigen.

Tolerogen: An antigen that induces tolerance.

Toxoid: Toxin rendered harmless but retaining antigenicity.

Transduction: Transfer of genetic material from bacterial strain to another by means of bacteriophage.

Transformation: Acquisition of genetic characters of one bacterial strain by a related strain grown in presence of DNA from the first strain.

Transport medium: A medium which increases the chances of survival of microorganism during transportation from patient to laboratory.

Turbid: Cloudy.

Typical: Showing usual features.

Undulating: Up and down, i.e., wavy.

Unicellular: Single-celled.

Unstable: Easily changed.

Urticaria: A skin rash caused by allergy.

Vaccinate: To introduce into the body killed or mildly pathogenic organisms to produce resistance against disease.

Vaccine: Material used in vaccination.

Variation: A change from the usual.

Vector: An insect which carries microorganism or parasite and is capable of transmitting this.

Viable: Able to live.

Vibrio: A comma-shaped microorganism.

Viremia: Presence of viruses in the bloodstream.

Virion: A virus particle.

Virulent: Harmful.

Working solution: A solution used in a test, made up from concentrated stock solution.

Yeast: A unicellular fungus.

Zygote: The cell formed by the fertilization of a female cell by a male cell.

Index

Page numbers followed by *f* refer to figure, *fc* refer to flow chart, and *t* refer to table.